THE **Thompson Method** OF **Bodywork**

D0912566

"Cathy Thompson had the rarest combination of experience, knowledge, and pure instinct. I only had to walk in the door for her to understand where I was at physically and emotionally. And the results were as unorthodox and surprising as her methods. She was one of a kind."

HUGH JACKMAN, ACTOR AND PRODUCER

"Cathy's extraordinary gift began in her brain, traveled to her heart, and continued through the tips of her fingers."

KATHIE LEE GIFFORD, TV PERSONALITY AND AUTHOR

"Throughout my professional operatic and teaching careers, I have been blessed with many who have supported and enabled my vocal strength and health. Cathy Thompson and now Tara Thompson Lewis have been instrumental in my success as a singer and teacher. Specializing in physical manipulation for professional singers, actors, and dancers, they are able to relieve pain, tension, and realign the body to achieve optimal health and performance. Here in New York City in my own professional voice studio, I am able to utilize their techniques to help my students understand the importance of proper physical organization as it applies especially to singing. I urge anyone who wants to be a better, healthier performer to read this book. I enthusiastically recommend their techniques, and I continue to be a delighted and grateful client."

CANDACE GOETZ, OPERA SINGER AND FOUNDER OF
THE CANDACE GOETZ VOICE STUDIO

"Tara Thompson Lewis has done a masterful job in completing this ambitious book begun by her late mentor and mother, Cathy Thompson, thus making these brilliant teachings available to anyone. *The Thompson Method of Bodywork* presents mountains of useful information (much of it drawn from Zen Shiatsu) and offers a banquet of exercises for healing the *kyo/jitsu* relationship within ourselves, whether the triggers happen to be physical injury, structural misalignment, or psychological, spiritual, or emotional pain."

KATHLEEN PORTER, AUTHOR OF *NATURAL POSTURE FOR PAIN-FREE LIVING* AND
HEALTHY POSTURE FOR BABIES AND CHILDREN

"I spent many years working with Cathy Thompson (and then with Tara), and reading this material reminded me of Cathy's very specific genius: her profound understanding of the body and, may I say, much more. Working with both of them had a profound effect on my singing, and indeed my life, and it's a great pleasure to be able to reconnect with Cathy's way of thinking and working while reading this book. I recommend it highly for anyone interested in changing, improving, and enriching their lives. It certainly did mine."

STEVEN LUTVAK, SINGER-SONGWRITER AND COMPOSER AND LYRICIST OF
THE TONY AWARD–WINNING BROADWAY MUSICAL
A GENTLEMAN'S GUIDE TO LOVE AND MURDER

"I first began seeing Cathy Thompson in my 20s, while starting on Broadway. Both my physical life and emotional life were quite demanding, and I needed all around custom-tailored care. After each and every session I've had, I've walked out feeling calmer, yet more energized, as well as open. As a vocalist and performer, being a clear channel is of the utmost importance."

DEBBIE GIBSON, AMERICAN SINGER-SONGWRITER,
RECORD PRODUCER, AND ACTRESS

"I began working with Cathy Thompson over 20 years ago, as a young singer with chronic throat tension. At the time, I thought her work was magical, her intuition uncanny. Over the years, I began to understand how the Thompson Method works and what Cathy was doing when she worked on my body and encouraged me to explore on my own. Now, two decades later, I am thrilled that Cathy's work is available to everyone who is interested in learning about how to take care of their bodies, voices, and minds. In addition to singing, I teach voice to a wide range of students. Access to the Thompson Method will add a great deal of value to their practice routines. In each chapter, Cathy explores and explains possible reasons for tension or lack of strength and mobility and then offers well-explained and illustrated exercises to address each of these aspects. Twenty plus years after being introduced to it, I am still reaping benefits from and learning about the Thompson Method, and I am grateful for it."

JAMIE LEONHART, SINGER, SONGWRITER, AND VOICE TEACHER

THE
Thompson Method OF
Bodywork

Structural Alignment, Core Strength, and Emotional Release

Cathy Thompson AND
Tara Thompson Lewis

ILLUSTRATED BY **Mike Saijo**

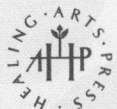

Healing Arts Press
Rochester, Vermont • Toronto, Canada

Healing Arts Press
One Park Street
Rochester, Vermont 05767
www.HealingArtsPress.com

Healing Arts Press is a division of Inner Traditions International

Copyright © 2018 by Tara Lewis

All rights reserved. No part of this book may be reproduced or utilized in any form or by any means, electronic or mechanical, including photocopying, recording, or by any information storage and retrieval system, without permission in writing from the publisher.

Note to the reader: This book is intended as an informational guide. The remedies, approaches, and techniques described herein are meant to supplement, and not to be a substitute for, professional medical care or treatment. They should not be used to treat a serious ailment without prior consultation with a qualified health care professional

Library of Congress Cataloging-in-Publication Data

Names: Thompson, Cathy, 1957-2008, author. | Lewis, Tara Thompson, 1987- author.
Title: The Thompson method of bodywork : structural alignment, core strength, and emotional release / Cathy Thompson, Tara Thompson Lewis ; illustrated by Mike Saijo.
Description: Rochester, Vermont : Healing Arts Press, [2018] | Includes bibliographical references and index.
Identifiers: LCCN 2017008794 (print) | LCCN 2017031505 (e-book) | ISBN 9781620556641 (paperback) | ISBN 9781620556658 (e-book)
Subjects: LCSH: Chronic pain—Treatment—Popular works. | Exercise Therapy— Popular works. | BISAC: HEALTH & FITNESS / Pain Management. | HEALTH & FITNESS / Exercise. | HEALTH & FITNESS / Alternative Therapies.
Classification: LCC RB127 (e-book) | LCC RB127 .T4974 2018 (print) | DDC 616/.0472—dc23
LC record available at https://lccn.loc.gov/2017008794

Printed and bound in India by Replika Press Pvt. Ltd.

10 9 8 7 6 5 4 3 2 1

Text design and layout by Virginia Scott Bowman
This book was typeset in Garamond Premier Pro and Avenir with Raleway and Avenir used as display typefaces

To send correspondence to the author of this book, mail a first-class letter to the author c/o Inner Traditions • Bear & Company, One Park Street, Rochester, VT 05767, and we will forward the communication, or contact the author directly at **www.thompsonmethodofbodywork.com**.

Contents

PART ONE
♦♦♦
Cathy Thompson's Philosophy of Bodywork

PART TWO
◆◆◆
Cathy Thompson's Exercises

Foreword

WHEN TARA ASKED ME to write a foreword to her book, written with her mother, I did not hesitate. I have known both authors for a very long time; in fact, Tara was conceived in my apartment! Her mother, Cathy Thompson, studied Ohashiatsu with me at the Ohashi Institute, which at that time, in 1982, was called the Shiatsu Education Center of America, at 52 West 55th Street, in Manhattan. I remember Cathy well for the intensity of her study. She always sat in the very front, staring at me with her piercing eyes. While at the institute she began dating Tara's father, Michal Pober, from the former Czechoslovakia, who was also my student. One summer we went up to our vacation house in Kinderhook, New York, and they asked to stay in our Upper West Side apartment. Nine months later, Tara was born. So I have known her since she was in the womb.

Tara began studying with me herself in the fall of 2012 and has been studying with me ever since. So the book that you have in front of you is the result of two generations of commitment and study. You will find many exercises within. In my own many years of practice I have found that "treatment is exercise given by the therapist; exercise is self-treatment." The Thompson Method gives you tools you can use to give your own treatment to yourself. Please approach the exercises the way that you would want a therapist to approach you, with openness and compassion.

I am so happy to see my students publishing with Inner Traditions, which has a long history of publishing excellent books, especially in the field of holistic health. Mr. Ehud Sperling, the owner, started at the Samuel Weiser bookstore in Greenwich Village and has dedicated his entire life to publishing.

I heartily recommend this work to those who work with the body or who are interested in healing and caring for themselves. It is a pleasure to see my students grow and expand the world of bodywork.

OHASHI

In Japanese, the name "Ohashi" means "big bridge," the perfect name for someone who has devoted his life to bringing Eastern modes of healing to the West. Ohashi lectures and teaches internationally and is the author of six books, which have been translated into eight languages, and eleven videos on his technique. In 2007, he was honored with a Cultural Bridge Award in recognition of popularizing the Japanese therapy of shiatsu in the United States and Europe.

Acknowledgments

I WOULD LIKE TO THANK Suzan Postel, who worked closely for years with Cathy and me, for her dedicated help and support with the entire writing process. Special thanks also to Joan Lader, Candace Goetz, Jamie Leonhart, Judith Clurman, Trebbe Johnson, Carrie Jacquith, Chris Simpson, Darren Aronofsky, Megan Frummer, Steven Lutvak, Ruth Williams Hennessy, Elissa Lewis, and Ohashi. I would also like to thank Mike Saijo, Michelle Joo, and Miguel (the three Ms!) for their dedication to creating the essential and beautiful illustrations to complement my mother's text, and all of our clients who have provided themselves for the development of the material. Thank you to everyone at Inner Traditions/Healing Arts Press for making the publishing process a pleasure. I'd also like to thank my husband, Brandon Lewis, for always supporting and motivating me and patiently helping me bring this project to you. I would like to thank my daughter, Adela, for giving me motivation and her wonderful nanny, Ariane, who made it possible.

T.T.L.

Preface

WHEN I WAS ABOUT six years old, I remember telling all my teachers that my diaphragm was tight and needed to be released, something my mother would have understood and helped me with. My teachers looked completely bewildered. Thus, early on, I realized my approach to my body and emotions was unusual. When adults asked me what my parents did and I said "Bodywork," I usually got puzzled looks and they'd say, "Car mechanic?" Now, finally, after thirty-two years of struggling to explain what to me is so natural that it is difficult to articulate, I am thrilled I can tell them to read our book.

I started working on this book with my mother in 2000. At the time, I did not imagine I would be finishing it without her. It has been an emotional and healing process; it was not until after giving birth to my own daughter that I was able to approach it in an open way, without being blinded by the loss of my mother. As I write this, I am grateful she left it in a rough form. It has meant that I too have embodied the work in the process of completing it. I have used every exercise in it, including befriending the jungle gym, and gained strength and insight into my body, as well as using the material in my practice.

Because I was so close to my mother, working with her on this from the beginning, I feel that what you have before you is what my mother wished, even though it has taken me years since her death and required a great deal of generously provided help to prepare it. Cathy Thompson left her essence in this work, and reading it is like sitting in the room with her, or getting a session. She continued to work on this book while undergoing intensive chemotherapy and radiation for a very aggressive cancer and experiencing extreme pain. In the mornings, she got up before me, and I would find her writing on little scraps of paper at her desk. Writing it was a source of joy for her, and I hope that you will enjoy reading it.

I have not been able to check over every point with her, so I have endeavored to stay as true as possible to her voice, vision, and style. I have changed very little, and my role has mainly consisted of organizing the material, rewriting and writing some chapters, editing, modeling the illustrations, and proofreading to make it accessible to you.

You will find biographical details and information about Cathy Thompson and how she developed her method of bodywork in the introduction. Here, I would like to add a little about our relationship and how this book was written. My mother was not only my best friend, but also my mentor. She was an exceptional bodywork practitioner and teacher. She began teaching me bodywork when I was about three years old for the simple reason that she got migraine headaches, and I was willing, free labor.

My mother was one of those rare people who completely embodied her work—it was a direct extension of her deepest self. Connecting with my mother also meant connecting with her work. She taught me how to work on her head, and then as the years went on, we spent many hours doing bodywork together. Growing up, I took it for granted that if you had any problem, the first thing to do was to start working on it! I could go to my mother with any ache or pain, or any problem at all (physical or otherwise), and she could almost always help me to lessen it or make it disappear completely. As I grew older, I became increasingly interested in how she did this with her clients. I learned that pain can be relieved through touch and conscious movement and it is usually a good place to start. It was a process of working through whatever was going on, delving into it, and exploring. It was never as though my mother was doing something to my body.

I also explored other types of movement and bodywork, mostly through her introduction. She was always open to learning different techniques and approaches. One of my earliest memories of this is from about age eight when a woman came and did stretches and resistance band exercises with my younger brother and me. I remember my mother coming out of a bodywork session in her workroom and my brother and I were on the floor howling from a hamstring stretch.

Sixteen years later, I assisted her in her private practice and gradually took over increasing responsibility as she became unable. I knew that I would take part in the writing of this book, and it is an honor to be able to present it to you. We started with brainstorming what form she wanted the book to take. We both took pleasure in the idea of creating a comprehensive and accessible explanation of my mother's ideas and techniques. She never typed or used a computer, so she spent many hours writing out each section by hand, and others typed them for her.

Her previous text, *The Bodywork Manual,* contains additional exercises, and it serves as a great introduction to how you can do bodywork on yourself. The book you have in front of you is a more personal look into Cathy Thompson's thought processes and method. It is the last word from her on her ideas about the body, which hopefully will serve as fodder for your exploration and for the future development of bodywork.

TARA THOMPSON LEWIS

Introduction

IN 1996, I WROTE *The Bodywork Manual*, which was primarily for the use of my clients, so I wouldn't have to repeatedly explain the basic premises of healing the body, to describe how they could work on their own, and also to give some specific exercises. Experience has taught me that most people don't understand the premise of bodywork; as a result, their intentions are inaccurate and they do any homework I give them slightly wrong. So the educational part of my work seemed to me to be the most important. As I delved into why it had proved so useful, I began to understand that the correct usage of our bodies is an issue that goes way beyond "good posture," "strong muscles," and so on. Our relationship to our bodies is challenged when we do any physical thing differently in a conscious way. This upsetting of the mind-body applecart can be profoundly disturbing and surprising as well as enlightening for many clients.

This second book is an exploration and an inquiry into the questions the earlier manual brought up for me. It is also intended to be used as a more complete and updated manual. It's also important to understand how to self-diagnose and self-treat your various physical issues, since, even if you have to have medical treatments, 99 percent of your recovery will be about how you work on yourself.

Now that we have such a plethora of systems of body use, it is difficult to know whether to do cardio, yoga, Pilates, or what? To aid you in finding your way, this book includes a general guide to working out, getting treatment for physical problems, and so on. The exercises in this book are designed to complement and deepen any exercise system.

My background, the part that I think is important, where my ideas formed, has more to do with experience than the various modalities I have learned. Mostly, I learned and practiced one modality at a time, which worked, with luck, for 60 percent of my clients (never more), and I kept wondering why the remaining 40 percent were not helped.

LEARNING TO
LISTEN TO THE BODY

My very first bodywork training was in England, when I was a child and suffered from terrible migraines. About one-half of the migraines were caused by food allergies; the remainder of the migraines seemed to be due to some kind of cranial injury. I had a number of whiplash injuries as a small child. A wonderful cranial osteopath, a Dr. Palmer, treated me so successfully with his cranial manipulations that I was able to live without any pain. I got really interested in the cause of my pain and the "magic" way his hands gave me relief. So from ages ten to twelve, I actually studied cranial osteopathy, English style. Cranial osteopathy became part of kinesiology and network chiropractic in the United States. Although it is effective, it is often not enough, and some people require deeper work. I developed the cranial fascia work that I use (detailed in chapter 19) partly from cranial osteopathy and partly from the original form of osteopathy, osteobionomy.

I was also studying art and later went to Oxford University, where I received a BA in fine arts. My degree is in sculpture. I enjoy painting and colors as well, but sculpting was what most thrilled me, and still does. Bodywork is the closest physical therapy to sculpture. My studies at university did have some relevance to anatomy, and I was able to perform dissections, but that's not the only thing that attracted me. I've always loved these two things, art and anatomy. My eventual decision to focus on the body studies that I have been preoccupied with since late adolescence was due to economic factors—I just couldn't make a living doing fine arts. It is remarkable how many bodywork practitioners have trained also as artists, writers, musicians, and so on. I believe that is because it takes a similar sensibility. When I first look at a client, I receive them, absorb them, and in that moment have the same feeling as when I looked at objects I was going to paint. Also, the surges of spiritual feelings, of oneness with the universe, that I sometimes have during meditation resemble how I feel when I create art and when I practice bodywork.

Just out of Oxford, I moved to New York and became a part of the then ungentrified East Village art community. I lived with a roommate at that time, and people in all stages of physical and mental disrepair kept showing up at our apartment and also talking to me on the phone about their problems. I'm sure it was very annoying to my roommate. No doubt to get some relief from this, she suggested I make a living, not doing art commercially, which I was very bad at, but instead helping people as a therapist of some kind.

That was one of those "aha" moments—and the next day I started at the Shiatsu Education Center in New York. I had the benefit of studying with the best shiatsu teachers in the country, including lots of time with Ohashi, the founder, himself. My ideas on *kyo* (need) and *jitsu* (behavior), which are the touchstone of my work, come from the ideas of Shizuto Masunaga, who was Ohashi's teacher. They are explained further in chapter 1.

Upon completion of my shiatsu studies, I realized that, again, I couldn't help anyone—I didn't know enough about muscles, joints, and structure. So I learned a kind of structural integration/Rolfing, privately, from a man who had trained with Ida Rolf. I took lots of other private trainings and many workshops. I studied dance therapy, yoga, Pilates, weight training, kinesiology, and so on. I learned all kinds of corrective alignment work, from subtle orthobionomy (osteopathic) moves to painful fascia work. I touched on polarity, *jin shin jitsu*, chiropractic, Muscle Activation Technique, and Body Mind Centering. I alighted for a while in Gestalt psychotherapy, completing a three-year training. It was all wonderful, informative, and fascinating. None of it taught me anything about healing.

That is an exaggeration, of course. I learned many techniques I've incorporated into my work, without which I could have no grounding. The real learning, however, came from my clients, not the theories. Through my experience, I put together the basic principles that I believe underlie all bodywork and healing.

Another important phase of my work came through working with a wonderful voice therapist, Joan Lader. I'm not a singer—far from it. Yet the small amount of understanding of the vocal instrument I gained fascinated me and enhanced my understanding of the body as no other work did. I think this is because after the body is relatively healthy and pain-free, the next natural interest a person develops is in expressing himself and his feelings. This expression can be through movement, breath, and the voice.

The understanding of the release of the vocal mechanism can help people reach a stage of readiness for self-expression more freely. So whether or not a client is a singer, I will usually work to free up her voice. It's also not difficult to work with vocal issues through bodywork, and chapter 10 in this book focuses on how this can be done.

What the learning of technique cannot give us is the ability to listen very precisely to the signals the body gives us. Our bodies really do have all the answers. The trick is to access that unconscious information. How can I tell, for example, when a client comes in, whether she needs an adjustment, psychotherapy, or deep tissue work? Generally speaking, the main question my students have is—"What do I do with this person?" They know lots of techniques and, if they are any good, can diagnose the client's imbalances correctly. What they don't know is where to start, which technique to use, and so on.

KEYS TO CHANGE

My intention in writing this book is to give you the keys to unlocking the hidden stuff in your body, in other people, or simply as an interesting exercise and study in human nature. The relationship between the bodyworker, who does deep, therapeutic work, and the client, who is usually working on a regular basis with the bodyworker, is complex and, I think, quite fascinating. I would like to convey some of the flavor of this journey, which I've never read about anywhere else. Clients can make huge life changes on the basis of the understandings they come to deep in their bodies through the work we do. In a way, the relationship is similar to that of the psychotherapist and patient—and yet I believe that the changes, because they are grounded in physical change, are even deeper and longer lasting.

Bodywork has to be the most direct way of helping us to overcome pain and grow as human beings. For example, it may be hard to believe that P.'s relationship to his brother is somewhere encapsulated in his right inner thigh. Yet this is exactly what happened with one of my clients—and changing P.'s thigh structure with awareness changed the family relationships. Like ripples in a pond, the softening and opening of the sartorius muscle allowed P. to begin communication with his brother, which led to huge changes in many lives. Amazing!

I have attempted to make the exercises in part 2 of the book—Cathy Thompson's Exercises—suitable for both the nonexerciser and the experienced athlete. Please don't be intimidated by the difficult exercises; just leave them if they don't work for you. You can use this book in the most basic way, to relieve aches and pains, or take it much further and learn to change patterns of emotion and movement in your muscles and nervous system. It's up to you. You will, to some extent, be changing deeper patterns, whichever exercises you choose, and the more consciously you can do this, the greater the long-term changes.

Chapter 9, Breathing, covers function more than structure. Since breathing is the bridge between mind and body and we can change our emotional experience through the breath, it relates closely to the material in chapter 3 on mind/body. It seems to me that the usefulness of breath as a psychological tool is greatly undervalued. It takes fifteen minutes—that's all—to change your feelings, your whole emotional experience, through a change in breathing patterns. So why not try that way first, before the medications?

This book is intended to be used as a practical manual, if you want to increase your body awareness and your health, decrease physical pain, and so on. It will be helpful to anyone working with patients, students, or clients in any of the healing arts. I am also hoping that the stories I include in the book, relevant to bodywork experience, will be entertaining at least and may give you an idea of how this approach could work for you.

FACING THE MYSTERY

There is one thing that cannot be excluded from this introduction. Since I began writing this book, about six years ago, my life has gone through a dramatic shift. In May 2006, the real-life drama started, and I don't mean marriages, men, or babies. I found a strange-shaped soft lump in my left breast, and then I started having terrible spinal/hip pain. This pain was so intense I sat screaming until my pain reliever patches kicked in; this was inflammatory breast cancer, a very aggressive kind. The excruciating pain was only the beginning, as my spine was eaten away by carcinoma and collapsed so that I lost about six inches of height in a couple of months and then had over thirty brain tumors—they stopped counting at thirty. These are just a few dramatic highlights. I did numerous alternative treatments of all sorts, from prayer to yoga, acupuncture to the most advanced alternative European treatments. I also utilized modern Western medicine, including chemotherapy, radiation, and surgery. The book you have in front of you has been a part of my own healing process, as it's something I've been able to work on even when I've been stuck in a wheelchair.

Everyone asked me why this had happened to me. I eat very cleanly, almost entirely raw and organic, have never smoked, exercise every day, and practice yoga. I do all the things to keep cancer away. I do have a few ideas: I live near the site of the former Twin Towers, and my balcony was covered in soot for weeks after September 11, 2001. I also took birth control pills for three months, and I have some emotional issues (don't we all?). But the reality is that cancer, and other illnesses, can be completely unexpected and without an obvious cause, or even any cause at all. I know of nothing that I did that created cancer.

Life is mysterious. You don't necessarily get the diseases you think you should. The ultimate answer I can truthfully give clients when they ask me about why or how they got a certain disease or condition is, "I don't know." I don't understand my own illnesses; how can I understand yours? I can often ameliorate them, feel into them intuitively, and use some of my knowledge to lessen them. It's still a mystery.*

---

*The "why" of my mother's cancer remains a mystery now, years after it caused her death, but this book is a generous sharing of the legacy of her insights and deep intuitive understanding about body-work, health, and healing. Cathy's life was cut short; however, in her life she touched the lives of so many others. They in turn were able to touch the lives of those around them, including millions who saw their performances. Through this book, her life and work continue to touch the lives of others. Ultimately, this to me is a life well lived.

PART ONE

૩૪

Cathy Thompson's Philosophy of Bodywork

1

Kyo and Jitsu

W. IS A SERIOUS ALCOHOLIC. He's been downing a bottle of wine almost every day since he was seventeen. Now he's started on whisky, and it's getting worse.

He's tried to stop. He's been to rehabilitation centers, outpatient programs, and Alcoholics Anonymous. Every time, he tapers off attendance because somebody annoys him or he doesn't like something about the program. Then he starts drinking again, one glass at a time, quite sure he'll stay in control this time. He can't imagine not wanting to drink. Sometimes he manages to control it for a few months, but eventually stress steps up, his drinking increases, and in a year or so, he's back in rehab. He knows he's in a desperate situation and his body, at age fifty, can no longer tolerate alcohol.

Everyone he knows can see what he needs to do—stop drinking, stay in a treatment program, and not fool himself into believing he can drink moderately. W. knows this too, in his moments of clarity. Yet he seems unable to use the knowledge he has. Some other factors are operating here.

A.'s neck hurts all the time. She's had lots of massages, chiropractic adjustments, and so on, which help for a while, but the pain always comes back. You couldn't say she was addicted to her pain—she hates it and would love to get rid of it—but some part of her requires it, or it would not persist so long after the initial cause.

Another client, P., goes through life trying all kinds of New Age therapies to cure his depression. Nothing seems to work for long. He's tried medication, but that didn't help either. The therapies have increased his awareness of his childhood issues and given him great insight into his personality. But his depression—though it ebbs and flows in ways that seem unrelated to his treatments—doesn't really get better.

I'm often a last resort. Like these three clients, many people, most of them quite sophisticated, come to me with what seem like intractable problems, after they've tried "everything else."

I got to asking myself—why does one very useful and valid treatment work for some and not for others? Why doesn't anything, apparently, work for some people? And why does the body hang onto symptoms and pain as though life depended on it? Do we have some strange need to be unhappy? None of these behaviors seem to serve any useful function.

Until recently, many therapists, especially those strongly influenced by New Age doctrines of personal responsibility, believed that there was some kind of "victim mind," which makes a person gain enough perverse satisfaction out of not getting better to warrant staying with their sickness. Actually, this idea goes back to Freud. He proposed that we are constantly stimulated and driven by a balance of two energies, represented by the mythical figures Eros and Thanatos. Eros is the sexual drive and creative force, while Thanatos is the death force of destruction. A person could be unbalanced, remaining in the self-perpetuating destructive behavior. The patient would resist treatment because of certain "secondary gains" of their illness, which could be physical, economic, social, and so on. The danger of this idea is twofold: It provides a convenient out for a therapist whose client isn't getting better, and it ends up blaming the victim while not identifying possible other culprits. It seemed to me, also, that at a biological survival level it makes no sense for an organism to be so self-destructive.

The same internal process—the body wisdom, which keeps our physical selves alive and more or less healthy—is responsible for addictions, intractable pains, and self-sabotaging behavior. The body wisdom is attempting to fill a need, but with limited or incorrect information. Since that part of us functions in a simple, binary fashion, and we are living in a very complex, civilized world, our needs become convoluted and distorted by what surrounds us.

WE ARE THE PROBLEM

Most of the people I see are smart and analytical enough to be quite aware of their own problems. But when they take steps to change things, these lower-brain, biological factors that don't think or analyze take over and control the out-come. All imbalances and ultimately all diseases originate in a real need that the organism is driven to fill, but for some reason cannot satisfy with what is truly needed. The environment may not supply it, or the individual may have the wrong information about what is available to him, whether his choices come from infor-mation encoded in his DNA, or from limited past experiences, or just incorrect perceptions.

For example, if W. has a genetic, metabolic deficiency in one or more of the liver enzymes that break down alcohol, he is more likely to have a body that perceives alcoholism as a solution to his emotional needs than someone who has different genetics. Another person might choose (unconsciously, of course) psychotherapy, love relationships, religion, or another kind of "addiction" to satisfy emptiness.

If the key fits the lock—in other words, if the object chosen to fill emotional hunger is truly satisfying and not a substitute for the real thing—the need is satisfied and balance is restored. If it's not the real thing, the needs are still there, untouched, despite the activity on the surface.

W.'s need is still there, and until he can satisfy it, he will remain an alcoholic or, at best, a "dry drunk"—someone who is still an addict with unfilled needs, who has to "white knuckle" through life and will probably fall into another addiction.

Unfortunately, the behavior of drinking and its compulsive nature creates its own problems. W.'s physical ailments and his inability to stand frustration or reason coherently come from the biochemical changes of alcoholism and also get in the way of his healing. He would have to access those unfilled needs—biochemical, spiritual, and emotional—perhaps by staying in Alcoholics Anonymous until he gains spiritual fulfillment and his emotional needs are met through the support of others—before his desire for alcohol will go away.

That's why willpower and conscious intention don't work in the long run; stop-ping the behavior without filling the real need creates resistance and even panic on a survival level. Anyone who has tried to go on a strict diet knows this.

The other reason our conscious efforts don't work when a problem is deep seated is that *we* are the problem. If we have created it, the attempts we make to get better will come out of the same tendencies and distortions, the same limited infor-mation, as the problem. Most of us know this on some level, and so we go to others for help, hoping an outside viewpoint will give us the extra energy we need to heal. But even our choice of healing modalities will reflect our prejudices. Somebody who is very physical and sensation oriented will try to help herself with exercise and sports, whereas a cerebral, analytic person will go to therapy and a spiritual person will turn to religion—all for the same problem. Often what's wrong with us—that blind spot—is obvious to those around us, since it tends to be out of our field of vision and directly in theirs. We know just what someone else needs to heal, but we can't fix ourselves.

KYO AND JITSU:
A STARTING POINT

So how do we help ourselves, given all these limitations? Eastern medicine provides a paradigm that helped me gain an understanding of this problem and showed me how to step outside the maelstrom of neurosis and imbalance to know at least where to start.

These ideas come from the work of Shizuto Masunaga and Wataru Ohashi, authors of *Zen Shiatsu, How to Harmonize Yin and Yang for Better Health,** who explain this from the Eastern point of view much better than I can. They wanted to integrate these ancient ideas with Western psychology. This is my interpretation of it. As Masunaga saw it, the need—emptiness, lack, deficiency, weakness, negative space—is called *kyo* (in Japanese); the behavior—symptoms, manifestation, pain, that which is active and conscious—is *jitsu* (see fig. 1.1 on page 12). The kyo (need) creates an imbalance in energy, which the organism will fill—either correctly (balance is restored again) or not (jitsu).

The jitsu, since it doesn't really fill the kyo, just sits there, unintegrated, and causes its own problems. The kyo still pulls us, drives us to fill it. If we try again, in the same misguided way we did before, we create another jitsu, which could be a habit or addiction. In the example we used earlier, W. needs emotional and spiritual nurturance (kyo) and drinks as a substitute (jitsu). Drinking provides him with excitement, relaxation, and a feeling of warmth but doesn't satisfy the real need (kyo). The glow wears off, he feels his needs again, plus whatever chemical and emotional problems the drinking created. Then, because he doesn't know how to fill these needs, he drinks even more (jitsu). Alcoholism is the most obvious illustration of kyo and jitsu I can think of.

---

*Shizuto Masunaga and Wataru Ohashi, *Zen Shiatsu* (New York: Japan Publications, 1977).

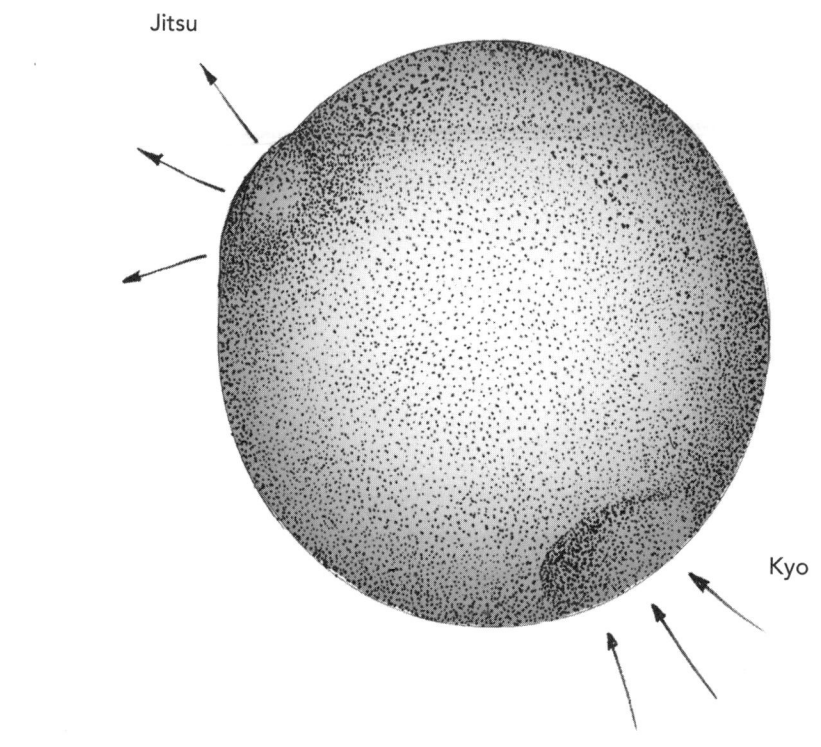

Jitsu

Kyo

Fig. 1.1. Kyo and jitsu

Let's go back to A.'s neck problem and see how the kyo/jitsu dynamic operates there. Her jitsu, of course, is the neck spasm. It's obvious, it hurts, and it's what she's most aware of. When she takes steps to remedy the neck spasm—goes for a massage, takes medication, buys a special pillow for her head, and so on—her neck stops hurting for a while. Then the pain comes back, just as severely.

So what is the kyo here? It depends on what point of view you look at the issue from. At a structural level, A.'s lower back muscles are weak and do not support her body correctly. She sits at a desk in front of a computer all day, with her head craned forward, the weight of her head falls onto her neck muscles rather than her whole back. Because her back is weak, as the day goes on, she slumps more and more in her chair and her head pokes farther forward, creating more pain for her. The unmet need in this case is to support her head correctly, with the muscles designed for the job.

From a psychological perspective, the neck pain could signal dissatisfaction with her job, which would be the kyo. She's not aware that she doesn't like her job—she does it mechanically, doesn't think about it—but her resistance and lack of energy about it show up in her slumped, depressed posture, which then creates the tension in her neck. Her unfulfilled need would be for satisfaction in her work life.

If you look into her situation from other points of view, you might find even more kyos. We might find that changing one of them helps a little, but not enough to completely cure her pain. Actually, this is the most common pattern I see in a client, because usually by the time they come to me, kyos and jitsus have interlaced and layered in a complicated way, reacting to each other until the origin may be quite obscure.

First Layer of Kyo and Jitsu

Kyo and jitsu function in layers. The first layer, the most superficial, and the one that changes the most easily, is the most recent. For example, if I do something that doesn't conform to one of my habitual patterns—suppose I garden or use a computer, things I never do normally—and I pull a muscle slightly, I might then go to a therapist, who will treat me once and I won't have the pain any more. That's the true first level kyo/jitsu. Children, since they haven't lived long enough to form habit patterns, recover quickly and dramatically if their first level of kyo/jitsu is healed.

As soon as we develop unresolved, compensated, and stuck tendencies, we have the possibility of a temporary slight injury hooking in to an old pattern. In this case, even if the stimulus is new—my gardening injury, say—my body will file it away neurologically as "pulled neck muscle, just like all those whiplash injuries I had when I was a child, so let's spasm up in the same old way." This injury will take longer to heal and will need more attention, since I will need to treat the unresolved whiplash too.

A.'s neck pain may be a recent "crick" in her trapezius muscle, which she pulled today as she was talking on the phone while she was on her computer. That's the first layer—the pain she acquired today, which will go away quickly after some bodywork. It might resolve on its own too, although it may create compensations. In A.'s case, though, the problem goes deeper and, even though she feels relief when she leaves me, her pain all gone, unfortunately, when she goes back to her office, sits at her desk at that same slight angle, and juggles the telephone and computer work, she feels a slight twinge again. We did not—could not in one treatment—approach the second layer, and that's what she's feeling now.

If her first layer is the relationship between her neck and lower back, it will correct easily. She'll feel much better right away and probably think her problem has gone. But it hasn't; perhaps it will reappear, less acute but still bothersome.

Second Layer of Kyo and Jitsu

The second layer is much more complex. This is the place where patterns are created and maintained, where compensation happens and there starts to be a struggle. It can be discouraging. The second layer is the source of the experience A. may have (it's a common one) when she feels she is "magically" healed after a few treatments or when she realizes that her lower back muscles, after she strengthens them, stop the neck pain. The pain recurs, perhaps not as badly or in a different location, but something is still wrong. One kyo is satisfied, allowing the other ones to surface. Depending on the complexity and duration of her problem, she will find a whole assortment of interweaving kyos and jitsus that may reveal that this minor neck pain is part of a system that reaches deep into every aspect of her being. If the problem clears up in a few treatments or if an exercise fixes it for good, that means the neck problem is superficial, that it has roots in the first layer.

Third Layer of Kyo and Jitsu

Most issues that bother you, that seem chronic at all, have roots in the second layer. If you keep going with the uncovering process, eventually you will hit the core, the third layer, which in many ways is a very difficult place to land. Change in the third layer can't be forced, and—since your body wisdom believes your survival depends on maintaining the imbalances within it—you will meet enormous resistance to these deep changes. If you don't find resistance, you haven't gotten to it yet.

The contents of that core relate to identity and self-definition, so if they shift, something radical is going to change that will threaten the person's fundamental sense of who he is, even if that change feels wonderful—what could be bad about being free of neck pain, not being addicted to alcohol, or not being depressed? Because of the threat to survival involved, there's still a mental reflex that we might recognize as resistance or feel as anxiety.

Kyo/Jitsu Layers in the Body and Aspects

The kyo/jitsu layers exist spatially as well as in time. People tend to be soft on the outside (kyo) and hard inside, through the deeper muscles (jitsu), or the reverse may be true. Dancers, for example, are often very flexible and have soft mobile tissue on the surface of their bodies. They might seem relaxed and fluid in their movements. But their structural issues are usually in the deeper muscles, which can grip with great force and cause a lot of problems. Other athletes, such as football players, have big, hard, tight outer bodies and inflexible joints, but weak, soft deeper muscles. Both these situations are unbalanced, and, ideally in any physical activity, the aim should be the distribution of energy through the body equally.

The first layer, in this aspect, would be the skin and the surface tissue—the part you can feel easily. It would also involve how a person looks and what you notice about her visually—the "skin deep" impression. The second layer would be most of the body tissue, the muscles you can feel without too much difficulty, and maybe some of the organs—the stomach and the esophagus are probably second layer.

The core contains the deep muscles: the psoas muscle, which, simply put, runs diagonally from the anterior lumbar spine to the groin through the body, joining the upper and lower torso (see fig. 7.1 on page 83), parts of the diaphragm, most of the organs, and the bones. It's hard to feel the core tissues, but they create and form our structure and our deeper emotional life.

Finally, there are the areas in which kyo/jitsu express themselves—the aspects. The dynamic can be structural, as in A.'s neck problem. It can be energetic/psychological, as in W.'s alcoholism. It can be expressed in a disease state, as depression (see below). It can also exist in relationships between people. You see it in disturbed families, where the "identified patient"—such as the family member whose crazy behavior troubles the other members—gets better and stops acting out. In this case the jitsu is quelled, but the kyo is not filled. So the jitsu will travel to another family member, who will act out the disturbance in his own way, creating another jitsu, until the deeper kyo of the family is healed. I've seen this in my own work where parents bring in their "problem kids."

L., for example, brought in his sixteen-year-old son, who had attention deficit disorder and had started getting headaches. It's usually a sign that the parent is involved in the kyo/jitsu dynamic when they come into the treatment room with an older child or adolescent. When L. and his son arrived, he told me all about his son's issues in a way that made it apparent that the son's problems were a strong focus for the father. In such a situation, where I'm not doing family therapy, my recourse could be to (a) ask the parent if I can work with the son alone, or (b) speak to the father about what I'm feeling, either directly or by expressing that what the son might need in order to get better is a certain amount of emotional space.

P. suffers from depression. He has a couple of dynamic jitsus. I learned this by chance when his wife came in for an unrelated injury. P. admired—even envied— his wife and told me often what a wonderful, dynamic woman she was, and how bad he felt that his depression was dragging her down. I did suspect that he might be angry with her, but conversation along those lines never went anywhere, and he'd been to so many therapists that he must have been aware of his anger by now, if he ever would be.

When I met his wife, she did seem like a very energetic sort of person whose positive energy more than made up for P.'s inertia. As she talked about herself and how she had come to the injury she had, what emerged for me was an impression of somebody who had experienced a lot of loss and trauma—far more than depressed P. had. So much, in fact, that she'd completely repressed the possibility of sadness— "I'm never depressed!"—and P. was expressing it for her.

His depression, in this sense, was the jitsu of their dynamic—it was the obvious, wrong thing that took up a lot of their energy—and the kyo was her denied depression. Her need, I would imagine, was for some kind of expression and nurturance of her sadness, some attention. But since P. was getting all the attention and all the therapy, her kyo never rose to the surface, and the closed system of their dynamic remained intact and unconscious.

Family therapists are very aware of this kyo/jitsu interaction between people, although they express it in different ways, such as "projective identification," "enabling," and so on. It can create a lot more sickness than intrapersonal kyo/jitsu, since the basis of an entire relationship may depend on it. For example, it's possible that P.'s recovering might allow his wife's depression to emerge. Then, if the basis of their relationship is not so healthy, their marriage might be in danger. Since P. doesn't want to risk his marriage, he can't allow therapy to succeed.

We can see from these examples some of the ways in which the kyo/jitsu dynamic can operate, and of course they all interweave in any given real-life situation.

Kyo/jitsu can exist spatially, within the body, as a weak (kyo) system creates an overfunctioning (jitsu) area somewhere else.

It exists in time, as in the most recent and superficial kyo/jitsu imbalance, which is easier to correct, versus the much older and more complicated kyo/jitsu patterns that only emerge after the recent ones are balanced.

It exists interpersonally, between people and in situations.

It manifests psychologically in conscious (jitsu) and unconscious (kyo) patterns.

P.'s depression, for example, as well as the jitsu for his wife's depression, could also be a jitsu for his own kyo feelings of anger and his unmet need to hit somebody.

FUNCTIONAL AND STRUCTURAL KYO/JITSU

Kyo/jitsu, on a more physical level, could be structural (weak muscle/tight muscle) or functional (unexpressed movement/overemphasized movement).

How do you move all day? A., the lady with neck pain from the beginning of this chapter, is sitting in front of her computer, tilted slightly at an angle. That's her movement jitsu—it's noticeably static and upper-body focused. Her kyo, those movements she never or seldom does, might be strong, fast lower body movement like dancing or sprinting. Maybe it would help her neck problem if she started becoming more active in this kind of way. A very active, athletic person, on the other hand, might be helped by sitting still.

Functional kyo/jitsu can be more specific than that. Various dance-based therapies analyze all human movement in terms of choreography. There are lateral (side-to-side), rotational (around), vertical (up-and-down), flowing, stuck, fast, and slow movements. As small children, we have access to the whole gamut of human movement and can learn movement skills very easily, just as our unconditioned mouths can form words in many languages. The culture and socioeconomic group we grow up in creates our first shaping of movement expression. If we grow up in an Italian or Spanish environment, for example, we may learn to use our arms and hands quickly and expressively when we talk, not held in close to our sides. Certain muscles then get more developed, and others don't get used so much, forming characteristic body shapes. We might also learn, or not cultivate, particular body skills as children. Perhaps we learn a sport, or maybe the movement skill we learn is just sitting in front of the TV for hours on end—these activities all create movement patterns that develop our bodies in particular directions.

Repetitive stress syndrome, tendonitis, carpal tunnel syndrome, and so on are created by a limited jitsu movement pattern. The therapist will give exercises that explore and strengthen different movement pathways—the kyo functions. At least one of these weak movements is likely to be the underlying kyo.

Doing something different, almost any change in movement patterns that isn't harmful, is likely to hit a functional kyo and correct a jitsu somewhere. But here's the catch: If you just move randomly, letting the body express itself as it chooses, you'll probably only repeat the same movements you are already strong in. You have to learn something different from the outside, a new skill.

The computer programmer with carpal tunnel syndrome takes up rock climbing, and the new upper body patterns strengthen muscles that she can then use to release the other, overworked muscles that are giving her pain. The football player learns yoga and starts to use extended, stretched muscle patterns, correcting the imbalances that create the contracted muscle paths causing his tendinitis.

What's the opposite of your habitual movements? What might change if you incorporate some opposite, unfamiliar patterns?

USING THE KYO/JITSU PARADIGM

We can see the kyo/jitsu dynamic in relationships, in structure, in organic functions (an overfunctioning stomach might be caused by an underfunctioning liver, for example), in psychology, in function and movement, and you can probably think of many other areas where it manifests. Now, let's look at how to use this paradigm. How can you find your own kyo? There is enormous power and the potential of healing if you can become aware of what in yourself is unconscious, weak, unfelt, hidden, and not used. The awareness itself invigorates the kyo and starts to wake it up so it can be available to you as energy.

Invigorate the Kyo

You have probably experienced some of this already in your life. Think of problems you've had that you "got over," whether physical, mental, or emotional. You probably didn't get over them by wrestling the jitsu into the ground—such as fighting the problem directly with willpower. You almost certainly transcended rather than won, bringing energy to other physical systems, learning a new way, having a life-changing experience, or doing something else that pulled awareness and vitality into what had, until then, been a kyo.

You can see this happen by chance when someone discovers a spiritual path, falls in love, or faces a catastrophe, and the flood of new input breaks the kyo/jitsu cycle. As we age and become embedded in habit and fear, we often stop the flow of new information, holding onto our jitsu and shutting off kyo from consciousness. So younger, or at least more youthful, people tend to fill kyo more dramatically and have fewer stuck patterns.

Let's go back to A. with her neck pain. First of all, I'll step back mentally from the minutiae of her problem in order to see the more general kyo/jitsu of her life. My first move is to go from the specific to the general, to see the biggest picture I can. I divide areas of emphasis into sections: relationships, environment, psychological, spiritual, exercise, diet, breathing, work, recreation, sleep, and so on. I look at her areas of emphasis. Perhaps A.'s area of emphasis is psychological; she experiences her neck pain as an emotional issue. Maybe she goes to her psychotherapist and talks about what it might mean, how her relationship stress might be causing it. Or maybe her work situation—she works sixty hours a week—is responsible.

What she never pays attention to is exercise. It never occurs to her that some type of movement might help her neck. So my first suggestion might involve her becoming physically active and perhaps doing some exercises to strengthen her back. My guess is that lack of movement is her neck pain kyo. Maybe she never pays attention to her diet, either. I pick movement first because it makes logical sense; her back muscles are weak and the sedentary nature of her work is making her compensate with her neck muscles. We have to start somewhere. I also have to find exercises for her that don't create too much resistance, aren't too opposite from her habitual way of being. Jitsu has to be placated! Also, I won't make them too complicated and "dancerly"—I used to make that mistake a lot. I'll explain them thoroughly—appeal to her mind—and emphasize the mind/body nature of movement.

Intensify the Jitsu

The other way we could work with kyo/jitsu is the exact opposite—intensify the jitsu to the point where her own nervous system recognizes there is an imbalance and corrects itself—a sort of vaccination process. In this case, perhaps if A. were completely and entirely still in her body and mind for a fixed period of time, as in some meditation practices, she might experience more deeply the nature of stillness and crave the movement that is its natural balance. There's a risk in this approach—not so much for A., but for W., who may have to "hit bottom" with his drinking before he realizes he can't fool himself any longer and may then seek treatment. Of course, the risk is that he will hit bottom and not come back up, that he may become seriously ill or die. So this approach is a little more risky than going directly to the kyo, because it presupposes some sense of natural balance that may not be there.

Working tight painful areas—jitsu—directly is our natural instinct, and usually a good one. We want to rub the areas that hurt and actually intensify the sensation there. One reason this works is that, when the energy is increased in the right place by rubbing or pressing on the area, the tension will naturally let go after a certain point. Lots of bodywork techniques work on this principle. If a muscle or joint wants to move in one direction too much, intensify the movement by compressing the joint into the favored direction. The nervous system may well readjust. Psychological jitsu can be increased by catharsis, exaggeration of the troubling emotion until the emotions balance themselves.

When a condition has just happened, right after injury or crisis of some kind, intensifying the jitsu will usually resolve the problem. However, in the course of my work, I rarely see people right after they have been injured. Compensation only takes about fifteen minutes to begin, at which time the patterns in the body shift, becoming complex, as the organism adapts to the insult. The only chances I've had have been when my kids have injured themselves when I've been right there and once when a client had twisted her ankle outside my building, just as she came in for her appointment. Then I've had the opportunity to experiment with this concept and worked directly into the injured area, with immediate pain relief. You can't do this, of course, if a bone is broken or the skin is open. Usually in these cases the pain is not right at the injured site anyway, or the person is in shock and numb.

You can try working immediately with a minor injury like a stubbed toe. Press into the sore part until the sensation of pressure equals the pain of the toe. The pain may go away, or at least greatly reduce, and you may limit later swelling or inflammation.

You can also practice by allowing jitsu to fully express itself through movement. You can explore this with chronic pain, any kind of bound, tight, or pent-up sensation. See if you can be specific about the type of energy locked in the tissue— is it gripping, pulsing and throbbing, angular, or sharp? Experience it as simply as you can, as held energy, rather than pain. Without fear and projection into the future, pain becomes sensation, and the body can unwind. Resistance and tightening around pain is natural—but it will only prolong it and make it worse.

Psychologically, this principle is being used in the technique of thought flooding. I always thought positive affirmations didn't work, and I was aware that I worried more, not less, after telling myself good things, surrounding myself with white light, and so on. Apparently, lots of people have this experience. A psychologist, Thomas Stampfl, has experimented with the technique of having a worrier think the absolute worst, most frightening thoughts they can (intensifying jitsu), without resisting them, for a limited period of time—say ten minutes a day. The rest of the time, the chronic worrier finds he automatically worries less and can control his thought patterns, knowing he has a "worry time" later to look forward to. It interested me how this practice gave me a sense of relief.

Some addictions can be handled this way too, limiting the time period they can be indulged in, and strictly refraining the rest of the time. However, the more powerful ones have a chemical component that does not allow purposeful indulgence, or are too damaging to engage in at all.

Finding and Filling Kyo

Intensifying jitsu is usually the first way I go with a client. It satisfies them—the issue they come with is given attention. It often works. If I have no success with this approach, we then need to begin the deeper and more profound task of finding and filling the kyo.

There are many layers, of course, and many kyos. However, there is always one deep and fundamental kyo underlying the structures, hiding in the third layer, the core. Finding this in oneself is usually a lifetime task. If you bring energy fully into your own blind spot, you will completely heal (make yourself whole).

Getting the Right Balance

D. came back to me for treatments after a hiatus of several years. She had had a car accident when we had last worked, and the resulting cranial injury from whiplash had caused her excruciating headaches. That was all fine now; the current problem was a strange tightness in her hips and hamstrings that wouldn't go away no matter how much she stretched. She had tried Rolfing, chiropractic adjustments, and two-hour-long deep tissue massages, but the pain always came back by the next day.

I looked at her hips; all that excellent bodywork had loosened up the muscles around that area so much that the tension melted away as soon as I worked into it. It was easy—too easy. Obviously, that wasn't the solution, since all her tension always came right back the next day. I wasn't sure why. The Rolfer and the deep tissue masseur had worked in the hip rotators and her gluteus—I thought perhaps the problem was coming from her psoas and quadratus lumborum. Sure enough, there was a bigger change when I worked there, as I would have expected. Working opposing, antagonistic muscles is often the solution to an intractable problem.

D. came back the next week, disappointed. "It all came back the next day, just like before. How many sessions do you think this will take?"

"Four," I said, out of the blue. For some reason, I always know in four sessions if this is a problem I can work with, and if so, how. That doesn't mean the problem is gone in four sessions. She understood that.

This time, I worked with the rest of her body, seeing if I could find some other factors that perhaps had been overlooked by the other therapists. She was extremely tight everywhere else in her body; the painful hips seemed to be much looser than any other area. I didn't find anything that seemed particularly related to the hip problem, and she left. I mulled over the conundrum all week—nothing came up for me that helped me identify what might be causing her problem.

The next week she came back, much happier. "The hips are much looser," she said. We were both surprised. "Now I can feel how locked up the rest of me is!"

Now her hips were looser and the original problems with whiplash were starting to show up. I continued what seemed to be helping, that is, giving her more of a whole-body treatment, and as I worked on her, I got it.

Her body was so tight from the car accident, and all the compensations since then in her spine, that her hips were the only mobile part. The rest of her body, though very jitsu to the touch, was functionally kyo—unaware, unmoving, not much energy in it. The hips, though loose and mobile, had become the functional jitsu—they moved too much, taking on the work the rest of her couldn't do. And in fact the tightening up was due to overstretching—even though the hips were tight, they were loose relative to her body.

Working the rest of the body (the kyo), and allowing it to be more mobile, meant those overstressed hips had to do less work, so they relaxed. Working into the hips and opening up the surface tension there might actually intensify the problem, since compensation would increase.

So paradoxically, the problem places in your body could be the most flexible areas that have to work too hard, and you may need to open up the rest of your body. Often, the tight places actually need to be strengthened and the rest of the body made more flexible.

2

Structural Health: Symmetry, Space, and Flow

STRUCTURAL HEALTH involves symmetry, space, and flow. Lack of symmetry shows up as imbalance in the right/left, up/down relationships of the body (fig. 2.1). Lack of space becomes compression and tension (fig. 2.2), and lack of flow manifests as restrictions in movement, poor circulation, and blocked energy (fig. 2.3).

The right/left hemispheric balance of the brain and heart should be reflected in a symmetrical appearance, which we usually consider beautiful. Most of us are born somewhat symmetrical and develop structural imbalances as we get older, through compensation, hemispheric dominance, injuries, and habit.

Compression happens as we get older too, and gravity starts to shrink us and pull us down, if we don't work hard to oppose this. Some people have naturally tighter joints and compress more, but we all tend to either collapse or tighten, which pulls us in, and we lose our natural space and openness.

Flow is a major function of the body, and rhythm is part of our being. Together they are expressed in the circulation of blood, lymph, and all the fluids that constantly pump through our tissues; the invisible electrical frequencies that create nerve force and meridian lines; and our emotional energies. We can block our flow by restricting movement, holding in mental and emotional energy, and contracting our bodies. Imbalance of symmetry and lack of space will create blocks in our flow.

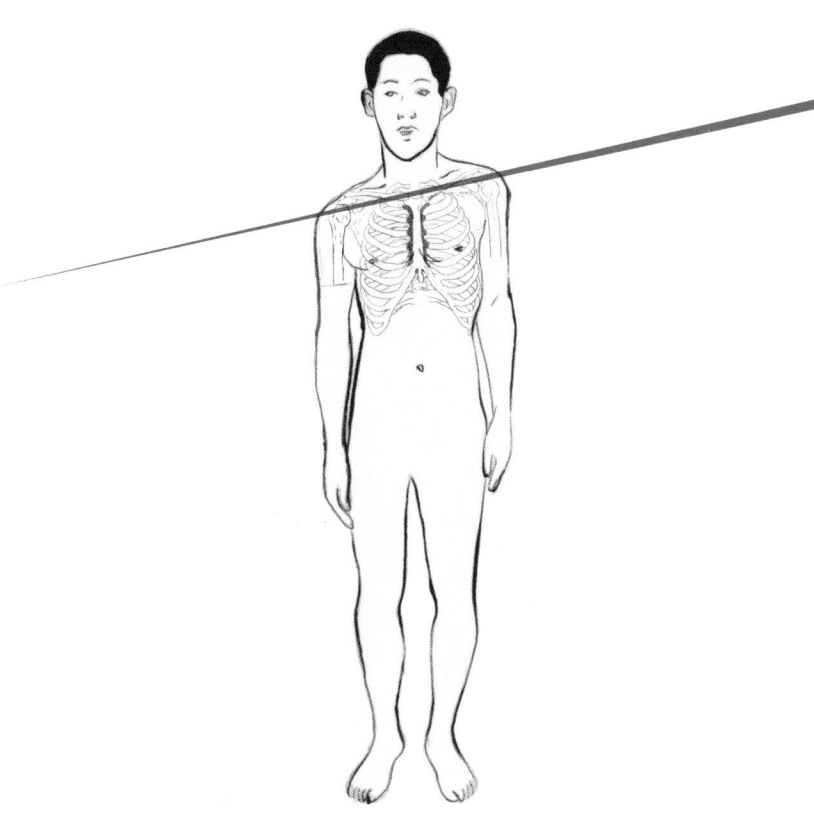

Fig. 2.1. Asymmetrical displacement and imbalance

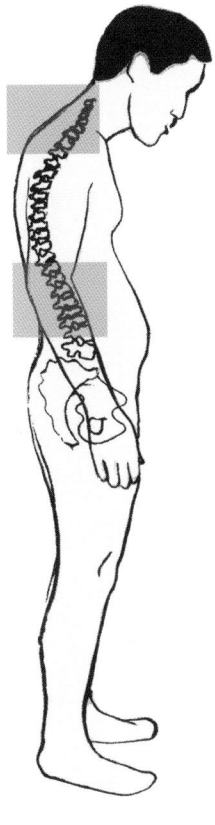

Tension
Compression

Tension
Compression

Fig. 2.2. Slouch profile:
compression and tension

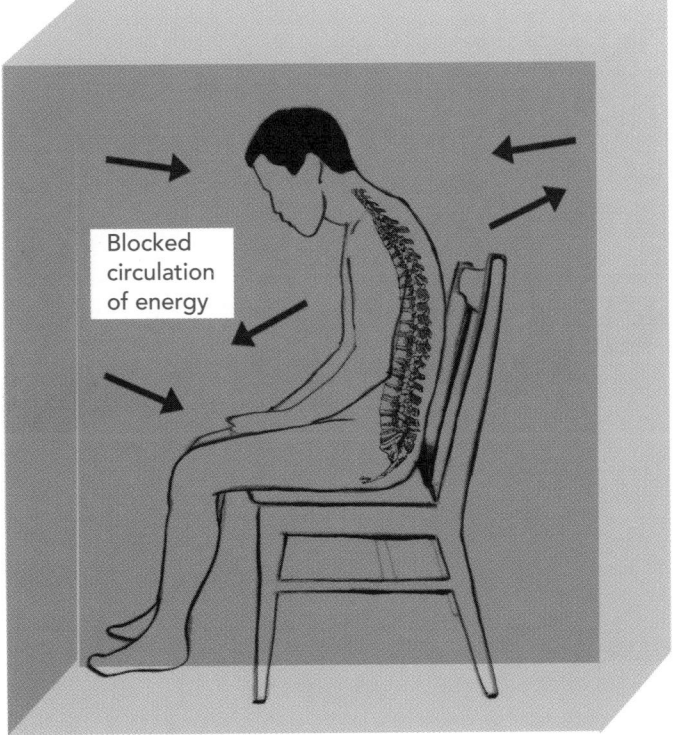

Blocked
circulation
of energy

Fig. 2.3. Poor circulation
and blocked energy

The perfect baby bodies in fig. 2.4 illustrate symmetry, space, and flow. As baby bodies change into child, adolescent, and adult bodies (fig. 2.5), they lose these qualities and become more different from one another. Individuality is gained at the price of distortion and probably pain. Some adult bodies maintain symmetry, space, and flow, yet still become distinct and individualized (fig. 2.6).

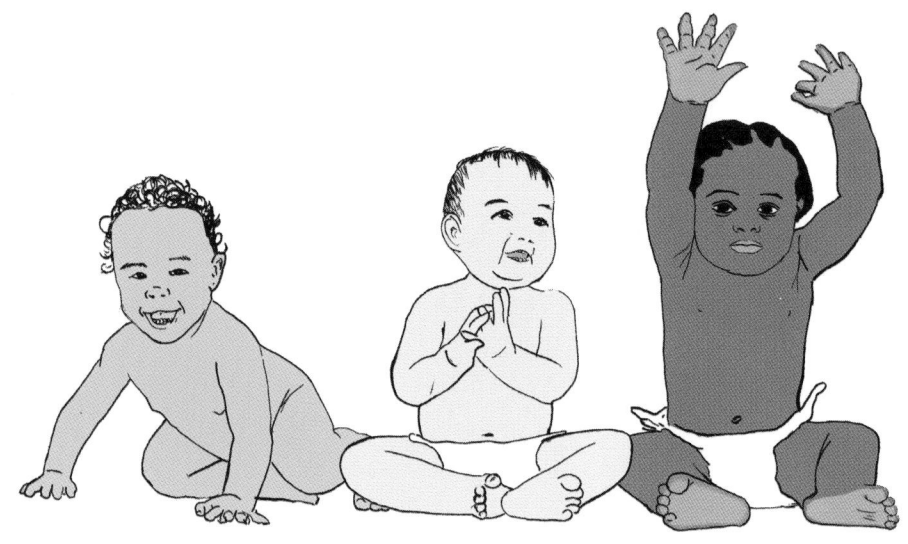

Fig. 2.4. Perfect baby bodies

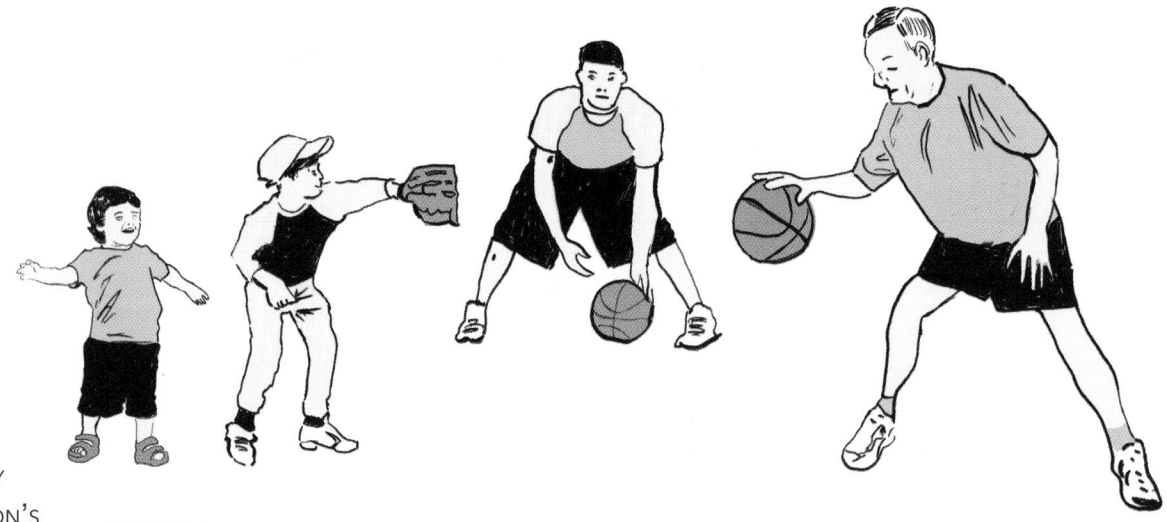

Fig. 2.5. Child, adolescent, and adult bodies

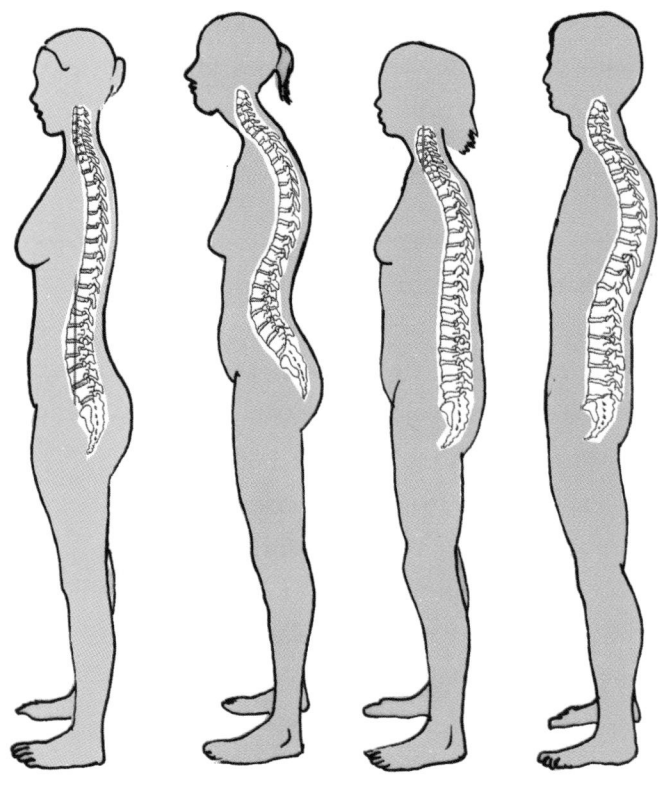

Fig. 2.6. Adult individualized bodies

GRAVITY

Gravity is probably the most important relationship we have of which we are unaware. Fortunately, it acts on us constantly and predictably, and yet that factor of constancy gets in the way of our consideration of its subtle effects on us.

Life on earth is unimaginable without the earth's force of gravity. We, as embodied creatures composed of carbon matter, share our body composition with the planet and all the organic (which means composed of carbon) life on it. We could not survive in our present form of life on any other known planet. Even at a short distance from the ground, we have to protect ourselves from removal from the earth's electromagnetic field.

We don't usually consider any of this consciously, though we know it intellectually. Furthermore, our artificial environments keep us even further insulated from awareness of our relationship with gravity. However, as our bodies progress through time, gravity forms our physical structure. Not only is gravity a ubiquitous force that pulls us downward, but we can play an active role in how we respond to it. It is this element of choice that we can work with to change our bodies.

Resistance

As upright beings we have a much more complicated developmental path than other animals toward a harmonious relationship with gravity. Human infants take a long time to walk on the ground, and lots of things can go wrong before we even succeed.

The womb, which is as close to a gravityless environment as most of us will ever experience, allows our unprotected beings to connect with the earth's surface through the mediating environment of our mothers' bodies. We're not ready, when we are born, to take on gravity full throttle. Of course, nobody expects a newborn human to walk. But we do expect them to lie on hard, flat surfaces, with gravity exerting a sudden unmediated force on their bodies. This is such a shock to a small body that usually a baby will respond by crying if left there for long.

If the crying fails to bring a response—and many well-meaning parents have left their children to cry it out, to learn to be alone—the infant will respond by tightening any muscles she can, probably in the abdomen or back, both to suppress the bad feeling and to create a sense of support, a false floor of hard muscle, inside the body, since it's not available outside. This sets the stage for later muscular armoring and an association of sensations of tightness and holding with security.

This is the beginning of a tension pattern most of us have to some extent, where the deeper muscles tighten up as we pull away from the ground and into ourselves (fig. 2.7). The emotions that go with this pattern are, first, a sense of alienation from the outside and an attitude of withdrawal into the self. The unwinding of this pattern, which is felt when the deep muscles start to release in a bodywork session, shows up when a person stands up after a session. They often say, sounding shocked, "I feel like I'm falling into the ground!" And as they move around afterward, the deep muscles of the abdomen, the inner core of the legs and feet, and maybe even the spine may begin to pull away from the ground again. It's such a strange feeling for most people, and nothing in the environment (shoes, floors, chairs, and so on) supports the release, so they usually can't maintain it for long. And yet this felt sense of connection with the ground is something we should be experiencing all the time.

The chronic state of anxiety most people live with is probably related to a severance from the earth's electromagnetic field, caused by incorrect and premature

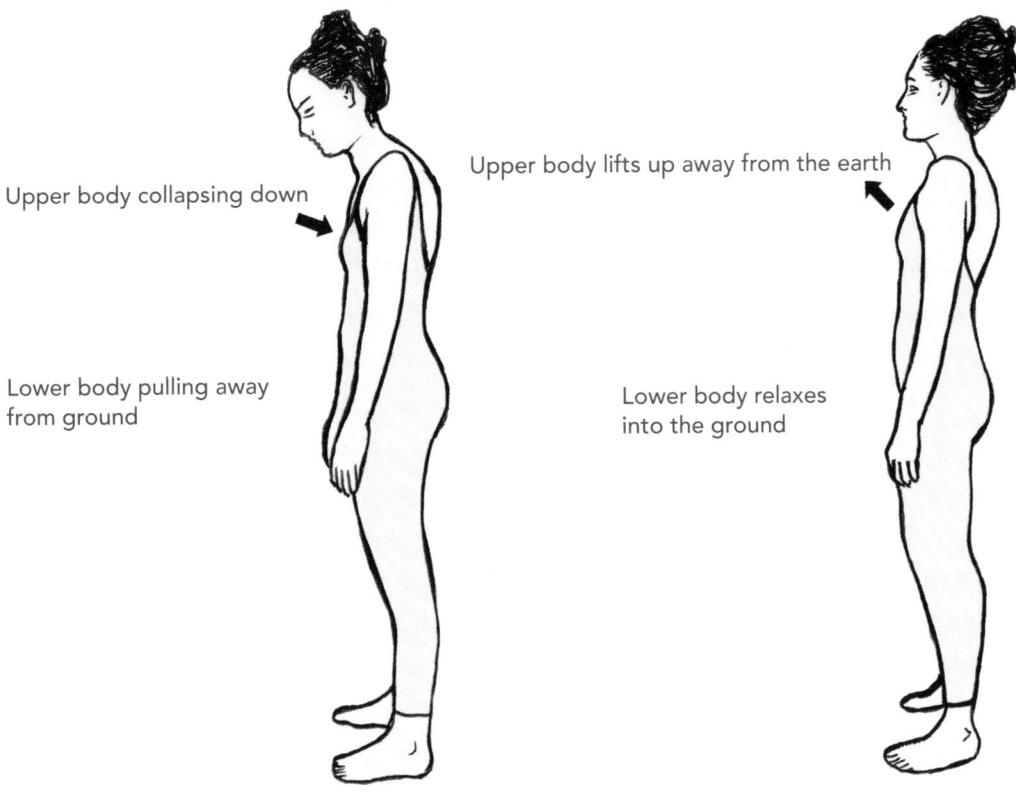

Upper body collapsing down

Lower body pulling away
from ground

Upper body lifts up away from the earth

Lower body relaxes
into the ground

Fig. 2.7. The effect of gravity on the body

exposure to the unmediated force of gravity. This abrasive and violent exposure leads
to deep tensions in the body as a defense, which later cuts us off even further from
having a proper relationship with gravity.

Collapse

The other, opposite pattern that expresses a distorted relationship to gravity is the
collapse into gravity. Usually, the pulling-away pattern uses up so much energy that
the person can't maintain a straight spine and starts hunching forward—giving in to
gravity.

We associate collapsing, hunching, and sagging with aging, and we do tend to
collapse more as we age, since it seems to require less energy to "give in" than to
resist. The inner feeling that is part of this pattern is that of defeat and despair, as
the pulling-up pattern reflects and creates mistrust. So we tend to see the lower body
pulling up away from the ground and then the upper body collapsing down. In fact,
the reverse should happen in a healthy body—the lower body should relax into the

ground to be supported by it, and the upper body should lift up away from the earth in order to move freely.

The movement pattern that would create this ideal posture is brachiation, which means the kind of diagonal swinging movement from branch to branch that monkeys do (fig. 2.8). That this pattern is part of our genetic heritage is shown by the strong grip a tiny baby has, redundant now, but useful when the baby needed to cling to its mother's fur (fig. 2.9). This grip develops later into the ability to brachiate. Children can still do this, as shown by the popularity of jungle gyms, but most adults never brachiate. Many would hurt themselves if they tried.

Notice how large the side muscles of the body are (fig. 2.10). These muscles are designed to brachiate, which works them in a stretched position, counteracting the pull of gravity by lengthening the spine. This is the kind of upward movement we need to do. We'd prevent, or cure, most back problems this way. See figure 2.2 on page 25 for a look at what causes most back problems.

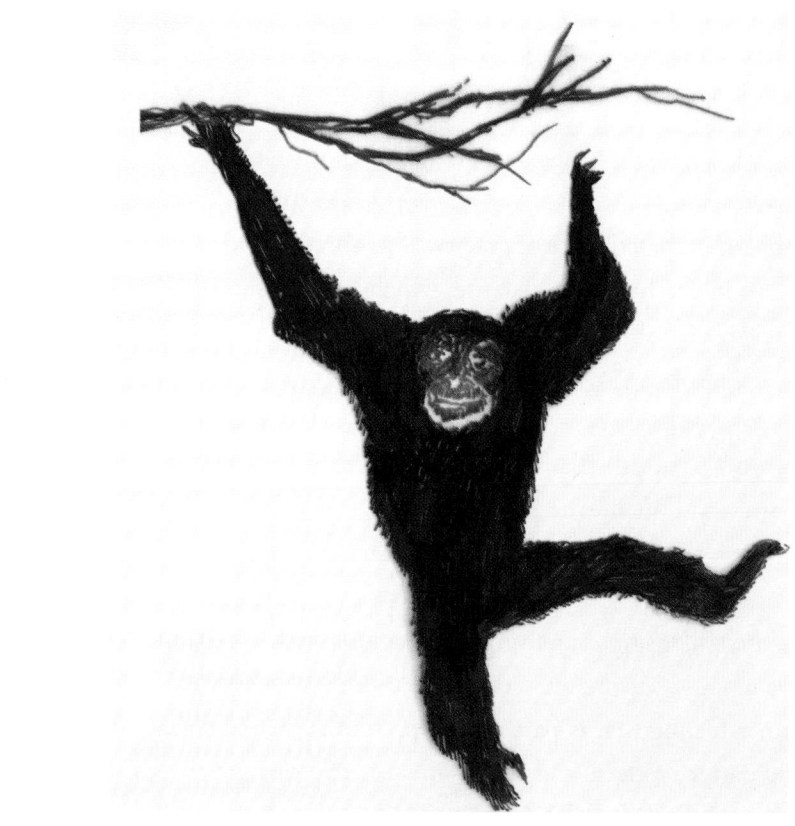

Fig. 2.8. Monkey brachiation

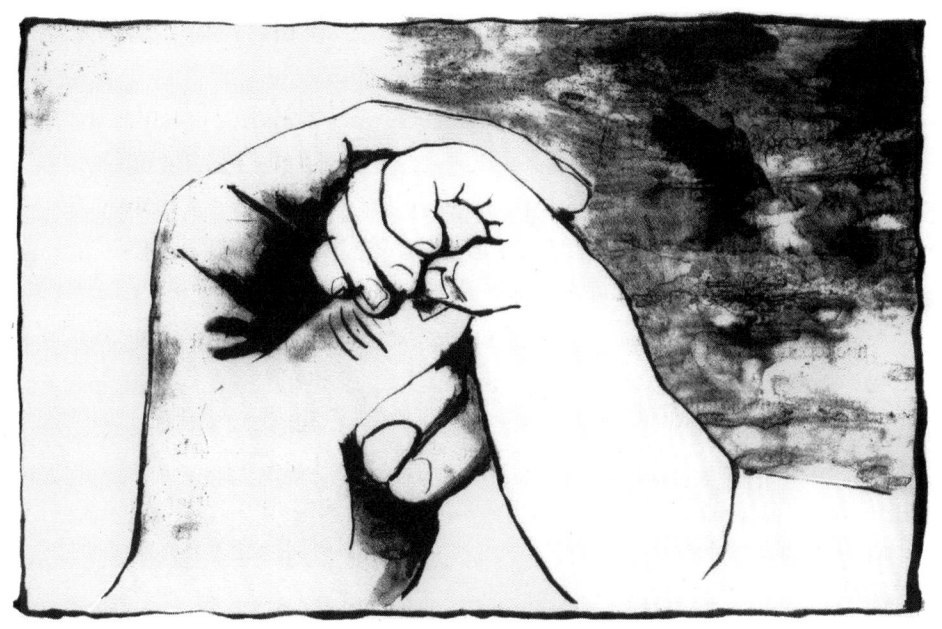

Fig. 2.9. Intense gripping from birth

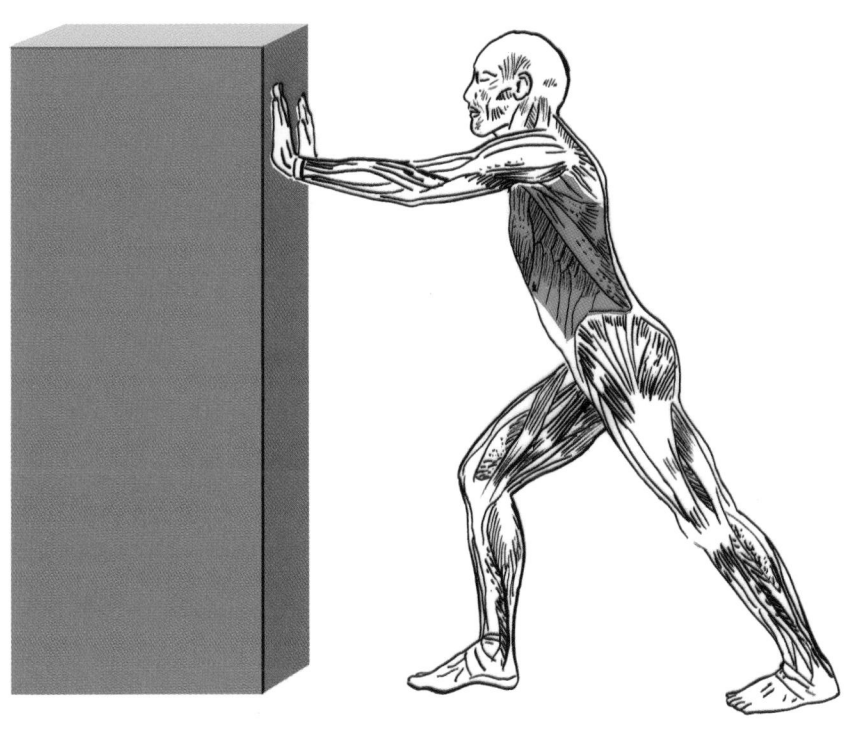

Fig. 2.10. Large side muscles

Most animals use their eyes as a source of information much less than we humans do. Humans in general trust their vision, even though it's not particularly acute compared with, say, a hawk. We also live in a visual culture, where we use our eyes all the time. Since our eyes are in front of us, this means almost all our activities have become forward facing—reading, painting, driving, watching television, and so on. In time, our heads and necks become stuck in a forward position, so the head is no longer supported by the entire spine.

The human head is so heavy (averaging ten to eleven pounds) that the tissues at the front of the body can actually start to pull away from the spine, prolapsing the organs and overstretching the back muscles, which can then tighten in order to correct the position of the spine. So we get back pain and spasms as one consequence of our troubled relationship with gravity.

This forward flexion posture, with the head pulled way forward off the central axis of the spine, the shoulders rounded forward, and the upper back forming a big hump, is almost universal in our culture (fig. 2.11). If you look at this picture more closely, you can see how the curled forward posture imitates the comforting curled-up position of the fetus in utero (fig. 2.12). It's a reaction to shock, curling in and around the sensitive organs and tissues in the front of the body. Without a balanced, mature relationship to gravity, you can feel unprotected and vulnerable walking in an upright position.

BECOMING CORRECTLY UPRIGHT

Being successfully human means resolving this problem in the body and becoming correctly upright. The design of the body at this stage of evolution actually will allow successful verticality—just—yet our lifestyles tend to mitigate it.

Look at people in the street, at work, from this point of view—how are they dealing with the challenge of gravity? Are they pulling away, collapsing and sinking, falling forward, or even locked in extension as a reaction to forward flexion?

What is a healthy relationship to gravity, and how can we achieve it? First, we need strength in the back and core muscles around the spine. The spine itself needs to be our grounding point, and its balance (firmly centered) in our body controls our relationship to gravity. The muscles of support are the back and core muscles, while the muscles of expression and movement are mostly in the periphery and front of the body. If we use the muscles of expression for support, we will have pain somewhere.

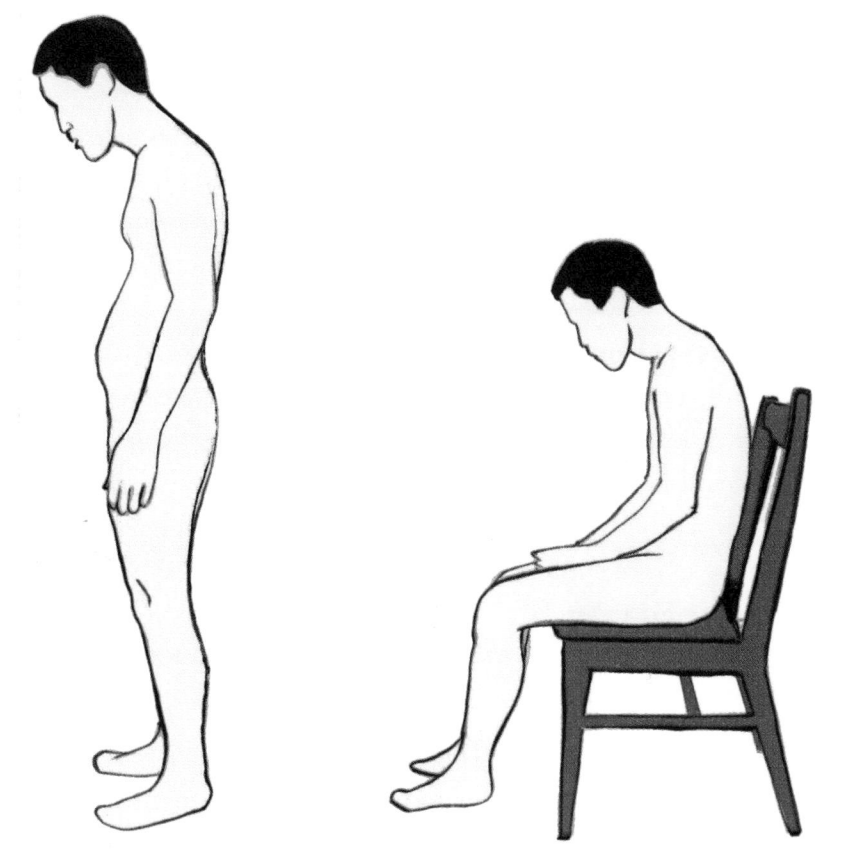

Fig. 2.11. Forward flexion posture

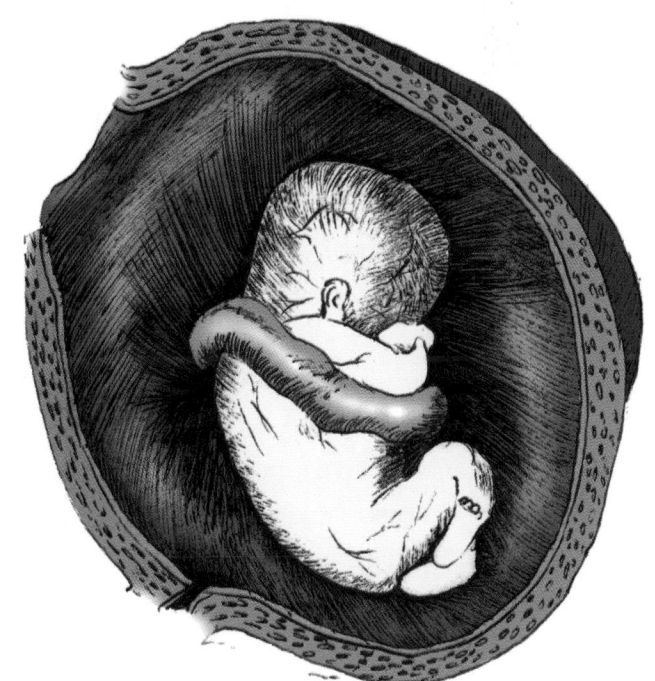

Fig. 2.12. Fetus in utero

When we are not using our arms, the hands should rest by the sides of the body, not at the front, and we should relax them when we walk so they swing naturally. Most people never fully let go of the tension that builds up in their hands and arms. When you are not using your arms, quiet them down; let them swing gently from the shoulder girdle, encouraging the free movement of the thoracic spine. If you hold the arms tight, your upper back will lock up.

When the legs pull up and away from the ground, the result is usually hyperextended, locked knees, and thighbones pushed too far forward in the hip socket. This results in stiff, weak feet with flabby arches and a rigid, high instep. Tension settles deep into the leg, as though right around the bones.

A lot of this has to do with the feet. Of course, our main connection with gravity is through the soles of our feet. The feet need to walk unshod on uneven, varied terrain. If you can't do this (and yes, I know most of us can't, or won't), then read the entire chapter on the feet (chapter 16) for foot help.

🍃 Correct the Position of Your Thighbones

This exercise should move the thighbones temporarily back into the right place, putting your legs in a more optimal relationship with gravity to support your spine.

1. Lie on your back with your legs stretched out and see how much space is under your thighs. There shouldn't be much at all. If there's more than an inch, your thighbones are too far forward.

2. To understand this, have a friend press down hard on your legs with her palms right below the hipbone for about a minute, exerting equal weight on both sides (fig. 2.13). Tell your friend she can rest her whole weight there. If she could balance, she could probably stand on that part of your leg and it would feel good. If it doesn't feel good, you either need a softer surface to lie on or your friend is pressing too low or too high on the leg.

3. To keep the bones in this corrected position, stand up and notice where your feet are on the ground, where the soles now press down, and where you feel the pelvis positioned. This is the right placement for your body. Walk around, and notice how you might need to use different sets of muscles now.

4. If you don't feel anything much, or if it's confusing, just notice where the hip joints actually are (fig. 2.14).

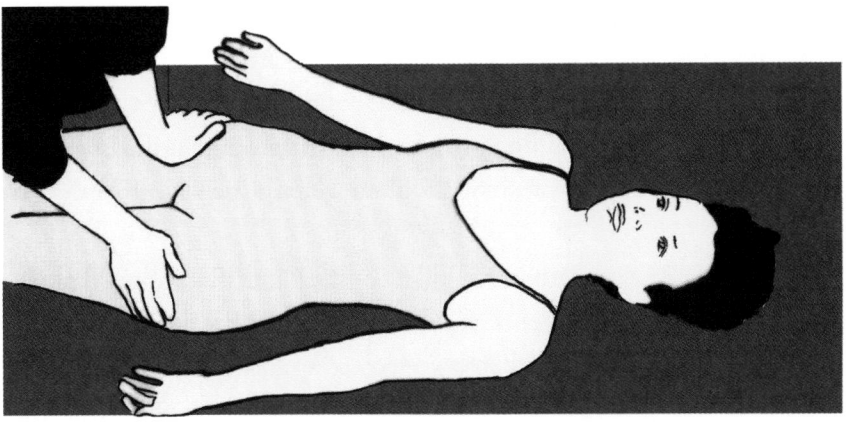

Fig. 2.13. Correct the Position of Your Thighbones

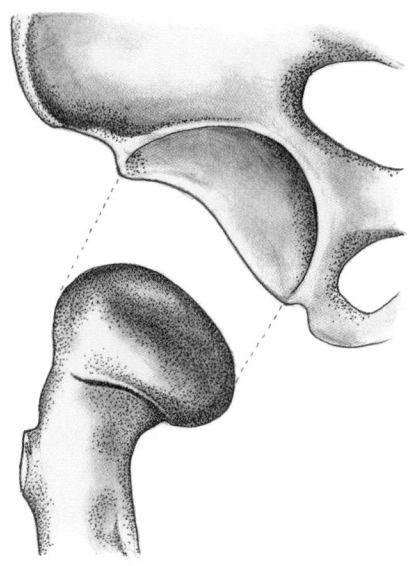

Fig. 2.14. Hip basin

5. As you walk, start the movement of the leg from a point as high as the hip joint, and slightly behind it. This will engage your psoas. Think of a kind of bouncy, up-and-down feel to your walk. You are playing with gravity, as though you are walking on a big bouncy ball. Imagine that the ground is springy and moves back at you as you walk. Feel a continuous, moving line through the center of your foot, your leg, and up into the hip joint. Imagine the springy ground is giving you energy as you move.

With this kind of movement, you probably won't be able to keep the knees locked. Soften them, even until it feels like you are bending them when you stand. Make sure your pelvis and knees stay fluid and mobile when you walk, and when you stand still, keep them free. You don't need to create two rigid poles beneath you to support yourself. Standing and walking should free up the pelvis, rather than encourage locking.

It's the muscular system, rather than fascia or the joints that should dialogue with gravity. This will give you resilience and bounce. Some very flexible people, whose joints are unstable, will lean onto their bones, creating all kinds of compression in the joints. You'll see this when people habitually stand on one leg, often with the other shoulder raised. Usually they pick the same leg to stand on, compressing the hip joint on that side more and more. These people will usually cross their legs when sitting—again, picking the same leg to cross over.

The core muscles of the body, especially the smaller paraspinals and the other connections into the spine, provide our dynamic resistance and release against gravity. The most important muscles to lengthen and strengthen, specifically in standing or sitting positions that work them in relation to gravity, are transverse abdominis, psoas, paraspinals, rotators of shoulders and hips, some neck flexors, all the muscles that support the arches of the feet, and the pelvic floor. Exercises for each of these muscles can be found in part 2.

STABILITY AND FOUNDATION

There are points of foundation in the body and points of stability. The foundational points are, simply, where your body touches a surface. If you are standing, your feet are your points of foundation—specifically, the places where your feet contact the ground, which would vary depending on the shape of the arch of your foot.

If you are sitting, your foundation points might be your feet, sit bones, and, to some extent, your back. Notice the position your body is in right now, probably sitting. The main points of foundation are where you rest most of your weight. Now press this part of your body—it's probably your sit bones—slightly into the chair. Think of pushing the chair down, away from you. Observe the differences in the rest of your body when you engage your points of foundation. Some areas relax and let go; others engage more. I feel my shoulders relax when I press my sit bones down, and my lower abdominals work harder. Automatically, I sit up straighter. I'm engaging in a relationship with gravity, rather than collapsing down into it or tightening up away from it.

When you press isometrically down through your points of foundation, you engage correct support. Foundation has to do with our relationship to gravity and that which is outside the boundaries of our bodies.

Stability, the way I'm using the term, concerns the inner intraphysical relationships of body part to body part. I've found three main points of stability. Of course, in any body position, there might be many others that vary as you move; stability interacts with free movement. These three main points are the ones that generally need to remain stable. They're navigation points with which you center and orient yourself.

The first is the soft palate, which is very close to the top of the spine (see fig. 10.1 on page 151). The second is the xiphoid process, at the bottom front of the rib cage (fig. 2.15). This is the place that Pilates instructors tell you to keep closed and slightly

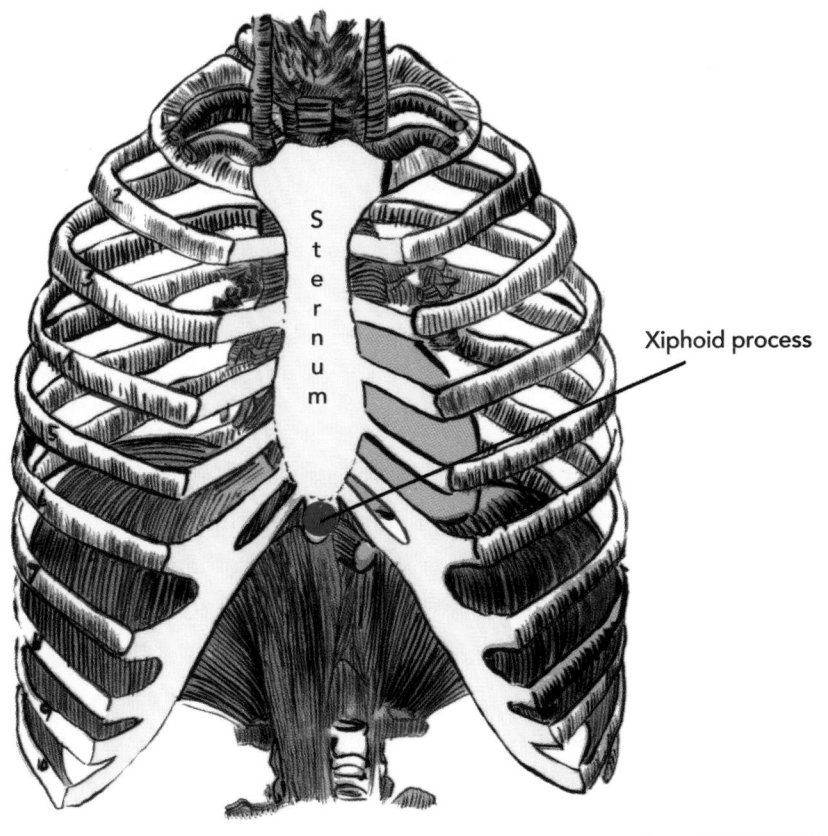

Fig. 2.15. Xiphoid process

tucked when you do abdominal crunches, to engage the deeper muscles and keep the back safe.

The third is the tailbone or coccyx (fig. 2.16). The stability of the very bottom of the spine creates the ease, or lack of it, in the hip joints and allows for easy balance when you are in alignment. The stability of the tailbone affects the inner ear; motion sickness and vertigo can be helped by correcting the position of the coccyx.

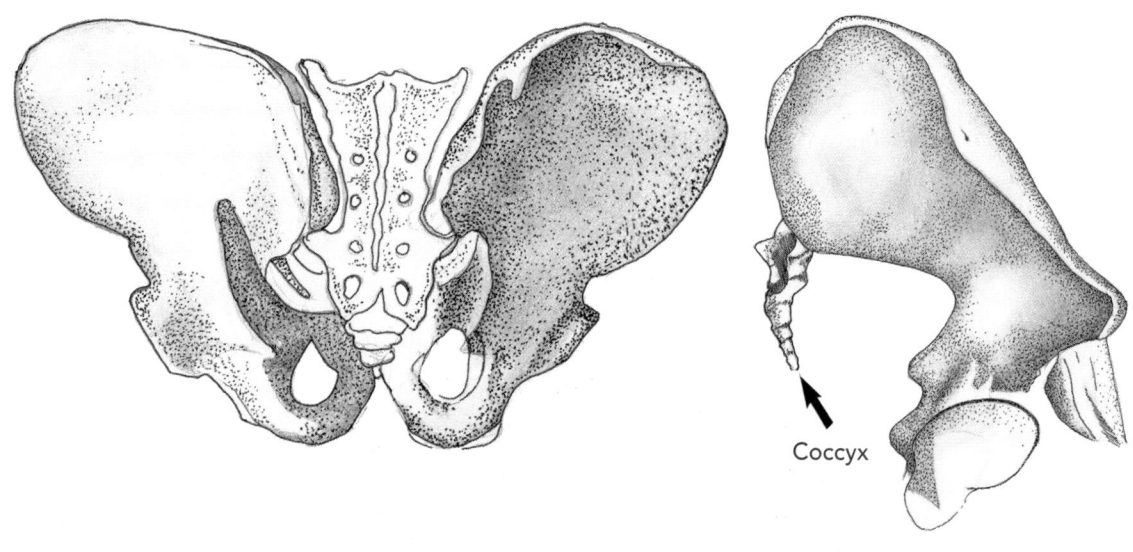

Coccyx

Fig. 2.16. Tailbone

You can also help to center your spine by using the tailbone in a balance posture, especially if balancing on your tiptoes, or on one leg, is difficult for you. Come into any balance position that's slightly difficult for you. Keep your tailbone fixed in one place. If you move in that balance position, as some yoga postures require, move from your tailbone and see how that changes your alignment.

Close to each point of stability, we have an area of the body that has a lot of movement naturally. If the stability point isn't stable, then that flexible area will compensate, and usually that's the place that will hurt. The correspondences are shown in fig. 2.17. For the soft palate, the corresponding flexible place is around

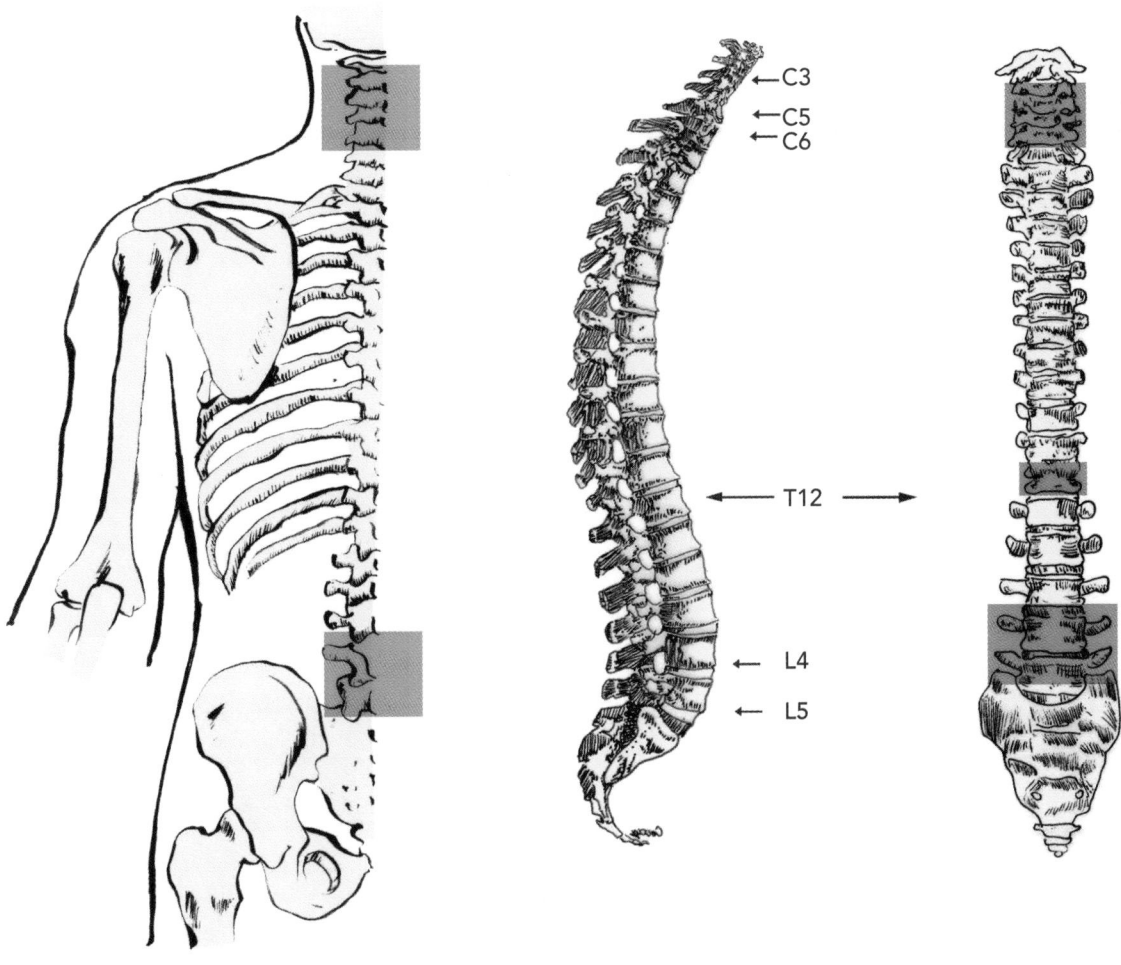

Fig. 2.17. The majority of disc problems occur in these three areas

C3, the middle of the cervical spine area. For the xiphoid process, it's T12, the hybrid thoracic/lumbar vertebra that can get us into a lot of trouble. For the tailbone, the flexible place is at about the junction of L4 and L5, where most lower back pain is experienced. The majority of disc problems occur in L4, L5, and either C3 or the stress point below it, at about C5 or C6.

3

Mind/Body

WE ARE BORN WITH, or develop soon after birth, a particular sense of living in our bodies that will condition our responses to the world for the rest of our lives.

Only we truly know what it feels like to live in this particular body, and we have no context for the feelings associated with the experience, since we have no clear idea of what it is like to live in someone else's body. We could infer that other people might have radically different experiences and assumptions—we might even be able to guess what some of them are—but we don't know why, or how, or what it is like to be another.

This very personal way of experiencing our bodies is different from the visual models of types and character that come from the outside. You might, for example, be a very short tight person, yet have a quite different experience of yourself from that of someone else with the same body type. It would depend on your nervous system, your genetics, and your early experiences.

For example, my hypermobility and weak core muscles resulted, as far as I can tell, in a feeling of inner emptiness, powerlessness, and general wobbliness that was based in the physical experience of having unstable joints that I couldn't trust to hold me securely. As I learned to walk, the paradigm for how we learn to move in and negotiate the world, the information I got back about myself and my relationship to my environment was, "Things are wobbly and uncertain. You can't trust yourself or other people. The ground may not be there when you put your foot down!"

I don't know whether the loose and shallow joint formation and the subsequent weak core muscles came from genetics, physiology, or something else—but they were there at such an early age that they formed my core beliefs and my basic view of the

---

world. The prevailing emotion I felt was anxiety and a sense of chronic insecurity. If you can't trust your own physical container, what can you trust? Even now I can't walk in the dark without putting one foot out gingerly to make sure the ground is there in front of me before I trust myself to step down on it.

The important aspect of this awareness is that changing the physical structure changes the psychology at the core level. I have experienced this and tested it out on myself. As I strengthened and stabilized those weak muscles, I became much more confident and less fearful. I stopped hating myself for being a wimp. It worked!

However, I had to be very specific about exactly which aspects of the physical structure were affecting me. Strengthening peripheral muscles, like biceps and legs, which was relatively easy, did not change my core experience. Only the deeper stabilizers actually seemed to connect with my sense of self. They were very hard to strengthen—it has taken years to understand how to do this—and I felt a strange inner resistance to the task, which guided me to the right kind of work for my body. I knew that this particular kind of resistance meant I was on track. Changing deep aspects of the self, on any level, including altering the structure of deep layers of muscle and tissue, threatens our sense of identity and our primary defense structures, so naturally the survival self will resist fiercely.

Other people, with very different types of bodies, have different psychological structures too. S., for example, is tight all over, and his joints hurt. I'm interested in this subject, and I ask him how he thinks his early body experience molded his physiology.

He answers, "My body is so tight I've only been able to feel my head—and maybe my penis—since I was a child. So I have been shut off from most of myself, especially my gut feelings, all that lower-brain stuff." Interestingly, S. was recently rushed to the hospital with acute diverticulitis (inflammation of the colon).

He continues, "What changed things for me was bodywork. As my body opened up, I felt parts of myself I'd never experienced before. I had been mostly unknown to myself, and my body was just a tight, painful nuisance." S.'s active tightness changed passively through being worked on, and my weakness changed through my own active work.

H. tells me her body has always felt twisted. Her spine is quite off center, and nothing wants to line up correctly. I ask her what that is like for her.

"I wanted to be a dancer," she tells me, "to feel that fluidity and grace in my body, as I could hear it inside when I listened to music. But when I moved, everything was all twisted and dammed up—I suppose like my emotional life was. I could never express myself freely. At least that's how it felt."

H. became a songwriter. She still looks wistful when she talks about dancing. Now she practices a lot of yoga. She talks to me often about her sense of something being in the way, standing between her and her goals. She doesn't really know what "it" is, but it's palpable; she feels it, and it does seem to manifest on the outside, as circumstances block her free flow of energy.

As we untwist her, and she untwists herself (her healing process being both active and passive), her life also flows in a freer and more directed way. People now seem more helpful, there are no sudden surprising setbacks, and success opens itself up to her. Still, her main conscious desire, for a successful relationship, is thwarted, just as the central axis of her spine is still subtly rotated.

I don't know whether she'd magically be transformed into someone who could have a good marriage if her alignment were corrected. Or, if she became that relationship-ready person, whether her scoliosis would untwist. It seems far-fetched—I think that the same factor in her that creates her inability to flow into relationship gives her the structural distortion. We could call this a neurological rather than physical or psychological issue.

Modern psychiatry has discovered the "biological base" of a lot of emotional illness, which it generally treats with medication. Despite many side effects and other problems with this approach, it's generally quicker than psychotherapy and often more effective. Because we are integrated beings, all problems exist on many levels (physical, psychological, and spiritual). However, it's often easier to change something on the physical level, because it's more tangible and therefore easier to manipulate.

So if you're depressed, I think it makes sense to start trying to correct the problem by using physical, harmless approaches, such as exercise, clean diet, and so on to normalize neurotransmitter levels. Nine times out of ten that works. Changing physical structures in a more profound way, as can be done through bodywork, will have much deeper effects on the mind and emotions.

MEMORY AND EXPERIENCE

The content of the personality is related to the experiences we have, and it is a little more conscious and under control than the structure of the body. Most of the defensive structure in the body is acquired, usually very early in our lives. The structure of the body influences not only the *form* that the personality will take, but also the basic way we engage with the world. As such, it tends to be very unconscious. Various types of "held energy" can be released from tissues without much verbal processing and still create major life changes.

Memory is not locatable in any particular part of the brain, nor can it be isolated in any part of the body. "Muscle memory" is probably a metaphor, yet I've seen thousands of people recall feelings, have déjà vu type experiences and flashbacks, when muscle and fascia release during bodywork. Perhaps that area of the body started to tighten when the experience happened, and the shock of the lengthening of the muscle somehow jolts them, triggering memory. We don't know the mechanism. However, there is a fairly predictable pattern to the kinds of feelings that are held in different muscles: The shoulders hold anger as impulses to hit are suppressed in the trapezius and in the gripping of hands and jaw; the hips and thighs tend to hold insecurity, sexual conflicts, and control issues (for example, toilet training). Feet and legs hold power and energy and express the way we connect to the ground.

How much of experience is memory? As we get older, memory becomes set into the physical structure and feels like our identity. Not all the memories that pattern us are conscious. Even if we were to lose all our conscious memories (i.e., become amnesiac), we would not lose all our habits, tendencies, or basic character. Multiple personality syndrome, where several identities are present in the same body, each with its own set of memories, illustrates this seemingly solid (because corporeal) and yet entirely insubstantial quality of the nervous system. One "personality" can have an allergy or some other physical condition, and the alter personalities can be quite free of it, even though they all inhabit the same body. So when identity Number 1, for example, ingests orange juice, and this identity is not allergic to it, there is no problem—but if the person shifts over to identity Number 2, which is allergic, while the orange juice is in his body, he can have an allergic reaction to it, even though he has no memory of its ingestion.

This demonstrates the power of the "mind" over physical reaction and also shows us how little the conscious, aware mind has to do with it. It's a very deep, unconscious level of the nervous system/mind that controls our body, and it is extremely hard to access. You can do affirmations to cure a disease until you are blue in the face, but nothing will change unless this part of the mind agrees with them. The chattering, externally focused part of our mind that most of us live in doesn't change our destinies much one way or the other.

THE POWER OF IMAGERY
AND VISUALIZATION

Imagery and visualization can help us contact that deep part in an indirect way. I've learned from teaching people that it's usually much more helpful to teach a complicated alignment adjustment (for example, Neck and Head Alignment in chapter 8) by actually stopping people from using certain muscles. Usually, we copy a movement shape by using the most available muscles we have, and the point of the alignment work is to use the very deep, subtle connections that we don't access.

So, if I say, "Absorb your C7 (see fig. 2.17 on page 39) bone into your body," most people will pull their shoulders back, stick their chest out, and so on. C7 doesn't move a bit. Whereas, if I say, "Don't move any muscles at all, just visualize or feel C7 moving into the core of your body," sure enough, the right muscles, the paraspinals, will magically engage. Visualization helped the body to correct in a way that was impossible with intentional physical effort. Some people are more visual, some more kinesthetic (touch and feeling oriented). For kinesthetic people, I might put my hands on their backs in such a way that they feel the right movement, and then say to them, "Remember how that feels when you think of C7 softening into your body."

You can use imagery yourself this way also. Visualize or feel each exercise carefully without moving—actually stop yourself moving—before you perform the exercise. Notice the differences between doing it this way and simply rushing right into the movement. If you can't visualize and feel yourself doing something, you will not be able to do it. The nerve connections are not hooked up along the muscle pathways to the brain. Work with the imagery of it, and you will eventually be able to do it.

Once our brains recognize something, we will start to process it automatically. Healing often does not happen because a traumatized area is shut off from the brain. We can reconnect it through imagery, feeling, and of course bodywork.

When I began to work on people, I didn't realize how powerful this simple reconnecting could be. I would put my hand on some part of their bodies, and they would start crying, sometimes even go into uncontrollable emotion, quite dramatically. It never seemed bad or even really frightened me; it seemed as though the nervous system was just unwinding and processing out some past emotions. Often the people did not even know what was triggering these powerful feelings. It did not matter. There was always both a physical change and an emotional relief, a sense that something that had been weighing them down was now gone. Moreover, this "something" did not return after the release was over. This seems to be how we can actually get rid of trauma. Animals, apparently, shake and emote for a while after a trauma and then are free of it. We are conditioned not to do this, so we hold in those natural responses, and years later, on my table, the release may finally happen. Too bad it takes that long.

THE EVOCATIVE POWER OF TOUCH

I was twenty-three and seeing one of my first regular clients, M. She wanted to "explore herself in a way that psychoanalysis hadn't done" for her. This was about 1981, when that sort of statement wasn't the usual thing I heard—now it's totally commonplace. I had started to work on M.'s rib cage, opening up the breath. I had noticed that when she wasn't breathing, not much that I did was very effective. Telling her to breathe usually resulted in a few overly deep breaths, as though she were trying to make up for lost time, and then a return to complete inertia. Breathing in an open way myself sometimes helped her open her breath, and of course it helped me maintain my energy, but the best way was to get the muscles that were so tight that they prevented her from breathing out of the way, by working the intercostal muscles between the ribs.

Despite her sincere intention to open up psychologically, M. couldn't let go at all. Oddly, she seemed to be almost levitating off the futon we were working on. I was poking at her ribs, she began to breathe, and then I said to her, "You know, it seems like you're not lying on the futon at all; why don't you just try feeling the surface your back is resting on?" She let go a little more, and then it was as though she had fallen way back away from my hands and somehow fallen through space into her body. She was moving back into something, and she started screaming, "Get *away* from me!" over and over. Forget about breathing—I was thinking, *What do I do? Who's listening to this? HELP! She isn't even aware I'm here.* It seemed appropriate to lightly rest my hands on her belly and wait. So I did.

She was sobbing, gasping, hyperventilating, then calming down very slowly, and then an upset would rise in her again. The rhythm eventually calmed her, and she lay for a while in complete stillness that I did not want to interrupt. Her breathing was flowing now without intervention. I waited, and finally she opened her eyes.

"Thank you," she said, and I was aware that I had done nothing.

"I remember it—I saw him standing over me—now I know it really happened." She had had a flashback of her father raping her when she was five. Despite all the therapy she had done, some sense of authenticity was missing for her because the memory itself was not there.

This was a very direct experience of the power of "muscle memory"—whatever that may be. It is empirically the case that releasing certain muscles and long-held tensions in the body can open up memories that have not been available before. Perhaps M.'s chest tightened to repress the terrible experience of incest at that young age, something her system had no language for and could not process. Maybe her father had lain on top of her, causing her chest to tighten in self-protection, and when I opened that area, part of her consciousness that had been locked in that chronically tight muscle was released and she could remember.

Touch can also operate on the deeper levels of the brain just as smell does, evoking the feel of a time and place in an undeniably powerful way. I don't know exactly how it happens, but it is a common experience. After that session I had a whole spate of other sessions with people who were abused or victims of incest, and who recovered memories as I worked on them. I was out of my depth. I didn't actually have any bad experiences, but I was aware that I might. And I had another, worse fear—that a perpetrator of one of these crimes might end up getting bodywork from me and recovering memories from his or her own perspective, and I was sure I couldn't deal with that.

On that basis, I decided to study psychotherapy, so I would be able to help clients effectively, as well as know what my own issues might be so I could keep them out of the sessions. The form I chose was Gestalt, because it is experientially based, deals with the present moment, and is nonanalytical, so it seemed to be compatible with bodywork.

✿ Working with Emotions through the Body

Here is a Gestalt therapy–based technique you can use with any uncomfortable emotion. I suppose you could use it to explore a pleasurable feeling also. You start by choosing a location in the body that you want to concentrate on; then you experience the emotion as a sensation in the body. You cannot feel any emotion without an equivalent physical sensation. It's impossible. Try it—you'll see.

1. Suppose the sensation you decide to explore is tightness in the chest. Suspend all positive or negative thoughts and judgments about that feeling, and focus, with your eyes closed, on the tight area of your chest.

2. Explore it with curiosity, sensing progressively deeper into the tightness. How are you creating it? Which muscles are involved? You could tighten it more to find out. Imagine this process as an exploration, as though you are taking a journey to a foreign land. You may see colors or images, hear a voice or sound, access a memory, think of a person, and so on. Don't judge; just keep going.

3. Go into the sensations of that area until nothing more happens, or until you find no further changes. Keep the focus. Breathe into the area. As you exhale, melt the sensations, images, and so on into the rest of your body, experiencing any tightness left as held energy that you are giving the rest of your body. Let that energy go to any place that needs it.

4. Become aware of your entire body. Then become aware of the space around you, about nine feet all around your body. Let any energy left over flow into that area too.

5. Open your eyes and focus again on the original emotion. Notice how experiencing it as physical sensation only, with no justifications or "stories" attached, allows the brain to process it in a natural way.

◈ Reverse the Process

You can work the other way too, starting with an uncomfortable, physical sensation, then breathing into it and experiencing all the feelings in that area in the same way. In this case, you may find locked-up emotions in the uncomfortable area. I do not find this a useful way to work with extreme pain, which tends to throw the nervous system off (at least for me) in such a way that calm focusing is not possible. It can, however, work for diseased areas of the body that don't actually hurt.

1. For deeper organs and systems that are giving you trouble, but not real discomfort, or for systemic conditions, go into the body and allow the organ or condition a voice. Listen with attention and respect. We generally try to tell our bodies all kinds of things and are so used to commanding them, that we don't take time to listen to what the body wants to tell us. Therefore, don't be discouraged if your body doesn't find its voice right away.

2. Again, the procedure is the same: Focus without judgment, breathe into the area, wait until there is no more change.

3. Then disperse energy through the body and nine feet around you, and reconnect with your environment.

MIND/BODY

RELAXATION OR *SHAVASANA*

Relaxation is a shift from sympathetic dominance to parasympathetic dominance in the nervous system. If we are not able to make the shift easily, we may have a hard time going to sleep or calming ourselves, or conversely, we may feel sluggish. Animals—wild ones, at any rate—switch from complete relaxation to total muscle activation, and back, very quickly and without difficulty. Humans deal with the obstacles of muscle memories, held emotions, and chronic stress. We may need to relearn the ability to switch autonomic dominance quickly.

Drugs that sedate or stimulate can interfere with this natural ability, and then the entrapment of the nervous system in one mode can lead us to use more and other drugs to soothe or enliven us. So let us learn this natural ability and bring our autonomic nervous systems back into healthy functioning.

Exercise, a prime example of sympathetic activation, can automatically bring us back into relaxation if our reflexes are healthy. The release of adrenaline, at a certain point, will actually relax us, as you may have experienced after intense stress, physical or emotional. There can be a wonderful feeling of physical calmness, tiredness even, and a mental softening, yet alertness. Chronic stress and fear let go for a while. However, this reflex works only as far as our minds can let go, and as we grow older and hold on more anxiously to ourselves, the stress/relaxation cycle can become less efficient.

🌿 *"Switching" to Relax*

Practice "switching" to relaxation after exercise initially, and when you get used to this you can use it to release mental stress, too.

1. Make yourself comfortable on the floor, any way that you feel good. Use pillows as needed. Get any fidgeting or tensions out of the muscles first. You can tighten all your muscles and then release them.
2. Amplify any distressing emotion by moving deeply into it, then expressing it as movement, discharging it as fully as you can through your muscles.
3. Then find a comfortable position on your back and completely cease all outer muscular movement. Focus on being very still. Involuntary movements, such as twitching, may happen, so simply wait until your body has freed itself of the need to move.

4. When your body becomes still on the outside, drop your awareness away from your muscles into your skeleton, the framework of your bones, as you lie on the floor without moving. Trace your bones in your mind's eye, starting with your feet, going up into the ankle joint, legs, knees, pelvis, spine, and so on. Don't worry about anatomical correctness; just feel the hard core of the body, paying attention to what you actually feel, especially around the joints. You will naturally still feel the deeper tensions as you shift your focus into the bones.

5. All tensions are in muscle or soft tissue, so instead of focusing on them, imagine the muscles dissolving like air and the soft tissues floating away from the bones, until you are just skeleton. Feel the properties of bone, living bone, which is pink as it exists in your body (bone only whitens on exposure to air). Identify with the part of you that is your framework, your skeleton.

6. When you feel this, shift your attention to your smooth muscles: heart, intestine, bronchioles (lungs), and the movement of your blood in the veins. When these sensations are strong, you will automatically shift into parasympathetic dominance, feeling a sense of calm and relaxation. At this point, you can either meditate or return to sympathetic mode.

4

What Is Tension?

THE MAIN FACTOR that gets in the way of our understanding pain and tension has to do with the process of compensation. The purpose of compensation is to ensure survival, crucial earlier in our history, but now mostly negative in that the healing process is inhibited by compensatory distortions.

Take as an example an injured knee. One knee hurts, so you stand on the opposite leg, causing compensation in that hip. Suppose the knee stops hurting, but you still stand on that leg because it feels familiar and is associated in your nervous system with relief from pain. It has become emotionally comforting to stand on that leg, so you do it more and more. The hip becomes tighter and tighter. You may even notice this and try to adjust, but the other hip has become weaker and unused to giving support so it feels uncomfortable and you forget about it. Maybe you end up with sciatica or a lower back problem from the compression in the tight hip. Even if you do not, or if you correct the pain symptomatically without changing the pattern, in more time the shoulders may start twisting to one side and the neck may twist to the other. All that is happening is your body is trying to find ways to keep you upright.

The compensations we use can be different for each of us, and they will be unconscious. So you can see how you could end up with a pain in the neck that comes from a pattern that is an adaptation to a knee injury. It is important to recognize that the painful neck is not caused by the neck but by the adaptive pattern. In order to work through the painful neck, the pattern itself must be undone. If the neck alone is treated, the pain will return, or shift somewhere else. When you start to work on a compensated area, such as the tight neck, the true causes will start to show themselves as the neck muscles unravel. At first, the shoulder may hurt, or

50

you may be aware that you are twisting it in some way. Then, as you start working with the shoulder, you may find out that certain areas in your back are tight, and so on, until you start to feel the knee and are able to work the original injury through and out.

It's not always this neat, of course, because there can be several processes of compensation happening in your body. Emotional stress, which is the suppression of a muscular response to a situation over time, can also lead to patterns of compensation that have little to do with their origin. The tensions in the compensating muscles will tend to create the stress over and over again by reinforcing memories and responses, in effect keeping part of the emotional energy fixed in a past experience. Understanding the emotional aspects of the patterns, even experiencing the feelings involved, often does not change the muscular holding patterns because of the process of compensation.

Work habits, like sitting at a desk all day and using a computer, create their own patterns just by engaging certain muscles over and over again and, equally important, not using others.

MUSCULAR TENSION

Muscular tension is the chronic contraction of a muscle. The contraction of the muscle is necessary for movement and weight bearing. A healthy muscle contracts and expands freely and equally. If the muscle contracts and does not expand to a sufficient degree to release the tension of the contraction, you will have a chronic imbalance and, eventually, pain. The pain may not be in the tense muscle, but the imbalance that the immobilized muscle creates will cause pain somewhere.

A chronically contracted muscle will become weak and nonfunctional. The sheets of connective tissue around and between the layers of the muscle will harden, because a healthy muscle functions as a pump, moving blood and lymph fluid and flushing out toxins. When the muscle is immobile, the metabolic wastes won't be pumped into the fluids of the body and will get caught in the net of the fascia, becoming granular, "crunchy." You'll notice that the muscles we move a lot, like the biceps, don't develop much granulation, and the less mobile ones can become quite crunchy (feel the tissue next to your spine, or on your head).

This hardening of the fascia may be the body's way of protecting a weak place by cocooning it with connective tissue to prevent motion and, therefore, injury.

You'll notice we don't have chronically expanded muscles. That's because inside each muscle belly is something called a Golgi receptor; that is, a bundle of nerves that tells us where we are in space—or to be more accurate, it informs the brain where the muscle is. When the muscle expands too far for too long, the Golgis set up a reflex where the muscle actually contracts to protect itself and to attempt to pull the body back into line.

For example, suppose you chronically tilt your head to the right to look at your computer screen. The right side of your neck will shorten and tighten first, since the muscles don't ever fully lengthen. Then the left side, which is always stretched, will contract due to the Golgi reflex. So you'll see that muscles can be "locked short"—the right side, or "locked long"—the left. Neither side will have full range of motion.

The nerve signals to the brain will also be blocked in time, and the Golgi sensing mechanism will dull, so you won't know any longer where the muscle is in space. You may feel like your neck is straight, and then a get a shock when you look in the mirror. One ear is probably higher than the other, one eye bigger and so on. All these asymmetries are signs that there is chronic tension in one group of muscles or more.

People often ask, "Should we be perfectly symmetrical?" It's a good question. The arrangement of our organs is not the same on both sides. Our heart and stomach are on the left and the heavier liver is on the right (fig. 4.1). So the diaphragm and the bottom of the rib cage, where those organs abound, are not symmetrical (fig. 4.2). The right side of our bodies is slightly heavier than the left. Aside from that, and what seems to be our natural right-handedness—which is not universal, of course—we are, for all practical purposes, symmetrical structurally. Think about how symmetrical—and alike—babies are. Part of the aging process is the gradual development of asymmetries. And they can cause, or indicate, problems.

THE INTERPLAY OF BONES AND MUSCLES

The bones, organs, and other tissues can also be out of balance structurally, and that will pull the muscles out as well. To paraphrase Ida Rolf,* think of a tent, the

*Ida P. Rolf, *Rolfing* (Rochester, Vt.: Healing Arts Press, 1989): 65.

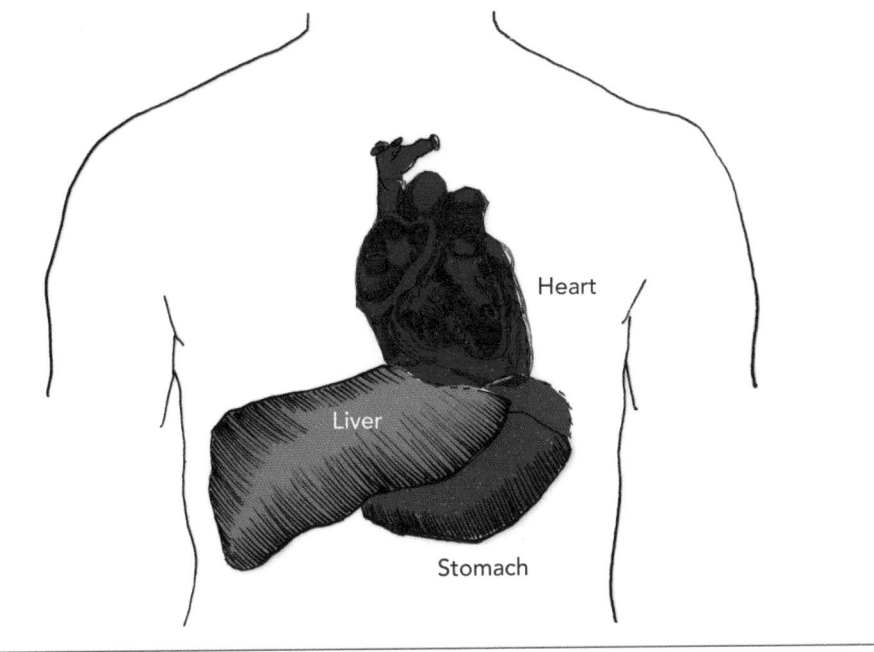

Fig. 4.1. Nonsymmetry of organs

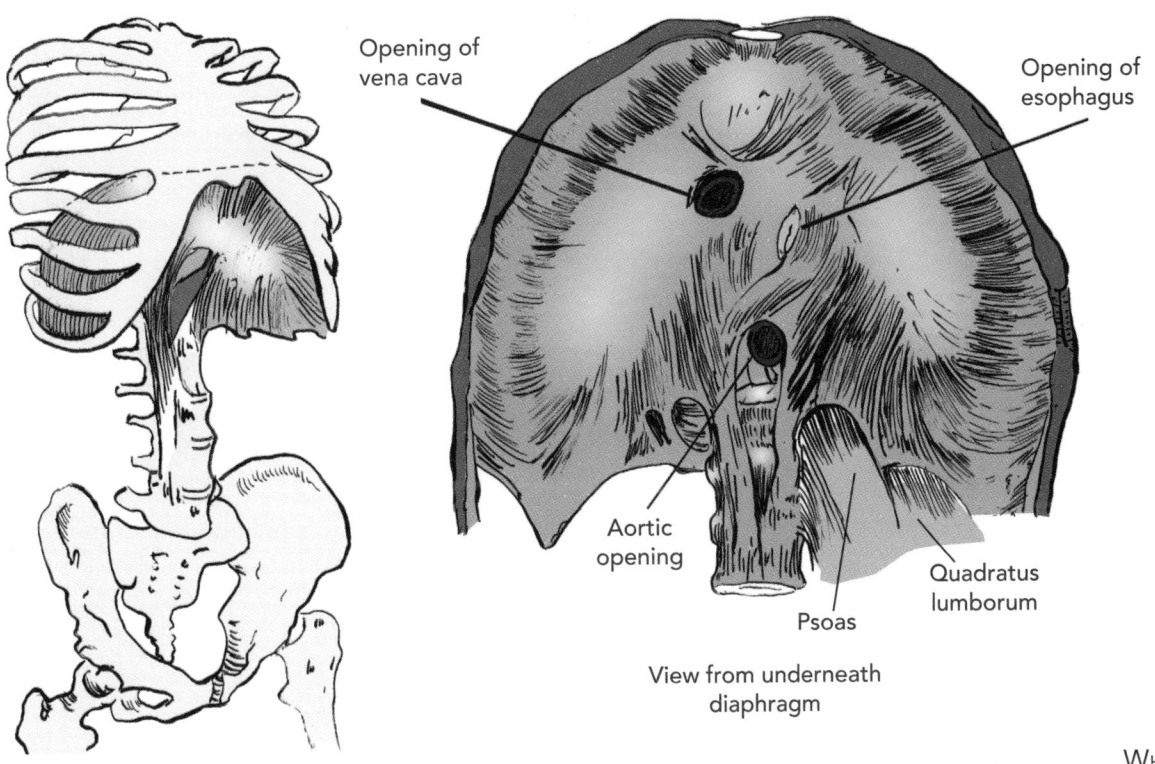

Fig. 4.2. The diaphragm

middle pole supported and centered by ropes; the bones are like the solid poles, the muscles are the ropes. The ropes can pull the poles out of line, and if the pole is leaning to one side, the ropes will be shorter on that side and more slack, longer and less taut on the other. Using this analogy with the body, you can see how the muscles would be affected if, for example, you have a curved spine. The same problems might happen if you have a habit of leaning to one side all the time. At some point, the bones will be pulled over in that direction because the attached muscles will shorten as I described. The bones can actually change their shape—in an adult as well as a young person—as the forces of muscles and fascia pull in one direction.

Tension in one part of the body can be caused by shortening in the opposite part. For example, most of us are very aware of tension in our backs and the back of our necks, while we are generally not as conscious of the pulling in of our shoulders and chest, the deep muscle contractions in our throats and abdomens that cause the tightness and pain in the back. The "forward flexion" posture (see fig. 2.11 on page 33) creates tension in the back of the body as our inner body intelligence attempts to balance us in space, making for an exhausting tug-of-war as the back muscles contract to straighten us up, and then the shortened frontal muscles tighten in reaction, shortening more. In order to free up the neck and back, we must lengthen and open those contracted front muscles, and the layers of hardened fascia that accompany them.

Since the "forward flexion" posture is so common, we can classify the probable relationships between front and back:

- Pain in back of neck, TMJ (temporomandibular joint) syndrome—chronically shortened scalenes
- Upper back pain—internally rotated shoulders, shortened pectoralis, serratus
- Lower back pain—shortened psoas, tight crura of diaphragm, calves, and shins (tibialis anterior)

And so on . . .

This is helpful to me, as a practitioner. For you, the concept of looking to the opposite side of the body for the origin of chronic tension can also be useful when you understand the various practical applications.

THE MAIN CAUSES
OF MUSCULOSKELETAL PAIN

For now, let's look at four main causes of musculoskeletal pain: compensation, compression, restriction, and biochemistry. All of these are the body's attempts to restore balance to an imbalanced situation.

Compensation

Compensation is a basic survival tactic that exists on the physical and emotional levels. Given a problem that can't be solved in the here and now, we will develop a solution that may stop us feeling the original pain and allow us to move and function more or less easily, but we have done nothing to solve the real problem, and the "solution" itself can create more problems than the original situation. Since the solution feels right, it tends to become habitual and fixed, persisting long after the original trauma should have healed and actually preventing healing. Psychological defenses and physical compensations work the exact same way—and of course correlate and cross over in real life, so that psychological issues create tangible, physical compensations, and vice versa.

Chapter 1 on kyo/jitsu explains the process of compensation more fully. For our purposes now, let's look at how this cause of pain operates in our lives. Suppose you have injury; say, you twist your ankle as a small child. You're jumping over a hole in the road, and suddenly you're in pain and can't move. The shock and trauma embed themselves deeply into your tissues. You never want to feel this pain again.

You get up and hobble around. Nothing's broken, so your parents just bandage up your foot, and you withdraw your nervous system from the foot. This part is important: You shut off the part of the brain that connects to some of the injured muscles in that area. You do this so it doesn't hurt, but the cutting off of sensation also weakens the muscles. This weakening may last your whole life if you can compensate successfully by using other muscles. Healing, complete recovery of all our capacities, doesn't happen in the normal course of things at all. What is restored is functionality, which we call healing. But functioning often means we come back to normal on the surface, yet we have lost big chunks of our feeling. We have lost our life force.

Now you, as a child, walk around for a while gingerly, not wanting to put any pressure on your injured foot. You learn how to play without using that foot at all. Eventually the ankle heals, and you could now walk on it, but you don't.

If nothing changes, you'll develop a habit of walking on the other foot. The extra weight you put on that side of your body will cause a strain in that hip. Maybe over time that compressed hip will start hurting, and you'll get lower back pain, which you will never connect—nor will anyone else—with the ankle you twisted as a child.

Because of the compressed, tight hip, your body now leans to that side. To balance yourself, you instinctively put your bag over your opposite shoulder. That stops you from overbalancing, but it causes tension in that side of your neck. You could be eight or eighty when this happens, and by then you've no doubt had many other injuries that will intertwine with this first one. With each succeeding injury, the life force shuts off more and more.

If you go to a doctor, you'll probably get painkillers for the neck pain. You can see now how this response, maybe necessary in the short term, can just cause more compensation in the long term. Compensation has to be undone before the trauma can fully heal. Again, we come up against the differences between "the mind of the body," which will not heal us, but will keep us alive and functioning, and the more conscious parts of ourselves that we must make an effort to use to heal.

Compensation comes from injury, habits and tendencies, emotional patterns, and other compensations. Undoing the compensation involves unraveling the layers of defenses on top of the trauma, and then providing the body with another solution—that's an important piece. Without the new, healthier movement patterns, we may revert to the old solutions.

Compression

Compression, the shortening of the tissues, collapsing of the softer structures, and hardening and pulling in of the tighter ones, tends to be seen as part of the aging process, as we give in to gravity and lose our childlike bounciness. Yet we see very little compression—sometimes none—in older yoga and tai chi practitioners. The length and space in the body can be kept open, no matter what our age, by opening up the spaces between the vertebrae and moving in such a way as to strengthen the muscles in a lengthened position. This is the secret of keeping length and flexibility in the whole body. We need to keep the spaces in the body open just as we should keep our minds open.

Sitting with the spine compressed, as happens when we sit in most chairs, locks up the bones, compresses the vertebrae, and thins the discs. The best chairs I've seen are the ones built around a physio ball—they look like the frame of a chair, structured around the ball. Bouncing on the round surface of the ball would be a perfect way of pumping up the discs and opening up those spaces. It looks like a lot of fun too.

Compression is often caused just by being sedentary, especially sitting for long periods of time. The large side muscles of the body are designed for brachiation—that is, swinging from the arms like you do on a jungle gym, or how you did as a child. Most adults don't continue this wonderful exercise. Maybe we wouldn't have so much back trouble if we did.

You can see that, from the evolutionary point of view, we are designed to cling to our mothers' bodies right after birth—everyone is born with a well-developed gripping reflex—see fig. 2.9. As we mature, this primitive muscular reflex develops into a lengthened, strong motion of supporting our spine from the large side muscles involved in swinging from monkey bars and climbing (fig. 2.10). This development would keep the spaces between the discs open, loosen and strengthen the shoulders and upper back, externally rotate the shoulders, and open up the chest—all the benefits of the jungle gym exercise. It would give our pelvis and feet a break too.

Pull-up-type exercises will give you some of the benefits of the brachiation (jungle gym) movement, but not the movement through three dimensions—they are straight up and down rather than diagonal, so they will only develop the muscles in one plane (fig. 4.3).

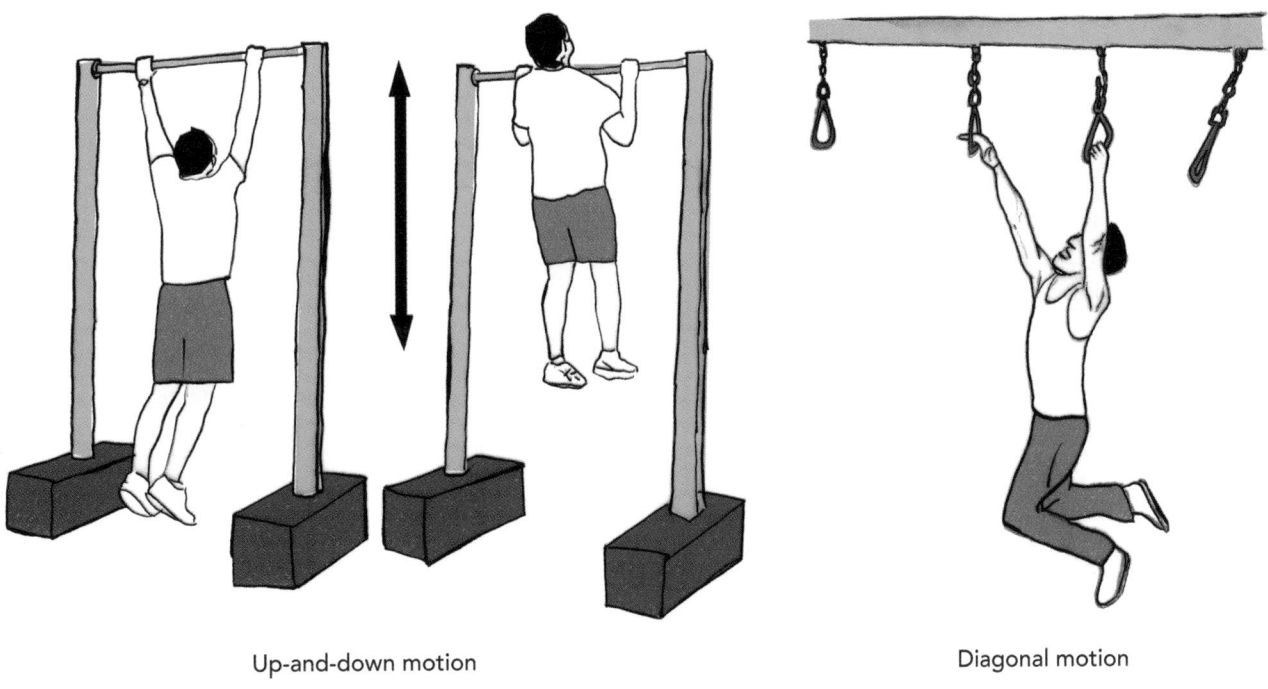

Up-and-down motion   Diagonal motion

Fig. 4.3. Pull up versus jungle gym exercises

If you can, and it does take a lot of strength, I suggest jungle gym exercises. You have to build up to them carefully, though, and not hang into the shoulder joint. The yoga position called the side plank will develop the lower parts of these muscles and can substitute for the jungle gym.

You can see how sitting at a desk has the exact opposite effect of brachiation. The typical sitting position, with the head bent forward, shoulders internally rotated and lower back slumped, flattens the spaces between the discs and compresses the hips. If we had thought about it, we couldn't have come up with a worse position. We are not designed to sit for long periods of time in a chair. If we have to, we need to compensate with opposite movements and also learn to sit correctly.

All positions that are held for a long time will have a profound effect on our bodies. They become, essentially, yoga asanas, changing our physiology and psychology. This is subtle and happens over time.

When children are first confined to desks, they suffer terribly and usually can't maintain this position for long. They squirm, wriggle, and become restless. We have to teach them to lose the natural disinclination to sit still. In the process, if they do as they are told, they will lose the mobility of their spine, the flow of lymph and blood to the torso, the openness of the chest and shoulders, and the natural breath. The organs are compressed in this position, the diaphragm can't move properly, and the pelvis loses its blood flow. Energy will tend to pool in the head and the eyes, which will feel like alertness at first but can become mental strain as the fluids congest in the upper body. Often the eyes are the first organs to feel the stress.

Restriction

The other factor that causes musculoskeletal pain is restriction of the rotational movement of the spine. We are so used to not moving the spine, we don't notice it much when we exaggerate this pattern, usually by carrying things on one side. The thoracic vertebrae are particularly prone to stiffen. It's the rotation of these bones, as we let our arms swing while walking, that helps keep the thoracic area open. Walking, which loosens the hips, letting the arms swing and positioning the head correctly, gazing straight ahead, is one of the best exercises there is to combat restriction. Yet how often do most people move this way?

I'm looking out of my window now, and below me on the street I see people walking—some fast, some slow. At least they are walking. If I were outside of Manhattan, they'd probably all be in cars (sitting in really poorly designed seats).

However, each of these people I'm looking at is carrying a bag on one shoulder, restricting the rotation of one side of the spine, or else they're clutching a cell phone to their ear or staring at a screen texting, creating an unnatural curve in the neck and shoulders. I see one woman walking without impediments, but what is she doing? Her hands are in her pockets, and one shoulder is hunched up to her ear.

When you are not using your arms, relax them, let them swing naturally from the shoulder girdle, and let go of any muscular holding in the hands. Feel how the shoulder girdle is supported by the rib cage and how the breath moves under and around the girdle. Instead of trying to relax and pull back the shoulders, let go of tension in the forearms and hands. If we are not holding onto something, or using our hands, perhaps we feel helpless—maybe that's why tension in the hands is so pervasive.

Experiment with walking like this, even if only around the house, and notice if you use your arms unnecessarily, bringing them up and against your body when you talk to someone, for example. This is a defensive position that closes the heart and chest. When the arms are relaxed, the chest is open, and you may feel more vulnerable. Use the breath around the upper chest area to relax the shoulders. This will also bring you back into self-awareness and make you feel less uncomfortably exposed.

Restriction, the holding in of a felt movement, can also happen when a desire to do something is blocked in the muscle and relegated to the unconscious. This is the body acting as the great garbage can of the mind, container of all the stuff we don't want and can't let go of, which then gets stuck in the tissues. I always think of the diaphragm as the lid of the garbage can, because all restriction of movement comes from a stopping of the breath.

Biochemistry

Biochemistry is another important piece of the puzzle. It is nearly always involved in pain but is never the only factor. In most cases, changing nutritional factors, improving breathing patterns, and exercise will have corresponding effect on biochemical factors. Structural resolution opens up the flow of energy, lymph, and blood. So they all interact. However, sometimes allergic and nutritional factors are the most important ones. The pain doesn't go away until an allergen is removed or the diet is improved. There are also genetic factors that involve biochemical differences and make some people more prone to pain.

It's complicated, so I'm going to simplify the description a lot. There are many new, interesting studies on inflammation and its chemical pathways, which you can read if you want more specific information. Arthritis just means inflammation, which is the body's response to increased acidity in an area. Acidity signals that something is wrong, since there are toxins in the area. Most of the natural metabolic waste products in our bodies are acidic—lactic acid, for example. Excess acidity is harmful, so the body sends fluids to dilute this, causing swelling, and immobilizes the area, causing pain.

Deacidification is really a better description than detoxification of the processes by which we eliminate toxins. Any prolonged departure from the natural pH of the body (which is a little different for each fluid) will create pain or disease.

The process of the body's attempt to resolve a balanced pH can also create damage. Most of the "aches and pains" we associate with getting older come from glycation, which is caused by an excessive carbohydrate buildup in the body. Actually, it can cause pain at any age, but it tends to build up in the tissues, so we often don't feel it till we get older. This excess carbohydrate, not used for energy, causes cross-linking and breaking of protein fibers.

People who eat a low carbohydrate diet will have less glycation, but if their diet is full of the acidity and the excess fat of a high animal protein diet, they too may experience glycation due to the effect certain fats have on insulin levels. The people I know who eat a lot of raw vegetables and fruits, the 80 percent alkaline, 20 percent acid ratio that's supposed to be ideal (most vegetables and fruits are alkaline), have very little body pain and rarely have arthritis.

The exceptions are if you have a biochemical "glitch," which is genetic, and can't metabolize oxalic acid, which is found in beets, spinach, and chard; citric acid, which is in citrus fruits and many supplements; or the compounds in the nightshade family, including tomatoes, eggplants, potatoes, and bell peppers. Salicylic acids can be a problem too; they are used in cosmetics, aspirin, antiseptic, and toothpaste, and small quantities are used as a food preservative.

Any specific allergies—food, environmental, anything—can trigger pain too, and it can seem quite unrelated. Headaches are frequently caused by the ingestion of allergic substances. TMJ syndrome can be caused by allergies; the nervous system is shocked by the substance, and a chain reaction follows. The flow and rhythm of cerebrospinal fluid is jolted by the shock, the covering of the spinal cord and brain (especially the outer layer, the dura mater) is affected, and this changes the positions of the cranial bones, which then affects the jaw, as a part of the skull.

Some minerals are very alkaline, calcium and magnesium in particular. Some minerals, especially magnesium, which is deficient in most diets, can be muscle relaxants and painkillers in large enough doses. You can experiment with taking magnesium as a supplement if you want. Start with doses of 500 mg and increase at 1000 mg per day until you start getting loose stools (bowel tolerance). Stay at the dosage that's just at bowel tolerance. It may take a month or so to see results. Use magnesium citrate for this purpose. You may also need to take calcium along with the magnesium in a 1:1 ratio to see a good result.

Magnesium in large doses (to bowel tolerance) is used as a treatment for migraine, in conjunction with riboflavin (B_2). In Europe, I believe it is used intravenously for this purpose, which makes sense, since that would avoid the whole issue of bowel tolerance.

You've Got Your Own Answers

J., 38, came to see me because of a generalized shoulder problem and chest tension. He was a personal trainer, very fit, and thought he might be lifting weights incorrectly, which would be causing his shoulder pain. He hesitated after he told me about his lifting style—something else was on his mind. "Maybe this tension is related to the heart attack I just had," he said. "Is that possible, do you think?"

"I don't know," I responded. "You're so young, you eat a low-fat diet, don't smoke. Do you have a family history of heart disease?"

"No."

Both of us were puzzled. Then I asked directly, "So why do you think you had it?"

He replied right away, "To leave my marriage. My wife didn't want to take care of me, and left. During my hospital time, I realized how much better I felt alone, even in the intensive care unit!"

He had fully recovered and divorced. We agreed that the heart attack had "worked"—achieved its purpose.

After this session I realized that there is a part of each person that knows what his disorder is about and also what would heal him. Sometimes (about 50 percent of the time), I can simply ask people directly, "What's the cause of this condition?" and they'll tell me, often surprising themselves. If they don't know consciously, if they resist or get angry, that's important information as well, and I can use it, so the question is always worth asking.

You can ask yourself—do it quickly so there's no time to think about it—"What causes my . . . ?" And see what you answer. It just doesn't occur to us that the answer is under our noses, and it's empowering when we understand we may not need to go to experts to figure out what is troubling us. Again, even if we can't access the information, it is good to know that the unconscious is keeping it from us, at least for now. The best way to ask yourself is by writing down the question at the head of a page, and then quickly, without thinking too much, writing down as many answers as come to you. Some people find it helpful to write the answers with the nondominant hand, which can help to bypass the conscious mind. (Or you might find it impossible or distracting to do this.)

Everything our organism does, at a biological level, is designed to ensure our survival. However, the "body wisdom" part of us, the instinct, is frequently out of sync with our egos, our minds. It doesn't comprehend that we live in the civilized world; we have complicated lives, technology, drugs, and so on. It still thinks it's on the African plains escaping from wild animals and struggling to survive. J.'s need to leave his marriage, which his conscious, grown-up mind might have suppressed from a sense of responsibility or guilt, or dealt with in more mature ways, such as therapy or discussion, was perceived by his lower "survival" brain as a threat to his life. Maybe, in some ways, the lower brain was right about the urgency of this—who knows? Anyway, J.'s lower brain responded to his need by shocking the nerves running to his heart in a violent, life-and-death way that may not have been the most appropriate for his ultimate survival.

5

Injury and Trauma

WHEN I WAS WORKING with K., who had a hip problem (and lots of other minor things), I noticed a relationship between the stiffness in her right ankle and the pain in her left hip. I thought she either wasn't using the right foot much, and so overusing her left side, or else leaning on the right leg too much for some reason and so causing some compensation on the left side. As I began to manipulate the right ankle, it became clear to me (and to her) that there was some pain there, particularly on flexion. It felt like an old injury. Usually ankle pain like this is an old sprain—lots of children twist their ankles in their exuberant running—the kind you've had for years and never really heal from, but that you learn to live with through the process of compensation. So the ankle pain was undoubtedly relevant to the hip pain. I asked her about it.

At first she wasn't sure. Then, as I continued to work gently into the ankle, she started crying quite hysterically. Obviously, something important was going on. "How did you injure this ankle?" I asked her again.

"Well, I remember now when it was," she said. "It was a beautiful summer day, I was at my cousins' house, and I was playing with my cousins outside. I was really happy that day. I twisted my ankle; it didn't hurt that much. I was busy playing, so I didn't really notice it till the next day."

"And then what?" I asked, expecting the mystery to be cleared up.

"Well, my aunt bandaged it up; it was okay. I was sad I couldn't run for a while, but no big thing."

K. asked me, "Why am I so upset?"

I didn't have any idea. Then I thought of something and asked her more about that time, the happy summer when she injured herself. I knew she'd had a problematic childhood, so I figured that something about the injury might be repressed.

But I was wrong. The day of the injury seemed to be without incident, just joyful childhood play. She liked her cousins—nothing there. She went on talking about that summer, a nice time away from an abusive father.

Then a memory surfaced, and it had nothing to do with the injury. That summer, her uncle, her cousins' father, had sexually abused her. Terrible memories and feelings coursed through her. She was crying uncontrollably. I continued working the ankle, assuming that there must be a connection I didn't understand, since the tissues of the injured ankle seemed to release a memory that was not directly connected to the injury. Also, K. was distracted by her emotional release, which allowed me to work the ankle in a way that it needed but would have been quite painful for her otherwise.

I noticed, in fact, how the ankle was regaining full mobility rather easily, and as the hardened tissues released, her emotional catharsis calmed. The ankle and the abuse were related. It didn't really matter how. K.'s ankle was better, and she also felt hugely relieved of a painful memory. Her hip was a little better too. But I was puzzled. I thought about it later, wondering how some puzzling thing had happened around an injury where the tissues seemed to hold memories that weren't connected to the injury but had occurred—that was it!—at the same time!

I got it. Injury and any trauma that occur more or less simultaneously are connected by the illogical lower brain. For example, a baby doesn't know, or reason, that the pain of a bitten lip isn't caused by the adult who is holding her bottle, but is coincidental to it. Her young, magical, mythic mind, the dreaming part of the mind, makes relationships and patterns where none may actually exist—simply because that is what the right brain does: It makes relationships, whatever the price. The brain delights in patterns as much as it can, and art, dreams, and imagination result from this unconscious tendency.

Therefore, other incidents that occur around the time or place of the injury have the same feeling as the injury itself. Unpleasant and traumatic events are connected in the muscle's memory and will be released, a Pandora's box, when the pain of the original injury is worked through the body. That is also why K.'s fun summer was not encoded in her ankle, since it lacked the feeling quality of the injury. Only the abuse contained the elements of shock and pain that allowed the brain to connect these two damaging events.

This is where I believe bodywork exceeds the possibilities of psychotherapy. K.'s contacting her abuse without also releasing the pent-up energy of the ankle pain would not have been a complete release of the entire experience. And K. did find that somehow her feelings about her uncle, his abuse, and the whole complicated mishmash of loyalty and hurt had lost their sting as the ankle healed.

THE LEGACY OF INJURIES

Think back in your life to the injuries you have had that still maintain some trace in your body, that are not 100 percent gone. See if you can remember, not just the circumstances of the injury, but anything upsetting or traumatic that happened at that time in your life. It's the element of emotional trauma, especially feelings of betrayal, that seem to get stuck in the tissues—maybe an injury feels like a betrayal of our body's integrity as much as an emotional loss of trust. Of course, you may find your brain comes up with quite different patterns; be open to whatever comes up. There are no simple answers to this one, and I rely on my clients to inform me about their particular tissue memories.

Chronic pains not caused by injury seem to connect less to other events in life. Perhaps the element of trauma is necessary for this phenomenon to occur. What it might mean for you is that the general atmosphere and events surrounding a persistent, unhealed injury may be part of what needs to be contacted before the injury—both psychological and physiological—can heal.

Here's an example from my own life. After I had Lasik surgery and was much less nearsighted, I got so entranced with my 20/20 vision that I didn't look where I was going, preferring to try to look into the distance, into people's windows, and so on. This new habit resulted in two very atypical accidents, one where a delivery bike ran into me and smashed my left hand and knee, and the other where I caught my sneaker laces in a grating and fell on my face. "Atypical" because all my other injuries have been head and neck injuries—I'm not normally prone to falls.

At the same time, I was going through relationship difficulties that I was not "looking at," and they too "tripped me up." The feeling of pain and betrayal and the determination to go on anyway color the injuries and are not fully resolved in my being. As I write about it, I see that one main feature of this time in my life was a kind of stoical persistence, which is a character trait that I find quite useful and probably hold on to because of this. So more than just the relationship pain, but also my defenses against it, are encoded in the tissue of my knee and hand.

Injuries also have a tendency to repeat themselves. As I mentioned, I have mostly injured the same parts of my body, my head and neck, over and over, although the accidents were not caused by me. Most were car accidents—and no, I wasn't driving. One was a fall from a horse. One was a physical assault. All resulted in the same damage.

Most people have this experience—always injuring one side perhaps. There's no logical reason for this if you accept the premise that an accident inflicted by an outside source is necessarily random. The source is not "your fault," of course. Your response to it, although instantaneous, is patterned on the kyo/jitsu model in an interesting way.

An injury creates a kyo—a weakness. Kyo, you'll remember, is a vacuum, an absence. Physical objects will tend to be attracted to a negative space, a vacuum—nature abhors a vacuum and wants to fill it. It's as though the incompletely healed injury created an energetic vacuum. The impact of a random accident will go to the part of your body that is energetically most kyo—least protected. Unfortunately we injure ourselves in our vulnerable spots, in all senses and all ways. Kyo must be filled to prevent this; that is, the need for healing and strength in the injured area must be addressed.

Often, just making the muscles strong in and around the injured area is enough to start the healing process. That should always be the starting place.

If that does not correct the problem, the emotional aspect of the injury (and all the related memories held in the tissues) needs to be addressed. Actually, there isn't a need to do much about the content of the memories and feelings, just feeling and re-experiencing them in a safe environment is usually enough. Letting the feelings run through the tissues and experiencing them somatically rather than physically is the key to fixing the "energetic gap," the propensity to reinjure the body. That isn't to say that the needs of the rest of the being, the emotional and spiritual self, are necessarily entirely filled this way. There may be more emotional processing needed.

The compensations in the body that develop as a result of injury are analogous to the psychological defenses we develop to protect ourselves against emotional trauma—useful at the time to keep us alive and functioning, but crippling and limiting when the wounds have (more or less) healed.

Physical injury is an emotional trauma too, of course, and it's more fruitful to see the structure of trauma and compensation as a law of nature, something that fulfills the overriding need to survive, to simply stay alive, that is our bodies' primary desire.

We need to understand that injuries don't heal. They may stop hurting, but the tissue memories and the compensation remain and actually worsen as the compensations create other compensations. The body's intelligence will bring us back to functioning and keep us vertical—but it will not heal us (make us whole). Injuries that happened years ago, that we haven't even thought about, pains we've completely forgotten still exist in the body, shadow us.

Eventually, we end up with so many cross-linkings of patterns of compensation, all interconnecting and sometimes triggering old feelings and memories, that we become weighed down by all this stuff. Bodywork can be a clearing out of the debris.

SPECIFICS OF INJURY

Most injury is not caused by muscle trauma. This is unfortunate because muscle heals in a few days unless completely torn. In my estimation, 80 percent of the injuries that really bother people and often stop them from playing their favorite sports are ligament- and tendon-related. Ligaments are the thin, rubber band–like structures that attach bone to bone; tendons are the thicker, gristle-like things that attach muscle to bone. It's rare to completely tear a ligament or tendon, but microtears are common.

Ligaments, tendons, and of course bones take a long time to heal—six weeks minimum. That doesn't mean you'll be out of commission for that amount of time, just that you'll be aware of discomfort and probably in some pain.

Most injuries to soft tissue should not be rested for too long. If you are in acute pain, use RICE (rest, ice, compression, and elevation) as soon as possible after the injury. Otherwise, stay as active as possible without hurting yourself. Muscle atrophies fast, and negative compensations will set in if you don't take steps to prevent this.

You should see a doctor if your pain is severe, there is swelling, you heard something "pop" when you injured yourself, or there is nausea, blurry vision, areas of severe muscle weakness, or bladder or bowel problems after the injury. A doctor can evaluate whether you have a broken bone, disc injury, or something that requires medical treatment. Very, very few injuries require surgery, and almost none requires emergency surgery.

Here are a few injuries that might require surgery: a slipped disc that presses on a vital nerve (you don't need surgery for most disc injuries), badly torn knee cartilage, complete bone fracture, and severe dislocations.

Surgery is getting more sophisticated all the time, so it behooves you to investigate the most up-to-date treatments you can find. Remember, though, that all surgery is another injury to the body and can set up even more trauma that you will need to heal from. Give yourself twice as much recovery time as the doctor advises to get fully better from a surgery. That way you won't feel bad when you still feel some pain after six weeks or whatever it is. It will take time to heal.

Now, let's look at the 99 percent of injuries that don't require that kind of intervention. You could have injured a bone. You can bruise a bone, have a stress fracture, a hairline or a complete fracture. Bone spurs are another source of pain. They are caused by abnormal frictions, as from shoes, and abnormal calcium metabolism. If the bone spur is small, working with the muscles and soft tissue around the area can actually shift it.

Bruised bone will heal over time; broken bone must be set properly or it will create more problems. Stress fractures and minor breaks in bone don't need to be set; they will require rest until healed. This is the common wisdom—from my own experience I'm not sure if it's true in all cases. I broke my left wrist—badly—and I didn't know it was broken. I was so afraid of losing function in my hand that I took anti-inflammatories, iced it, and went straight to the gym to work it out. My hand was functional and stopped hurting in about a week, but I noticed it didn't look right; there appeared to be a hollow area in the wrist. About a year later, I had an X-ray, which revealed a badly broken wrist—one of the small bones had been shattered and reabsorbed by my body. The doctor who saw the X-ray told me I should have had surgery.

I'd never recommend to a client that she treat a broken bone this way. My guess is, though, that stress fractures might be well served by the appropriate exercise.

Bones, especially the small ones, like the ribs and cranial bones, are really part of the tissue structure of the body and not so separate as we tend to conceive of them. If you could look inside your body right now, as a living organism, pulsing with the rhythms of life, you'd see your bone as a pink vibrant substance connected to all the other living tissues of the body. That's why exercising really helps bone regenerate, as the pulling of the muscle tissue away from the joint stimulates the cycle of bone growth.

In general, of course, a larger broken bone should be set and rested completely till it heals, usually six to eight weeks.

Even though ligaments look a bit like muscles, they should function as extensions of bone, and therefore as stable structures. Tight ligaments can be compensated for by loosening the muscles, but hyperextended ligaments can't be tightened up. Hyperextended ligaments are a cause of joint instability, which can lead to muscle spasms or even a tear of that ligament.

Torn Ligaments

How can you tell if you have a torn ligament or just muscle tears?

1. Time of healing. Ligaments take six to ten weeks—muscles a few days.
2. Pain on passive stretching. Generally, it will feel okay or good to work the muscle involved, but stretching the ligament will feel painful and not okay.
3. Poor healing. Ligaments tend not to heal well and leave lots of internal scar tissue. This will feel stiff and "bunched up," and it can also get in the way of natural movement, dragging out the healing time.

If a ligament is completely torn, especially at the knee or shoulder, it may require surgery. Minor tearing is common and can be healed much less invasively.

One of the most common causes of lower back spasm that "comes and goes" is torn ligaments, usually sacral area ligaments that have healed as scar tissue. I would treat this just the way I would any other back pain—by strengthening weak muscles and stretching tight ones, bodywork, and so on. There is one holistic medical treatment for torn ligaments and incompletely healed ligaments, and that is prolotherapy.

Prolotherapy is the injecting of an irritant saline or dextrose solution directly into the injured ligament to help it to heal. The irritant solution can cause the ligament to strengthen (proliferate) in response—or not.

Client reactions to this treatment have been mixed—from, "What a life saver. No pain now!" to "What a nasty painful treatment, and it didn't help at all!" I know of no useful studies of this therapy. Personally I think it's worth trying—it's not really that painful—and it has no serious downside or risks that I know of.

Torn Tendons

A tendon is the big, whitish, fleshy thing that attaches bone to muscle. Most of us are familiar with the Achilles tendon at the back of the calf.

Tendons can be torn through sports, accidents, and so on. You can see how difficult it would be to rip through a tendon (fig. 5.1). However, since, like ligaments, tendons do not stretch or contract much and have little blood supply, they heal poorly (also just like ligaments).

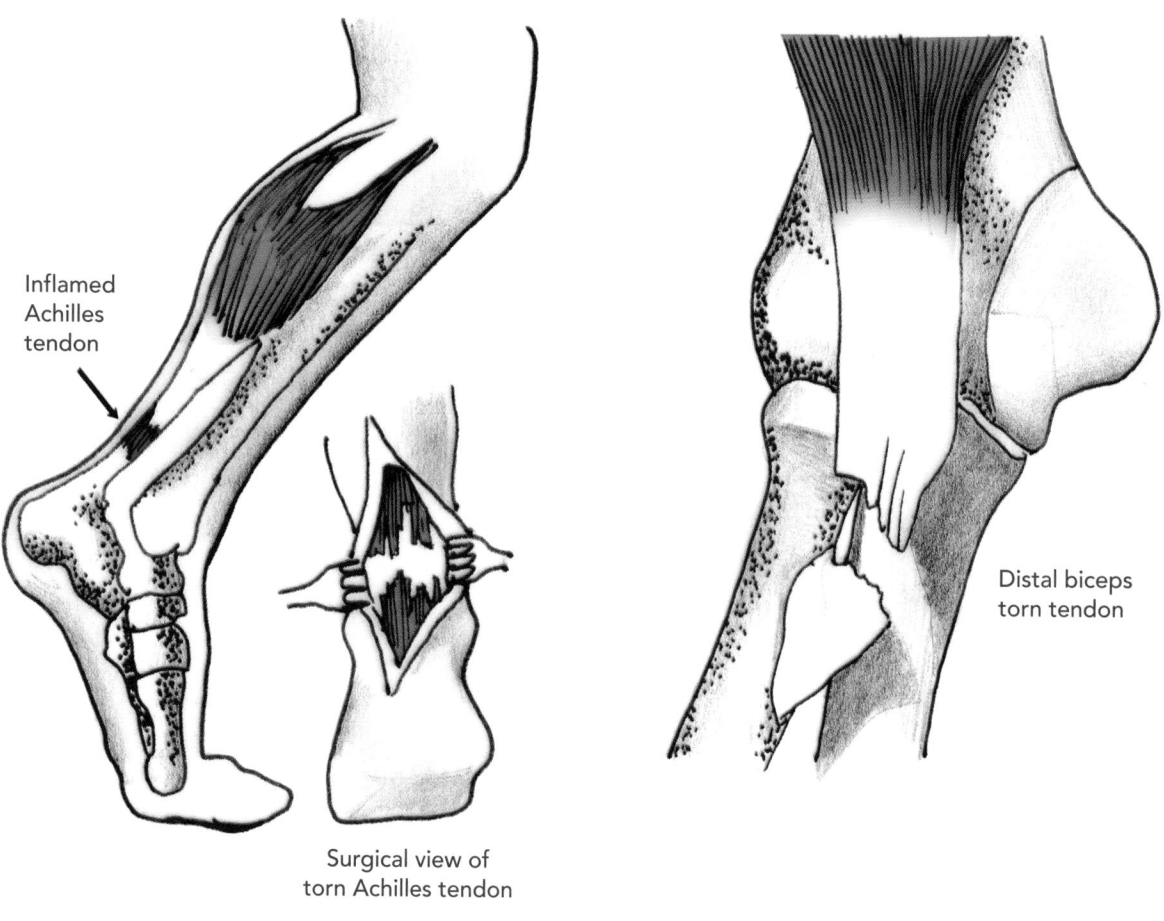

Inflamed Achilles tendon

Surgical view of torn Achilles tendon

Distal biceps torn tendon

Fig. 5.1. Torn tendons

Even slight tears, when only a few fibers in the tendon structure are actually injured, are still very problematic, because the whole tendon and the muscles it attaches to are weak and vulnerable to reinjury. Tendinitis, a very common diagnosis, just means "inflamed" tendon and usually refers to a partial tear. Tenosynovitis, a common running injury, is usually caused by repetitive stress rather than by an accident; it afflicts the sheath around the tendon itself. This can cause all sorts of interesting crunching, grinding sounds.

The key to healing any tendon injury properly is:

1. Increase the blood supply through massage, bodywork, alternate ice and heat (when appropriate), and some gentle movement. Just doing cross-fiber rubbing around, not on, the site of injury will help.
2. Don't let lumpy scar tissue form. The cross-fiber rubbing will prevent this too. So will correct movement.
3. In the long term, strengthening the surrounding and attached musculature will help. I would look for a muscle imbalance that could cause an unequal pulling at the site of attachment—for example, if the calf muscle is developed unevenly, the Achilles tendon could get pulled much more in one place than another, causing an imbalance that would render it vulnerable to injury.

6

Pain

PAIN IS A BAD THING. The human nervous system is unfortunately supremely sensitive, and wholly inaccurate. As you have certainly realized, pain isn't always proportionate to the degree of damage. A hangnail can feel excruciating. Migraine pain is the worst I've ever felt, and terminal cancer can give us no pain at all. I won't go into the reason for this here but will instead talk about how to stop severe pain.

Clients often ask me if it is better to struggle through pain or take a painkiller. Pain itself creates horrible compensations in the body, and walking around in pain, aside from being stressful and tiring, will create bad habits that will not necessarily resolve when the pain goes away.

So should you take a painkiller? Painkillers, on the one hand, all have side effects, and they have a rebound, so when you stop taking them, your pain is worse. They will also dull the whole brain and nervous system to some extent.

So neither state, sedated or in agony, is ideal. There are some harmless natural ways to relieve pain, though, so try these first. They will not completely numb pain, which I think is actually a good thing. Pain is actually doing us a service by letting us know that something is wrong. Most of us can stand mild pain (discomfort), not acute pain.

If these remedies don't work, and you have a diagnosis of your problem, take something relatively safe to numb the pain and take as little of it as you can. But don't suffer more than you need to. Suffering may be good for the soul, but it's bad for the body.

Short Cut 1: If you cannot, or don't want to take medications, you can use turmeric or ginger or both as natural, safe anti-inflammatories. Turmeric works

---

72

quite well for arthritis and bursitis, and both herbs have antioxidant and other good properties. You will need standardized turmeric, containing at least 350 mg of curcumeroids, per day. Of course, consult your doctor or health professional first.

Short Cut 2: Use a negative electricity charge. This is an old remedy that also works quite well. I knew it from years ago as a kid in England and saw it mentioned in *Alternatives* newsletter in an improved version. You can make your own negative electricity charge in this way:

Go to a plumbing supply store and get a thin piece of PVC pipe, about 1 inch in diameter and 1 inch long—it doesn't matter that much exactly how big the pipe is. Then create a good static charge by rubbing the PVC pipe against a piece of fake fur or similar synthetic for thirty seconds or so. The pipe will be crackly and hot when it's charged. Place the static (negative) charge on the painful area. Pain and inflammation have a positive charge, so the negative charge of the homemade static device will cancel out the pain temporarily. You don't need to rub the pipe on the area, unless it is a big area; just leave it there, tucking it inside clothing or tying it to the painful place, for at least ten minutes.

This is a much better method than the one I knew, which involved rubbing shoes against carpet (!) and was impractical.

STRUCTURAL METHODS

If you feel a pull in some part of your body that is beginning to tighten up, your tendency is probably to stretch away from the pulled area. If stretching loosens it up, fine. It often doesn't, sometimes causing more pain later on (remember the Golgi tendon reflex?). We can use the stretch reflex to our advantage.

Move into the pull, maybe stretching the other side. At a certain point, the muscle that's pulled will not hurt or have any sensation at all. Beyond that point, you may experience a feeling of compression. You don't want that, so stay in the place of no sensation in that area, focusing your mind there and imagining blood moving into it. Then gently ease back, perhaps not all the way.

The pull is a jitsu. Moving away from it intensifies it, creating more jitsu. That jitsu may travel full circuit and release into kyo. Leaning into it decreases sensation, giving us the kyo, which is also the hidden, opposite movement under the jitsu. The kyo fills (imagining blood flow, focusing on it), and the jitsu releases.

To be specific, consider these structural methods:

1. If the left side of your neck hurts, move your head toward the left. Try to move into the angle of the pain—diagonal, lateral, or whatever—until you feel the compression. Move slightly toward neutral, and in the place of no sensation, stay for 90 seconds (muscle memory time, page 43).
2. If the pain is in a muscle that has an identifiable opposite—such as the inner and outer thigh, calf and shin, back and front of body, sides of body, inner and outer wrist—and you can move into the painful place without an excessive increase in pain and also find the right spot of "no sensation" fairly easily, use this method.
3. If not, you can try "sandwiching"—that is, working the muscles above and below or opposite the painful area. Use weights or other strength resistance systems that can effectively isolate these muscles.

So for neck pain on one side, you use resistance on the other side. Or you could use the upper back muscles. For upper back pain, try the chest muscles. For lower back pain, the abdominal muscles are the obvious choice, but the stretching of the lower back involved in forward flexion may hurt, so I would go to hamstrings and upper back.

If you know anatomy, you can use the agonist/antagonist relationship. Strangely enough, sometimes stretching the opposing muscles works, so you could try both ways. This can also be a more permanent method of addressing pain, and some of the exercises given in the second part of this book use this principle.

HOW WE REACT TO PAIN AND WHAT WE CAN DO ABOUT IT

The natural reaction to pain is to fold into the painful area, to protect it. This reflex does have a useful function when used purposefully, but most of the time collapsing and sinking into a painful area will make it hurt more, create compensations, and cut off the blood, nerves, and lymph flow needed for healing.

For example, if you have low back or hip pain, your tendency will probably be to sink and sag into your lower body when standing and sitting. Instead, try tightening your abdominals and stretch the lower ribs away from the pelvis. You can walk this way if you have severe lower back pain or sciatica, and you will find that you have created a lot more space for the hip joint to move in. You may be able to move your legs more freely, perhaps even without pain. Lift up out of the painful area with muscle contraction, actively stretching the spine away from the ground.

Wheels and Spokes

D. came to me with horrible pain in her shoulder. I explained to her what a rotator cuff injury is: The shoulder joint is like a wheel with four spokes, each of which is the four rotator cuff muscles. It's a shallow joint so we can move it around extensively. The arm bone (humerus) is primarily attached by muscles. If one of the rotator cuff muscles is tight, is weak, or doesn't move properly, it's as though the wheel has one spoke shorter than the others. What would happen to the movement of the wheel if one of the spokes was broken? That's what happens to your shoulder joint as it moves around—it's the axis of the wheel. This image is not anatomically that accurate—look at an anatomy book! It's actually much more complicated than that, but the image works well to give a feeling and understanding of the movement. D. "got it" and started moving her shoulder around, sensing the movement of the joint, tuning in, shifting it. It was actually in a slightly better place when she rested it again. The image of the wheel and spokes got her to connect to her shoulder again, beginning to heal it.

Sending awareness to an area, as opposed to thinking about it, literally sends blood and nerve energy into a painful place, and that alone will start to heal it. I think a lot of the healing power of bodywork functions in this way. The brain "forgets" traumatized (injured or painful) places after enough compensation has set it. Just as in psychological trauma, healing can't happen until feeling is restored. When the brain acknowledges and reclaims the deadened places, the connections that are re-formed will, on their own, bring healing.

Awareness is different from thinking about, or worrying about, a pain. That removes consciousness from the pain and attempts to control it. Awareness is the placing of consciousness in the area and is neutral and somewhat open ended in focus. A very simple working knowledge of the basic structural mechanics of the body and its logic helps us connect with painful areas. We are empowered when we are in the body, not outside judging it, worrying about it, or getting mad at it.

D. was worrying about her shoulder when she came in; she was not "in" it. I opened the arm back behind her head as she lay on her back (if necessary, I would have supported her elbow with a pillow) and worked the ribs in the armpit and the inner aspect of the shoulder blade. This position allowed me easy access into the joint itself. If the joint is not positioned correctly, it feels like there is a little ledge, a step, at the inner-upper part of the shoulder blade—that's the part of the shoulder joint winging forward. After loosening the rotator cuff muscles and the general area, I gently pushed the small "step" back into place. This is a type of "nonforce" adjustment, called nonforce because it is slow and does not use momentum (unlike most chiropractic adjustments). It is an adjustment because it does move the joint directly, involving bone as well as muscle. After this adjustment to the shoulder, D. could feel the "wheel" was tracking better. And instead of worrying about her shoulder, she now had awareness of it.

You can move the "step" back into place yourself by stretching the inner part of the shoulder (page 150) and working the rotator cuff muscles (page 160). Because of its shallow nature and mobility, the shoulder joint is easier both to correct and to damage than the other joints.

7

About the Exercises
in This Book

THERE ARE LOTS of excellent and easy-to-follow exercise books and programs you can buy; they seem to multiply daily. The intention of this book is not to add to the collection but to make any other books and programs you choose easier to follow.

The exercises you'll find here are all corrective in nature; in other words, their aim is to balance and realign you. That is why I have written so extensively on the specific way you should do each one and have suggested lots of props. It's really important that you do each exercise correctly. That may be tedious, but the payoff will be that you'll feel a lot better, and hopefully, you'll reduce both pain and your risk of injury.

I'd much rather you do one exercise exactly right than lots of them with poor alignment, so please follow along and do them *as prescribed*!

How are these exercises different from core exercises—that is, programs that are designed to strengthen and stretch deep postural muscles? Well, there is a certain amount of crossover, because postural muscles do determine a lot of your alignment patterns. But take a look at any very simple core exercises and you will see how easily they can be done wrong.

For example, consider the "swimming" Pilates exercise, where you lie on the stomach lifting the legs and arms simultaneously and fluttering the legs. I'm looking at a photograph of a very well-proportioned, well-aligned model doing this exercise. She's doing it correctly and will no doubt reap the benefits, a strong, evenly developed, and pain-free back.

But imagine what happens if one of this model's hips is higher than the other, one shoulder is tighter, or she's pushing up the back of her neck with her jaw pushed to one side. Well, she probably wouldn't notice because it would feel right to her; after all, she's used to this alignment. However, it would change the way the exercise affects her. She would work her muscles quite unevenly, actually making her condition worse. She might give up on it and wonder why it's not helping, or the exercise might just feel bad and she'd stop anyway. She certainly would miss the point of it; without correcting her basic alignment, the exercise wouldn't help her.

FAMILIAR IMBALANCES

Most of us have numerous imbalances that are reflected in everything we do. The imbalances feel right to us over time because they're familiar to us. Anything we're used to starts to feel right, even to the point where the correct movements and more balanced alignment feel wrong. And mostly it's these chronic imbalances that cause pain and aging. It can also set us up for injury.

So somebody may come to me for an injury that she thinks just happened out of the blue. She just bent down to pick up a book she dropped, for example, and her back went into spasm "for no reason." Many of us are accidents waiting to happen. How can we prevent all these and correct them once they've happened? First, by becoming more aware of our habits in an objective and distanced way.

You can take one typical day and notice every single thing you do, how you wake up, what position you are in, how you get out of bed, which foot goes onto a stair first, which hand holds the toothbrush, what position you're in in the shower. Do you sit most of the day or stand? How do you sit (are you twisted at all)? What do you look at? Where is it? And so on. You can reverse everything you have control over. You don't have direct control over your waking position in bed, for example— or maybe you do. Picking a different spot in the bed to go to sleep in or using a different pillow gives you some control over how you sleep. Concentrate on shifting your habitual patterns. Use the other foot to go upstairs, shift onto the other buttock or leg as you sit or stand, change hands to dress, wash, and so on. What does that feel like? It could feel liberating, opening up a different part of your brain, or maybe it just feels awkward and annoying. Anyway, you'll learn what your habits are, and you are bound to come up with some insights.

Perhaps you chronically stand on one leg—no wonder that hip is tight. Or you sit all day at a desk with your head tilted to see the computer screen; that's why you have a neck pain. More subtly, you see better with one eye than the other, so you keep your head at the optimal angle for seeing but not for structural health. You may be able to change some of your physical imbalances just by realizing how your habits create them. However, the chances are that even though you become aware of some habits, you don't know how to correct the imbalances they set up. You may have not used certain muscle groups for so long that your brain doesn't register them, and you don't know how to engage them consciously. This is not a lack of physical strength—it's a neurological blind spot; we generally develop more and more of these as we get older and accumulate injuries and compensations. Some people, healthy in all other respects, end up with only a few restricted movement patterns. This is where the corrective exercises come in.

If you go to the gym, you'll notice that each machine has an illustration showing you (usually in red) which muscles you are using when you do that exercise. Unfortunately muscles don't work that way. Your body under stress will naturally use whichever muscles are already strong and you are accustomed to. The weaker, less used areas and the weak side of your body will be employed as little as possible. This is your body's wisdom to avoid injury by not stressing the weaker areas and so preventing injuries, but in the long run this pattern may lead to damage since the weak areas will get weaker and the strong areas will get stronger.

🍃 *Using Kyo and Jitsu to Increase Body Awareness*

1. Lie down on your back, and scan through your body mentally, from your feet to your head. You will notice that some areas—your jitsu places—are much easier to feel than others. They may feel tight, sore, hot, cold, anything—but not numb or dead.

2. Normally, your attention would gravitate to these places. This time, do the opposite—place your attention on the hard-to-feel areas. Of course, as soon as you pay attention to the less aware and sensitized parts of your body, they'll change. Maybe you will locate some places that you can't feel at all, no matter what you do. Don't force it. See if you can find the edges of the kyo area—the places where you can just begin to feel something.

3. Now, forget all that, and still lying on your back, pay attention to both feet. Equalize the sensation in the two feet. Whether you visualize, imagine heat, whatever, just concentrate on making the sensation equal in both. Do the same with your knees, hips, hands, elbows, eyes, and ears. Again, don't worry if you can't get it—just imagine you have done it.

4. Now, relax and notice the kyo/jitsu relationships all through the body again. Have the kyos changed at all since the beginning?

This is a good way to increase body awareness, begin your exercise sequence, and just relax. Sensing the kyo like this will automatically shift the nervous system into parasympathetic mode, which is a necessary preliminary to achieving any kind of positive shift in the physical state.

The most difficult aspect of working with yourself in any way is the quite natural unawareness of your own kyo, which means you may never become conscious of your underlying energy patterns. A simple exercise like this can help you experience the unfelt, inexperienced, and unconscious patterns that underlie what may be troubling you.

THE IMPORTANCE OF CORRECTIVE EXERCISE

If you work hard at correcting your alignment without specific corrective exercises, you will get somewhere. Your muscles will probably feel more relaxed. But your job will not get easier—you will have to keep correcting yourself consciously, and it will get progressively more difficult as you become aware of all your compensations.

For example, say you notice your left shoulder is higher than your right. You change the position of your computer, the way you carry your bag. You keep reminding yourself to drop the shoulder. You will definitely help your shoulders, but then, since the underlying muscle imbalance is not corrected, your neck may start tilting more to the left, or your right hip may start compressing. Your body will find another way to attempt to balance itself, and it will struggle as hard as it can to avoid using the weak muscles. So I suggest at least trying the corrective exercises—they will actually make you work much less in the long run, since only through isolating the weak and stiff areas progressively will you correct the underlying imbalance.

Corrective exercise is different from other types of exercise in that it targets the specific muscle pathway you need to activate. This isn't easy. A compound exercise, like a push-up, uses a lot of muscles, and if you have some "switched-off," that is, inactive, muscles, your instinctive body wisdom, wishing to avoid injury, won't let you use them. Unused muscles tend to be hard to feel and use, not only because they are weak, but because the nerve pathways that conduct the impulses from the muscle to the brain are not developed. They are not damaged, but exist as potentials rather than being available to the conscious mind. The instinct to not use them is so profound that you can do almost anything while using almost any muscles. The push-up of a person who has injured his shoulder is going to be quite different from the push-up of a person with a lower back injury. So most exercises won't, on their own, correct muscle imbalance.

On Changing the Reflex to Avoid the Inactive Muscle Pathway

It takes careful attention to the placing of your body, your alignment, focus on the area you want to help, and a slow pace (usually) to change the reflex to avoid the inactive muscle pathway. Mental focus will send blood and nerve energy to the area, helping to connect the nervous system to the muscle. The exercises in this book will force you to use the weak muscles and not any others, which can be very hard to differentiate on your own. It may take some practice to do them easily, but with patience you will. You will then be able to transfer this feel for the muscle to your everyday life.

When the muscle group has truly engaged, you will probably be able to use it in compound exercises also. Don't underestimate your body's desire to avoid the muscles you want to use. That's why I give repeated instructions about how the exercises should be done.

Learn to distinguish between unnecessary discomfort in a position, which you must alleviate to have a good result, and the kind of satisfying or productive discomfort of working an underused area. You should not be able to drift off mentally when doing corrective exercise. The mental focus should always be slightly greater than the physical.

Go five times more slowly and with smaller movements than you want to. This is the correction I make for almost everyone, so I'm assuming you will go too fast and too big also.

The shape of the movement doesn't matter, for now. Let that come from the inside. Feel the movement deeply in the nervous system, and focus your mind on it. Your gaze, usually straight ahead, should not wander or become blank. Your eyes and your breathing control your mental focus, so keep both open, receptive, and deep.

On Correcting Alignment

I've learned this one through experience, so I pass it on to you. Don't work the body in asymmetrical and one-sided ways to correct alignment. Many advanced exercisers make this mistake, and it's a subtle and tricky problem.

To elaborate, don't start standing on one leg because you've noticed you always stand on the other. Balance your weight in the middle. Otherwise, you will create another imbalance. If you carry a bag over one shoulder habitually, alternate shoulders or wear a backpack. The tricky aspect is when you correct more complicated patterns that have several parts to them. For example, a client of mine tried to correct her neck alignment by using all but one of the steps I outlined, leaving the natural curve of the neck. She changed her upper back, absorbed C7, used the hyoid smile and a yawning technique to relax the occiput—but she continued to flatten her neck. As a result, she tightened her larynx to such an extent that she could hardly breathe.

The general principles—staying relaxed, listening to your body, and understanding the purpose of the movements—are more important than the details. Being mindful of the larger areas, such as the general curve of the spine, matters more than knowing exactly where each bone is.

Also, remember that distortions are always related to movement, so you should experience your body as a moving, living being, with pulses and rhythms, not an object that you can mold into shape like a sculpture.

🍃 Taking a Kinesthetic "Photograph"

If you can both visualize and feel a movement—that is, if you can sense the muscles and other tissues involved—you will be able to strengthen and stretch those areas so you can do the movement (eventually). If you can't visualize it, that's where you start.

1. Pick some movement you want to do and visualize yourself—not somebody else—performing it.

2. Now put yourself in the picture kinesthetically. Experience as fully as possible in your body how it would feel to make this movement, all the way from the starting position to coming out of it. Which muscles would engage, where would your eyes look, how would the various pressures of the points of foundation feel? See if you can slightly engage these muscles.

3. Then, if possible, put yourself in a modified, supported version of the posture or part of the movement. For example, if the movement is a split, you come into this position *only* as far as you can with good alignment and no strain. Give yourself support under your legs with pillows and under your hands with yoga blocks, remaining comfortable. Then stay there. Align yourself, engage the appropriate muscles, feel like you're doing a full split. Actually, you are—full for

yourself at this moment. Relax and feel pleasure in the position. You have to be comfortable enough to stay in the position for at least two minutes.

4. Then come out of the posture, memorizing the feeling of how this felt, the sense of the muscles and tissue expanding and contracting. Feel the whole body as well as the working areas.

5. Then file this kinesthetic photograph away in your brain for future reference. That way, you can work the neurological connections between brain and muscle, which will open up the movement channels from the other end.

HOW TO STRETCH

Muscles need to expand and contract fully to be healthy. Some of our muscles, for example the biceps, get a good workout in our everyday activity and need less stretching in general. Others, like the psoas (fig. 7.1), are deep, run close to the organs inside our bodies, and often get very stiff. A chronically tight muscle will also become weak, even though it may look and feel strong. It becomes prone to injury and, even if not injured, will form fascial buildup around it as a protection, which restricts movement further.

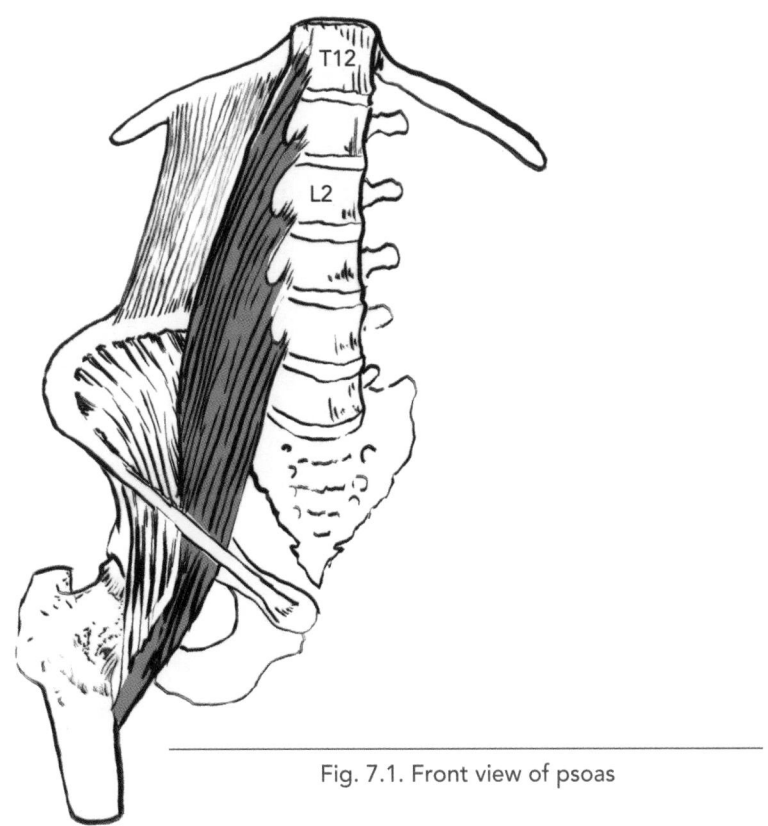

Fig. 7.1. Front view of psoas

Flexibility, our natural range of motion, has little to do with how much we need to stretch. Flexibility is determined primarily by genetics and is created by (a) the length of ligaments and tendons, which cannot be stretched safely and which control the types of joints we have, and (b) the density of our tissue. Some people have muscles with bigger, thicker, and closer fibers than others, and they will be naturally less flexible. Our body proportions have something to do with our measured flexibility. If you have a long torso and short legs, for example, it will obviously be easier to touch your toes. If you have very long arms, it will be even easier. So the markers of flexibility aren't that important.

What matters is that our muscles are evenly stretched, long, and elastic. To understand the place of stretching in our exercise routine, it is important to know what kind of natural flexibility we have, because it will change how we approach it. There is a continuum of mobility, with hypermobility at one end—that is extreme contortionist-type flexibility—and hypomobility, poor range of motion, at the other. You probably know where in the continuum you are. Hypermobile people tend to have trouble developing strength, especially in the core muscles and upper body. They have joints that "pop" or even dislocate and may have muscle spasms if they go beyond their safe range of motion.

In my practice I have found most people (especially men) to be hypomobile. Hypomobile people will have better balance than hypermobile people, who have wobbly ankles. Some joints can be either hypermobile or hypomobile in the same person, and some joints are happier with hypermobility, such as the hip joints, which are deeply set in their sockets and tend to stiffness. Others do less well, especially knees, which can be injured easily if they go out of alignment.

The hypermobile person should concentrate on stretching muscle only by stabilizing the joint and focusing on isometric contractions of opposing muscle groups to release safely. The temptation to "show off" and fling into hyperextended postures must be avoided. Postural muscles are likely to be both tight and weak and will need extra attention.

Timing and Taking Time

Hypomobile people should focus on stretching slowly, taking the muscle through its full range with care. They tend to bounce in all stretches, because that way avoids the discomfort of stretching. For the types of stretches in this book, don't do that! There is a good system of stretching, the Wharton Method, that works well for hypomobile types and does involve somewhat bouncy movements. But the system presented in this book, where we go into deep muscles and work alignment, must be done very slowly. So go just to your edge (the place where you feel discomfort but not pain, and your breathing stays open), support yourself with a pillow or bolster as you need, and stay there—three minutes if you can. You'll get much more out of this than bouncing around.

Stretching is more effective when the muscles are warmed up with some type of activity, or if they're done at the end of the day. Hypomobile people must warm up before stretching; the hypers don't need to do as much. But it can be discouraging to stretch "cold"—you won't go nearly as far, and the desire to go farther can cause injury.

These stretches require time, about one to three minutes each, so you need to go to your edge, whatever that is for you. The stretch should release after a while, not feel more uncomfortable. It is better not to go far enough than to go too far and back out.

Make sure your breathing is slow, even, and relaxed. Check the rest of your body to make sure no other muscles are working. Do a body scan—you'll have time—and breathe into each part of your body, releasing it, including the muscles you are stretching.

If you cannot stay at your edge without effort, if you're tightening your body in some way, then support yourself with pillows or a bolster, anything fairly soft that allows you to let go and also open the muscle.

Which Areas to Stretch

I'd like to share with you a stretching routine that works for me and may work for you. It goes like this: (1) Stretching the Back and the Neck (chapter 12), (2) Wall Hang Stretch (chapter 12), (3) Advanced Psoas Stretch (chapter 13), (4) Shoulder Stretch Series (chapter 11), (5) Wall Hang Stretch again.

I hold each stretch until I feel a significant change in my body, from one to three minutes. If I skip it or even change it very much, I've noticed I tend to lose the advantage of working my whole body in a fairly general way. After I do that, I can focus on other, more specific stretches.

My experience has been that it is not a good idea to focus on opening up one area without a sort of general stretching and releasing sequence. An overly precise focus in one place can lead to destabilizing the structures there and result in injury. I've done it!

So after you have stretched and warmed up your whole body in a more general way, you could focus on your "problem area." Here's a rule of thumb if you are not sure what your problem area is:

> If an area won't strengthen, no matter how much you try to strengthen it with focused resistance exercise, you need to stretch that area.
> If muscles don't stretch, despite your diligent efforts to stretch them, you need to strengthen those muscles.

TYPES OF STRENGTHENING EXERCISES

Most of the exercises in this book are strengthening exercises in the same way that lifting weights, and even yoga and Pilates, can be. I give attention to postural muscles, whereas most strength exercises will target mostly the phasic, active muscles, although there is some overlap.

Lifting weights is a common cause of injury, just as lifting anything else can be; so many people shy away from it and go to the subtler, gentler exercises. Yet I have found in my own practice and through observation that a simple improvement in overall strength can correct a lot of physical problems.

Shoulder and neck tension come from weakness in the supporting muscles of the back; it's amazing how these tensions melt away when the back gets strong. Stretching a tight muscle is our instinctive response to discomfort, and it helps short term (calming the jitsu), but the tension originates in a weak muscle somewhere else (a kyo), and probably won't be resolved until that area is strengthened.

Weight lifting has a significant disadvantage, though, aside from its injury potential, and that is that it usually works the concentric part of the movement (positive) much more than the eccentric (negative). For example, the effort of a biceps curl is in the curl itself, rather than the lengthening down of the muscle as the weight moves away from the body (fig. 7.2). This can result in shortening the muscle. It is not necessary to shorten or bulk a muscle to strengthen it—ideally the muscle should be long and strong.

Therefore, the eccentric (negative) part of the movement needs to be strengthened equally. You can do this by using TheraBands; the cable machine, which uses a similar kind of resistance; certain types of weight-lifting machines; or the super-slow strengthening system.

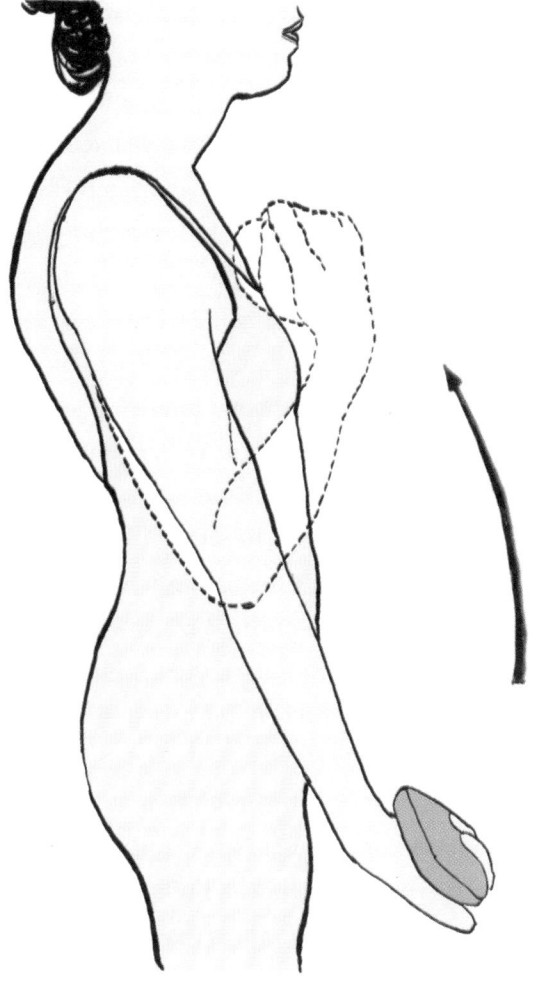

Fig. 7.2. Bicep curl

Trainers seemed like a luxury thirty years ago when going to the gym started becoming so popular. Now, the industry is booming, as people have realized that weight lifting, for most people, requires instruction to be safe. If you do lift weights without a trainer, and even if you are working with a trainer, follow the alignment rules I've outlined for the exercises here, pay attention to the parts of your body you are not using, gaze straight ahead, and focus on what you are doing. Work very slowly, and do not use the momentum of the weight to complete your movement. Work through the "glitches" in your movement; don't rush through them. Make each move slow and continuous, and don't stop moving until you can't work any longer.

When you go to the gym, don't just use the machines you like. Usually these favorite exercises will strengthen us where we are already strong—that's why we like them. Instead, concentrate on working your whole body.

One client of mine was having knee trouble, though she used the gym regularly. Her hamstrings and gluteus muscles were so weak that she was having trouble going up steps. These muscles are easy to work in the gym, so I was at a loss to understand how she had not strengthened them more. On further inquiry, I found out that all the hip and hamstring machines in her gym were up a flight of stairs that she didn't like to negotiate, so she had never used them. The result was an even greater imbalance between her strong quadriceps muscles and her weak hamstrings, giving her even more of a propensity to lean forward and injure her knees.

That said, if a machine doesn't feel good at all, and you don't seem to be targeting the right muscles in the right way, don't use it. Find another way to use the same muscles. Some machines are just going to be wrong for your body dimensions.

There are also different types of strength, and again, we will tend to gravitate toward working the areas that we are already strong in because that feels good. It's important to develop the capabilities of our bodies as evenly as we can, so pay attention to which types of strength your body doesn't naturally have and then what might shift if you could develop them.

One type of strength is aimed at by building muscle through weight training. This kind of exercise targets one particular type of muscle fiber, the fast twitch, which everyone has. If you're the type of person who bulks up quickly, then you were probably born with more of it. The types of moves that develop this part of your muscle are contractions against resistance.

Another kind of strength training is isometric exercise, which is static contraction against resistance. The parts of the tissue that can hold difficult positions for a long time, such as in yoga, are included in this category. This has to do with the strength and size of the tendons and ligaments—again, that's probably genetic, but can be developed. The reason to do isometric work is primarily therapeutic. If you think about it, all the postural muscles do isometric work all the time, supporting your body in a static position upright, which is effortful. Including isometrics in your workout will help your alignment and "use" of gravity and space. You can also increase your flexibility safely with the right isometric contractions.

To an extent, isometrics in the muscles will increase endurance (the slow twitch fibers). The other type of endurance work, aerobics, uses the slow twitch fibers, of course. Aerobics, running, biking, swimming, anything that brings up your heart rate and forces your body to use more oxygen is vital for good health and stress relief. Aerobic exercise will benefit your heart, your lungs, and your body chemistry and will improve your mood. It does not build muscle. The slow twitch fibers are not the same ones that lift weights. Aerobics may give you stamina, however, so you can lift weights for longer periods. Prolonged aerobic exercise, like marathon running, actually breaks down some muscle fibers, so you should always balance aerobic exercise with strength training of the same muscle groups. In other words, if you are a runner, you need to strengthen your legs with resistance exercise. It will help you run faster, too.

The other type of exercise that we need for most sports is plyometric; that is, forceful, explosive moves like jumping (fig. 7.3). Many people, myself included, hate

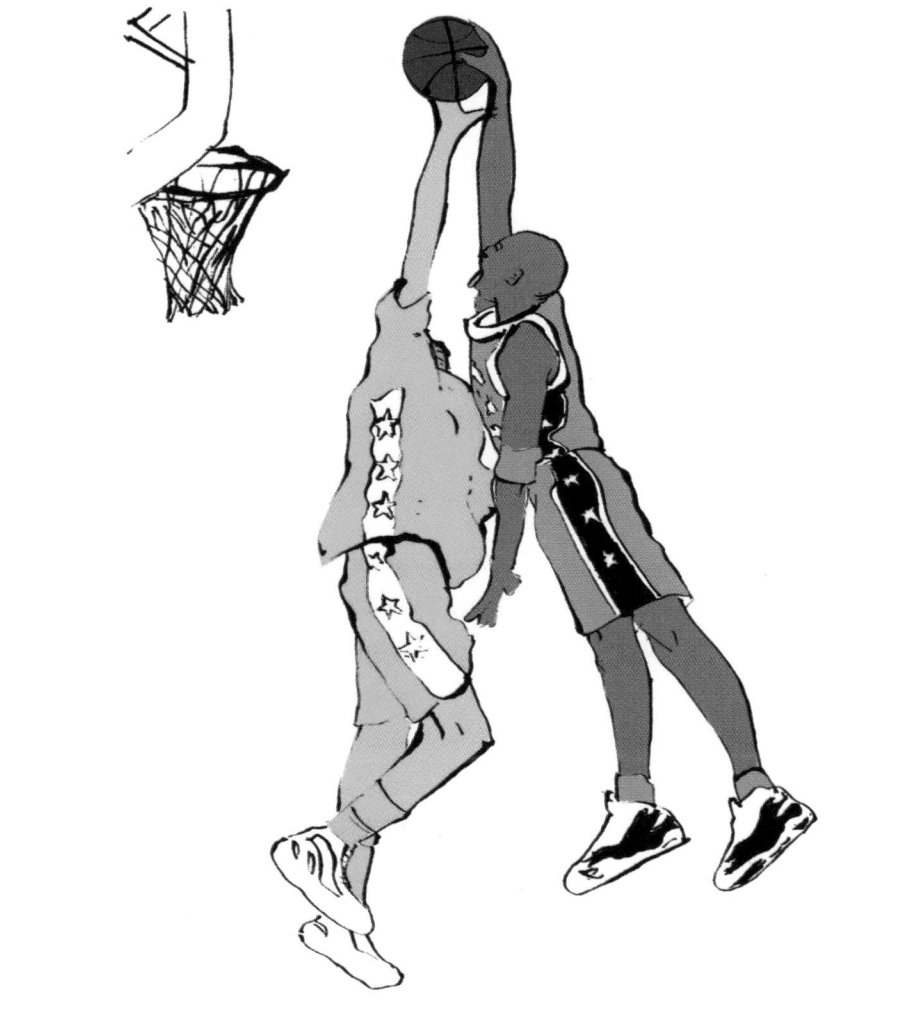

Fig. 7.3. Plyometric sports

this type of exercise because we've hurt ourselves doing it. If you have alignment problems, very loose joints, or damaged cartilage, approach plyometrics with caution. But don't give up on them! Jumping is an interesting example. The only way to use the muscle pathways involved in jumping is to jump. You could jump just a little, on a soft surface, or run, or use a trampoline.

Surprisingly, yoga can be plyometric—inversions, lunges, and balance poses have plyometric elements. Ashtanga yoga is extremely plyometric. The better your balance is, the easier these types of explosive moves will be for you.

Sometimes we need to move fast and reflexively in life. For example, we use plyometric moves in emergency situations and in playing with children, who are relentlessly plyometric themselves. Grandpas, or even dads, who have long given up all sports and their neurological components, injure themselves time and time again playing with their bouncy grandkids.

AVOIDING TILTING AT WINDMILLS

Our bodies can be subject to various structural idiosyncrasies, which can impact our capacity to change. They can occur in our skeletons, in the positions of nerves, and in the placement of organs. It is important to understand these kinds of idiosyncrasies so we don't end up tilting at windmills, so to speak. There's not much point fighting what will not change. Most aspects of physical structure will strengthen, however, if we pay attention to the obvious, and let that guide us to work around our natural difficulties and exploit our genetic strengths.

Yoga is great for teaching you the limitations of your body structure and how to work around them. It amazes me how some "easy" yoga postures are very hard for me, and some so-called advanced or difficult poses come naturally to my body. A deeper understanding of the body can be gained by reflecting on the reasons for the ease or difficulty of a move—is it a true limitation, to be worked *around*, or a malfunction, to be worked *through*?

Skeletal Structure
Your skeletal structure may prevent you from performing certain moves, or types of moves, with ease. You can change your skeletal alignment to some extent. If you get very strong and find there's still some exercise you can't do, no matter how you approach it or how hard you try, the fault is probably in your bones.

For example, the Pilates roll up and roll down (abdominal flexion in slow motion) is impossible for people who cannot round their spines properly. There will not be enough space between some of the vertebrae to create room for the flexion. You can see from the illustration (fig. 7.4) how the scoliotic distortion of the spine could cause this condition. Understanding ths is only the first step toward changing it. In this case, the same flexion exercise performed while sitting will change the spine enough to allow the muscles to strengthen. Or the roll up/down can be repeated with support. The difficult part of the move can be held isometrically, also with support if necessary. And the distortions in the spine can be worked with separately.

Straight spine

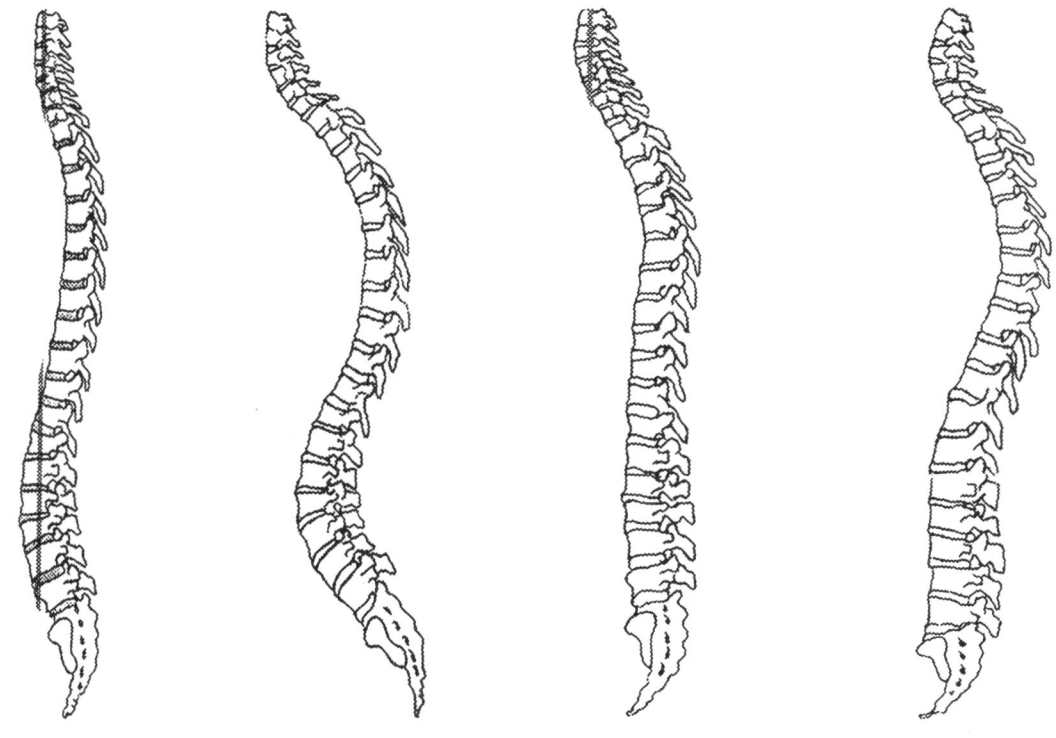

Fig. 7.4. Spinal distortions

The placement of the hip joints can create a problem with pelvic stability, which affects balance (see fig. 2.14 on page 35). Obviously, if one joint is placed farther forward or back, or more to one side than the other relative to the pelvic girdle, any kind of balancing and, possibly, coordination will be negatively affected. Strengthening gluteus medius and the hip rotators evenly may help. Keeping the pelvic girdle deliberately still when balancing or lifting one leg will also assist.

Natural differences in body proportion will make a difference in how you benefit—or don't—from strength training, and of course these can't really be changed. Small feet are harder to balance on, as are small hands. A long torso means touching your toes will be easier, and abdominal work will be harder since the torso will be longer and heavier relative to the legs. Petite, compact body structures will generally have fewer structural problems.

Nerve Position

Then there are the quirks of nerve positioning. Sometimes, a nerve bundle will be placed so that there's uncomfortable pressure on it in certain positions. The ulnar nerve is often a culprit for some reason (fig. 7.5). If your arms "go to sleep" easily, you may have some compression along this nerve pathway, or the nerve may simply be positioned in a touchy place. The former can be changed, the latter probably not.

I was always told in yoga class that if I got used to sitting cross-legged, after a period of time, my legs wouldn't go to sleep as they invariably do. I can easily sit cross-legged for hours with a straight back—but my legs still doze off after five minutes or so. I think the tendency for limbs to fall asleep is mostly due to nerve positioning, superficiality of nerve bundles, and density of tissue. People with loose, open connective tissue seem to have more nerve sleepiness than the tighter, denser-bodied types. These things don't change, no matter how long you sit or how much strength you develop.

Organ Placement

The relationship of organs to structure can also affect the ability to do an exercise. The following section will be confusing to anyone who isn't familiar with the energy meridians of Oriental medicine. For a much more complete understanding of this fascinating system, read *Zen Shiatsu* by Shizuto Masunaga with Wataru Ohashi or any of Ohashi's books (see bibliography).

If a meridian (energy channel) is blocked, the muscles along that pathway will be tight or weak or both. Since the meridians correspond to organs and

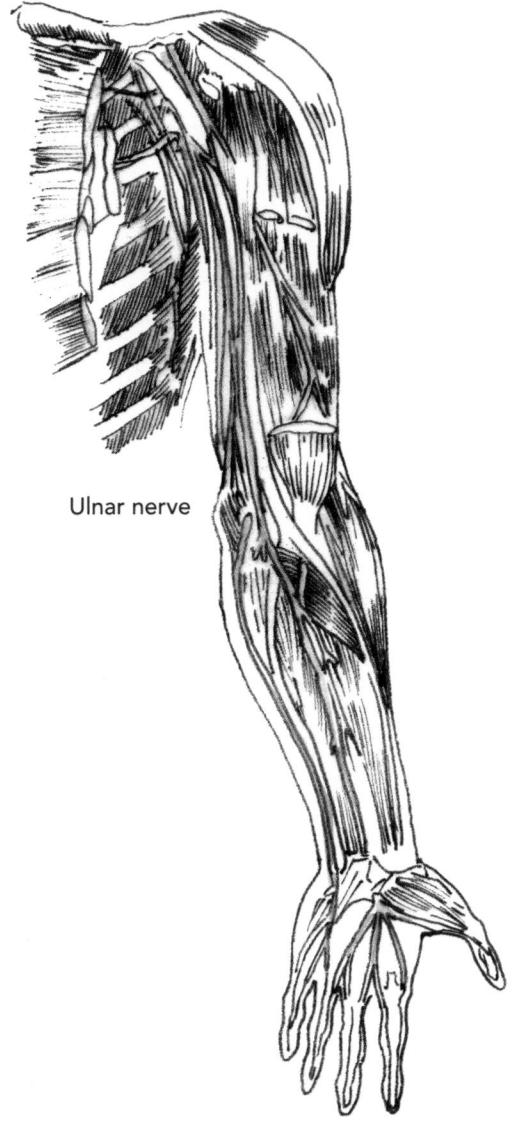

Ulnar nerve

Fig. 7.5. Ulnar nerve position

physical systems, you can both identify and treat internal problems with certain exercises.

Some of the paired organs may seem strange, but that's how the Chinese, who developed this system, did it, and it makes sense if you study it. Briefly, here are the correspondences:

ORGAN MERIDIANS AND
ASSOCIATED PARTS OF THE BODY

Organ Meridian	Related Parts of the Body
Lungs and Large Intestine	Pectoralis major and minor, sides of neck (Upper Chest Stretch is beneficial; see page 165)
Heart and Small Intestine	Triceps, rotator cuff muscles (see Rotator Cuff Muscle Exercise, page 160)
Bladder and Kidney	Hamstrings and spinal erector muscles, Achilles tendon (Wall Hang Stretch is beneficial; see page 190)
Stomach and Spleen/Pancreas	Quadriceps, front of body in general (Supta Virasana is beneficial, see fig. 7.6)
Liver and Gallbladder	Iliotibial band (ITB) abductor muscles, sides of body, sides of neck especially
Triple Warmer and Pericardium (these have to do with the endocrine and immune systems)	Inner thighs and inner arms

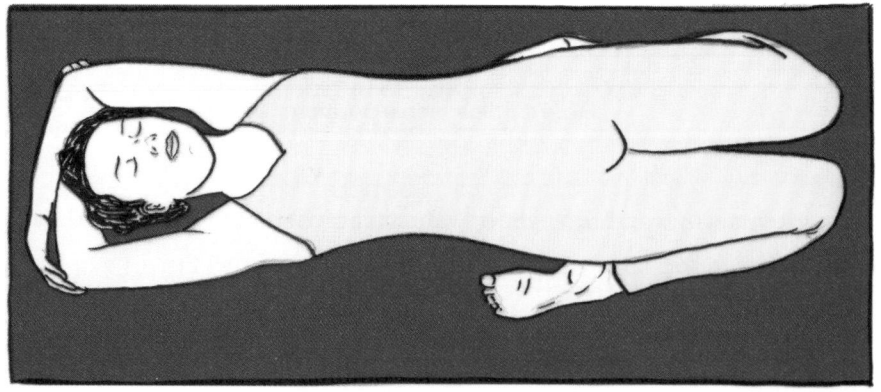

Fig. 7.6. Supta Virasana pose

POPULAR MISCONCEPTIONS

You may get bored with and not need the material in this section, in which case, skip it. However, in thirty years of practice I've found that certain misconceptions come up again and again. So even though these themes appear throughout the book, I'm giving them some extra space to emphasize their importance.

Myth No. 1

The first myth is the one about "functional" exercise. That's the idea that you can do sports and other strenuous activities to build strength. This misconception also includes the belief that to do better at a sport, you need to do it more. There is some truth in this, of course—an athlete is going to be stronger than a sedentary person in a general way. And a manual laborer will develop muscles undreamed of by the person who sits at a desk all day. So why do I see so many dancers and athletes who have serious physical problems when we know strong muscles are healthy muscles? And why do some muscles actually get weaker over time in active, strong people?

I decided to explore this question very thoroughly, testing muscles in athletes for specific imbalances, and sure enough, lots of skilled athletes are very weak in some areas and have developed extreme imbalances between very strong and very weak muscles. What happens over time, as we do our favorite activities in our favorite ways, is that our tendencies, whether healthy or the converse, increase. If we favor our biceps in a sport, perhaps because of compensation for an old injury or a genetic quirk, our biceps will get stronger and we'll gradually use them more and more, because it feels good to use a strong muscle and it feels bad to use a weak one. This is a natural tendency of the body to avoid injury—but we have to outsmart it. Otherwise these imbalances get worse over time, and we end up with a problem.

Generally speaking, gym exercise is used more as a corrective type of movement (changing the body so it functions better, feels better, and, maybe, looks better) than as a sport (exercise for its own sake). On the other hand, few people play golf, for example, because it aligns their bodies—it usually does the opposite; they do it because they enjoy it as a sport.

This is how it works. In an unbalanced activity, or any activity performed with an unbalanced structure, some muscular and neurological pathways get stronger, and those pathways that are not used will weaken. The body, to avoid injury, will continue to strengthen the strong ones, so the strong get stronger and the weak get weaker. Eventually, the strong muscles will tighten until they can't move enough to maintain strength. Then the entire system will weaken to a place where injury or pain is felt, somewhere in the body.

In my own case, for many years, I worked on people in a very body-damaging position: my clients lay on a futon while I worked on them with my knees, forearms, and hands; I was working hard and crawling around on the floor. After doing this for twenty-seven years, I started to get lots of pain. An unrelated injury caused compensation, and I ended up with constant pain in my back.

I understood then why people panic when they experience pain while doing familiar movements, such as in the sports they love and their work. I knew which imbalances I had developed, but not how to correct them. The corrective exercises that follow in this book come out of my experiences with my own pain, mostly the trial and error approach. It took me many errors, some more pain, and about a year of time. The result was that I could work as much as I liked, with a few minor positional adjustments, while continuing some of the exercises two or three times a week.

I want to share these with you so that you will not have to give up any of your favorite activities as you get older, as long as you balance out your muscles over time. My goal here is to enable you to work with your body enough that you can enjoy your favorite body-damaging sports indefinitely. This probably means changing how you do the sport and also doing some corrective exercise.

Myth No. 2

The second myth is that doing an exercise correctly means copying some preexisting shape. This misconception comes from a mental state in which one is focused almost exclusively on appearance, where one is outside of the body, looking at it as though separate from it, and probably judging it in comparison to an idealized image. Dance and many sports exploit the use of the body toward ends that may not be in its best interests. For those movements that focus on making the body function and feel better, we need to focus internally on the feeling of the exercise and the internal visualizing of movement in order to gain benefits and also not to injure ourselves.

The difference between a great dancer or athlete and a less than great one is that the best dancers and athletes integrate mind and body in their work. They have mastered their form to a point where they inhabit their bodies fully all the time.

Remember that corrective exercises work on the nervous system too, so if you don't feel the stretch or the contraction of the muscle, you miss half the equation.

Myth No. 3

This myth relates to the first one; it is the idea that muscles function as isolated units and that they will necessarily be strengthened by using, for example, the weight machines that are designed for that purpose.

Most isolation exercises don't work because muscles don't work the way we imagine from looking at diagrams or the illustrations of what muscles you will use that are on the sides of weight training machines. You might get the result you think—or you might not. This is because muscles do not operate as named units—that notion is just a convenience for the sake of understanding their locations and functions. In real life, pathways of muscle tissue involving areas of named muscles are used. These are complicated and obscure in origin, probably neurological in nature. You may have to isolate a pathway—one particular part of one or more muscles—to really strengthen a function or area.

For example, abdominal crunches don't necessarily strengthen the abdominal muscles, even though they are considered an isolation exercise. You could do them in a convincing way (by that I mean they'll look right to an untrained eye), using your back, hip flexors, even legs. The only way you would know that this is happening is if you try another movement that requires abdominal strength—you won't be able to do it. And of course, once again, our psychological tendency is not to use the weak pathways because it doesn't feel good, and that discourages us from trying further.

Electromyography, the measuring with a machine of the firing patterns of different muscles in exercises, does not (cannot) take into account the parts of the muscle being used, their relative depth, and so on.

This is starting to sound very complicated and possibly discouraging. The good news is that you can effectively isolate these pathways with controlled, modified movements, and you can try out various exercises to find out where your weaknesses lie. Many of the exercises I share with you in part 2 have modifications, so you can do them even if you are very weak in the areas that they utilize. You can do all the muscle pathway exercises to see which pathways need strengthening.

Correcting Misconceptions

The first misconception mentioned above is illustrated in the story of M., who had hip dysplasia and could not decide whether to have hip replacement surgery. In the meantime, to optimize her chances of recovery, with or without surgery, I gave her a series of isolation exercises for the hips and worked carefully with her on them.

I could tell it was a bit of a struggle for her to focus so intensely on small movements, but that reaction to isolation exercise is quite common.

Anyway, a month later, M.'s hip rotators felt just as unbalanced to me as they had before. I asked her if she'd done the exercises. "I've exercised a lot," she said. "So do you think I should have the surgery?" I would probably have advised her more strongly toward the surgery if I hadn't asked her to show me how she'd done the exercises. That's when it turned out she hadn't done the exercises I gave her at all—she had just exercised. She had been swimming every day. That was wonderful but would not help her hip directly.

So the first misconception is that all exercise is the same. All exercise can be useful, and of course, movement is essential for health, but to fix a specific problem in the body, generally speaking, you need to isolate (identify) the weak muscle and then work *only* that muscle. That will mean suppressing all the natural protective impulses the body has to use strong areas so you don't injure yourself.

So please move, swim, dance, whatever you enjoy, but remember, all compound movements (movements where you use a variety of muscles) may increase health but will not correct imbalance in the body.

Psychosomatic Illness

Finally, let's look at the idea of psychosomatic illness. This whole concept comes from another era before we really understood anything about neurotransmitters, neuropeptides, and all those chemical and neurological properties of the body, which really do affect emotions. I think Candace Pert's book, *Molecules of Emotion*, published in 1997, changed the way the general public regarded the mind/body relationship.[*] People began to understand that the mind and body are one functioning unit, not two separate entities that might have a relationship.

It is useful sometimes to separate in our minds "the body" and "the mind" for the purposes of understanding both. However, don't forget the reality, which is that body events, injuries, and so on, affect the mind, and changes in the mind and emotions profoundly influence our denser, more visceral functions.

I find it more useful to see the self as a being composed of various levels of density, from the physical, through the emotional, to the invisible layers of spirit.

[*]Candace Pert, *Molecules of Emotion* (New York: Simon and Schuster, 1997).

HOW LONG WILL IT TAKE?

"How long will it take?" is one of the most common questions I am asked, often by people I have not yet worked on. This is, of course, a legitimate question—they are spending a lot of money and want a clear sense of the benefit they will receive in return. I may be able to give them some idea of how long it may take to get some relief from the pain, but that's different.

The only true answer I can give to the question of how long it will take is: "Probably a lifetime of changing deeply entrenched physical habits. Because, once you correct the habits it has taken you years to create, you will uncover even deeper spiritual and psychological issues, and once you start to unravel those—well, your whole life could change. I think this shift is a fascinating journey through the self, and I love it, but you may not want that."

I chuckle a bit when I think of all the stories of all the people who came in to have their little toe fixed, or something equally inconsequential, and ended up, through the exploration of this work, leaving a mate or finding one or changing their inner and maybe outer lives profoundly.

Or you could just take a pain killer. . . .

PART TWO

ༀ

Cathy Thompson's Exercises

How to Do the Exercises

For all of these exercises, here are the checkpoints, unless I specify otherwise.

1. Gaze is straight ahead, in the direction the spine is facing—imagine a spine with two eyes.

2. Head is in line with the pelvis. Almost everyone will pull the head forward. The head usually should be one to six inches farther back.

3. Don't thrust the chin forward when you bring your head back! The face should be parallel, with the spine, forehead, and chin on the same plane. The natural curve in the neck remains—don't tuck the chin in either, which over-straightens the back of the neck. Align the head by moving it from the back.

4. Hips are square to whichever plane they are facing. Check by feeling the hipbones where they project forward.

5. Center the weight on both, or all, of the points you are supported by—hands, feet, thighs, whatever. If one foot is the foundation point, center the weight over the four corners of the foot.

6. Use the supporting surface—ground or wall—to push down into in order to achieve dynamic stability.

7. Remember that an exercise is a means to an end. The point is not to "do it right" if you thereby engage the wrong muscles. You can "do it wrong" or barely at all, as long as those muscles get the appropriate work. My emphasis on alignment changes the exercises from sports type activities to corrective exercise. If you follow the alignment pointers carefully, rather than forcing yourself into a shape, you will correct your alignment. Don't get upset if you can't do them "properly." You are still getting the right work for yourself.

8

The Head and Neck

ONE OF THE MOST DIFFICULT TASKS you have to accomplish as a human being is to support your head. It weighs ten to twelve pounds and is poised on top of a rather vulnerable neck. If the weight of the head falls onto muscles that are not designed to support it, the result can be a lot of tension and pain throughout the body. The support of the head is not the job of the neck. In fact, all the muscles in the neck that carry the weight of the head originate in either the rib cage or the back, so that the weight of the head can be relayed down the whole spine. Extremely heavy weights, such as jugs of water, can be carried on the head without hand support at all if the weight is aligned correctly with the spine. In traditional cultures, people carried heavy objects on their heads and upper backs so they could use their whole spine for support.

Correct alignment means that the top of the head and the tailbone are in a straight line with each other. The back of the neck is long so the muscles at the front and side of the neck are left free. Every time we move our heads, the whole spine all the way down should move slightly to adapt to the shift in weight; the head and spine should move as a functional unit.

🍃 Neck and Head Alignment

The movements in this exercise are incremental. Isolate each movement as completely as you can.

1. It's particularly hard to feel your own neck alignment, so first of all align yourself in front of a mirror, checking that your shoulders, ears, and eyes are level. Bring

the tips of the ears back and slightly up until they are directly over the tops of your shoulders or at least as far back as possible without causing strain.

2. The next step is to absorb your C7 vertebra (the big knobby bone at the bottom of the neck) slightly in toward the center of your body and slightly up, without engaging your shoulder or your jaw. Place your hand on your collarbone in the center to keep it still. With the head and neck in the same position, pull in C7 in a tiny, almost invisible movement. Think of the inside of the seventh cervical being sucked into your body about an inch, and moving diagonally up toward the crown of your head. Relax the shoulders, don't bring them back deliberately, but notice how they naturally fall back, the collarbones widen, and C7 moves into place.

3. Then feel for the hyoid cartilage in the throat (fig. 8.1). It's about where the Adam's apple is, a free-floating semicircle of cartilage that contains the muscles that support your larynx and thyroid. Absorb the hyoid cartilage into your anterior spine and slightly up. Keep the chin parallel with the ground and the jaw relaxed.

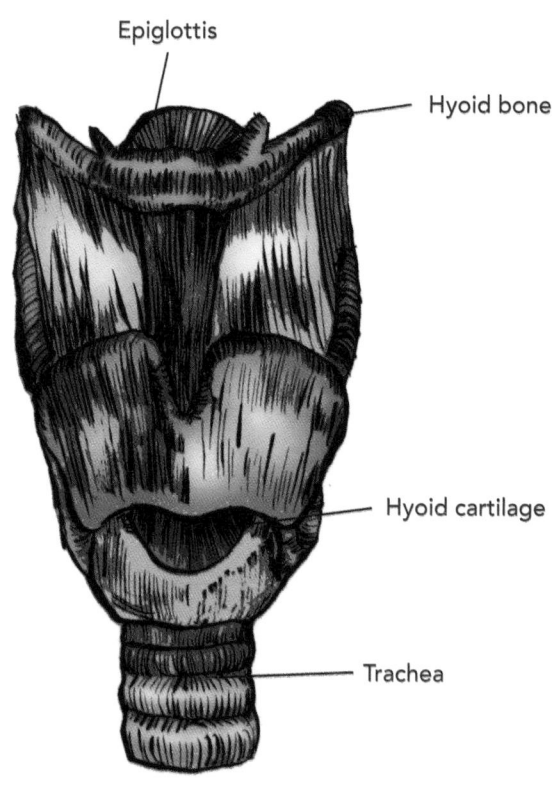

Epiglottis

Hyoid bone

Hyoid cartilage

Trachea

Fig. 8.1. Hyoid cartilage in the throat

The cartilage will "smile": imagine the corners angling up and back, as though you had smiling lips where your hyoid bone is. Feel how the back of the neck releases as the bone draws in.

4. Now run your tongue back along the center of the roof of the mouth until you feel the hollow area at the very back. This is your soft palate. It's actually just in front of the very top of the spine. Most people don't realize that the spine ends at the level of the ears and cheekbones, so the skull is fitted carefully into the surface that the top vertebra creates (fig. 8.2). This allows for a much more balanced distribution of the weight of the head over the spine.

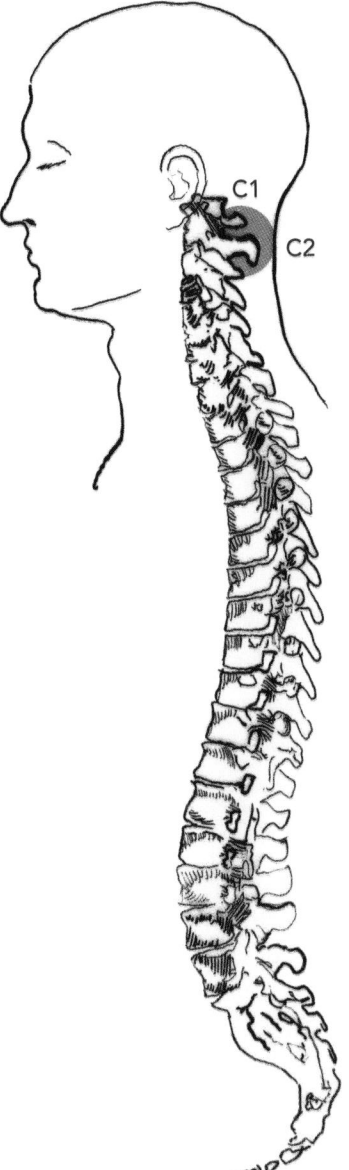

Fig. 8.2. The skull is fitted carefully over the top of the spine, level with the ears and cheekbones.

5. Now find your pubic bone (direct line below the navel to the top part of the triangle of the groin)—you should feel a thin, horizontal bone. Put one hand there and the other on your tailbone. Visualize the point directly in the middle of your two hands—the very center of the pelvic floor. Line the soft palate up with that point. This will align your head correctly on your spine.

6. Imagine someone is lifting you up, holding the sides of your head, and that he lifts you high enough so that your feet come off the ground. Feel how your spine would dangle in its natural curves, as you hang there from your head. Move your head slightly in all directions. You should feel a sense of freedom and "lift" in the neck and head.

7. Then imagine you have an inflatable rubber ring around your upper neck. As this ring inflates it expands up, down and out, but not inward (your throat does not compress). As you inhale, the ring expands farther, lifting your chin and the base of your skull evenly, slightly raising your ears. Feel the space around your upper throat and upper neck. Keep that spacious, airy feeling, and drop your collarbones and scapulae down.

8. Come into a forward bend from standing and notice which parts of your neck may shorten. Imagine blowing up that rubber ring again, and move your head toward the floor from the soft palate, the top of your spine. As you move the palate, feel how the rest of your spine lengthens and moves from it.

9. Make circles clockwise and counterclockwise from the soft palate as though drawing them on the floor. Is it easier to move clockwise or counterclockwise? Is it easier to move forward or backward?

10. Close your eyes, and move the soft palate in the most difficult direction. You can explore this movement using the whole spine, drawing circles around the perimeter, or keeping the spine below C7 still while moving the head. In the latter case, imagine your circles moving around the inside space of C7. Keep the feel of the rubber ring inflating with your inhale, deflating slightly as you exhale during the movement.

GAZE POINT

One of the most common causes of neck pain has to do with the gaze point, something I don't think I've ever seen mentioned in relation to this common problem.

People who have neck pain tend to look downward habitually. It's part of the forward flexion defense pattern we have talked about (page 32). This habit goes with myopia—if you can't see very far ahead, it's much safer to look down. Emotionally, it has to do with drawing into yourself—withdrawing—low self-esteem, and shyness. Just notice where you habitually look as you walk along the street. If you do find yourself always casting your gaze downward, try looking straight ahead for a while. What is that like for you?

I tried looking ahead after noticing that I always look down. The first thing I was aware of, of course, was that I was making eye contact with a lot more people. This is disconcerting for a shy person. I also became aware that I always carry a book or magazine around to read when I'm on the subway or just waiting for something. Part of this is a desire to catch up with my reading. The other part is, if I don't look down and into the world of a printed page, I feel overwhelmed by sensory input from my peripheral vision. The reading and the downcast glance feel like a defense against people, against meeting their eyes, and encountering a possibly hostile environment and overwhelming sensory stimulation.

Notice how you habitually look at the world; see how you feel if you change your glance—perhaps you look up habitually if you are a short person. That can be a strain on the neck in a different way. People with neck pain have also often been told not to look up, to relax and lengthen the back of the neck, but this results in the muscles getting "locked long" and the deep inner neck muscles "locked short."

The natural head position is not the one we use for reading or computer work. It is this: gaze straight ahead with a strong awareness of peripheral vision, so that there is a visual awareness extending in a wide arch across the front of the body. This would also be the safest head position for a primitive human in the jungle—if you look down, you won't see predators coming.

So gaze straight ahead, neither to the right nor left, but be aware of both sides in a relaxed way. When the back of the head lifts, the chin is parallel with the ground so the neck doesn't shorten. Try this for a while, and notice how you feel and how your neck feels.

"Cracking" Your Neck

Lots of people ask me if it's okay to "crack" their necks. The cervical spine has lots of mobility and a complex structure, so it's easy to move the joints over each other and crack them. The cracking sound is actually caused by air pockets (carbon dioxide) that get trapped in the joints. But cracking isn't a good idea, because the problem that makes people think they need to have their neck cracked doesn't actually come directly from the neck itself. It has to do with the relationship between the upper thoracic vertebrae, which are much less mobile vertically, and the flexible cervical spine.

When the upper thoracic vertebrae are jammed, we often overcompensate by twisting the neck around—on the principle that we can do that more easily. But this actually makes the situation worse, as it increases the discrepancy between the thoracic and cervical spine. So the solution is generally to strengthen the neck and increase flexibility in the upper spine.

CHANGING OUR MOVEMENT VOCABULARY

We can often find clues to our mysterious aches and pains in the way we do certain common movements, such as walking, writing, driving, moving our jaw, and so on. One reason pains clear up on a weekend or a vacation is not because we have a break from the stress of work, although that may be part of it as well, but because we have stopped moving in a way that causes tension. These are good areas on which to focus attention, because there can be large gaps in our movement vocabulary, which we may never notice or connect to a chronic pain.

🌿 Jaw Release

In order to release head and neck tension, the jaw must be released. The jaw is not connected to the head muscularly in front of the ears, but under the cheekbones, about four-fingers-width from the ears. Run your fingers from your ears along your cheekbone, toward underneath the eyes, and you will feel the connection at the inner edge of the cheekbone. This awareness can help you keep the jaw relaxed because you will use the strongest part of the masseter muscle (chewing muscle) if you think of using the inner, central part of the jaw when you chew and talk. There should be some space between the top and bottom molars when the jaw is at rest.

1. Begin by stretching your tongue out of your mouth as far as you can, then pull it even farther with your fingers. You can use a piece of gauze to make it easier to hold the tongue if you like.

2. Now, keeping your shoulders relaxed, bring your right ear as close to your right shoulder as you can comfortably. Feel what happens in the jaw and tongue as you move your head. Does the jawbone move closer to the shoulder than the head, or does it stay in the same relationship to the head as when both are straight? Can you feel your tongue move with your head, all the way down to your throat?

3. Now bring your left ear to the left shoulder and see if the left side feels different.

4. When your jaw is completely relaxed, it should feel as though there is a hinge at the opposite side of the jaw (by the right ear if you are moving to your left shoulder). That hinge opens as you move your head. Let your chin relax completely to help you feel this.

5. Try moving your head forward and back, moving it on a diagonal, and twisting it. Notice what happens to your jaw.

6. Also be aware that opening the mouth can involve lifting the head from the cheekbone as well as opening the jaw downward. Try opening your mouth while holding your chin with your hand so the lower jaw does not move. Think of using your nose to lift your head away from your jaw. This simple movement can relieve a lot of jaw tension, by throwing the constant up-and-down movement of the mouth onto stronger muscles and a larger area.

⚘ Correcting Head Tilt

The position of the head on the spine is one of the most important factors in neck tension. Because we are almost always facing forward, the weight of the head tends to be supported by the side and front muscles of the neck, a position that tightens the sides of the neck and the rotators just under the skull. Most people also have a significant tilt to the right or left. In this series of exercises, we'll explore the sideways tilt, which, again because of the weight of the head and the amount of mobility it has, can throw off the rest of the spine and the hips. So let's correct it and find how the spine can release and strengthen without our having to struggle to balance our heads.

THE HEAD
AND NECK

1. Sit in front of a mirror, on a chair with legs uncrossed or on the floor. You need to be in a position in which your pelvis is stable and square to the mirror. Bring your arms straight out to the side, palms facing down and in a straight line through the body, both hands in line with the shoulders.

2. Now close your eyes and turn your head from side to side. Feel where your ears are in relation to your shoulders and where the top of your head is in relation to the lower spine; the hands, arms, and collarbone are still. Only the head moves.

3. Now, with your eyes still closed, find a place where your head feels completely centered. Open your eyes. Notice: Are your ears and eyes in a straight line? Is your head tilted or turned in any way? Are your hands and arms still even? Probably not!

4. Notice this, reposition yourself more evenly, and then repeat the exercise. See how your body can absorb the information your eyes have given you. Keep correcting yourself until you can feel the center position with your eyes closed.

🍃 *Enhancing Side-to-Side Balance of the Head*

Without moving your shoulders, turn your head from side to side. Keep the ears even and the crown of the head over the spine—don't lean the head forward at all. Keep the face parallel to the wall and the eyes moving with the head.

1. Rotate your head slightly, with no forcing or effort at stretching, turning the chin first toward the right shoulder. You will notice that at a certain point in the twist, the head will automatically shift upward very slightly, the shoulder you turn toward may want to rise up (don't let it), and you will probably feel a slight "glitch" at the side of the neck. This is the place where the two top cervical vertebrae (remember the spine starts at the level of the ears) shift slightly in their relationship to each other, and a gentle movement becomes a more effortful stretch. Notice this place on the right by looking at it in a mirror if you can, or just noting with your hands the position of the head relative to the body.

2. Then turn to the left, and locate the "glitch" where the movement shifts on that side. What we are interested in now is the difference between those two places. It is likely that the head will turn more easily to one side than the other.

    Most right-handed people can move farther to the right because they look at things and write turning to the right (the opposite pattern is true for most left-handed people). The left side of the neck usually tightens to pull the head back into line, and the left shoulder rises up to compensate. There is usually a bigger space between the inside edge of the right shoulder and the ear to compensate, and a bigger space between the inside edge of the shoulder blade and the spine on the left side than on the right. You can experiment with this by placing books, the computer screen, and so on, at an angle that is different from the familiar, probably more to the left, and see how that changes your alignment and your focus and connection.

3. To correct the habit you have, turn to the side where the "glitch" is closer to the centerline. If this is to the left side, you are probably chronically tilting your head to the right. Stay in the glitch. Relax and drop both shoulders, making sure the collarbone is straight. Lift the soft palate to lengthen the spine.

4. Now move your head back and forth over the glitch about 1 inch to either side of it, feeling the twist in the whole spine. Move your eyes all around, loosening up your field of vision—look as far in the direction you are turning as you can without moving the head more than an inch. Keep lengthening your spine for about two minutes.

5. Now turn your head back to the center. With your eyes closed, move your chin in a half-moon shape, swinging slowly from side to side, keeping your alignment. Even out the movement. After a minute or so, come back to center and notice any changes. Rest.

🍃 Moving Your Skull over Your Neck

This exercise has a lot to do with how we use our eyes, the coordination between them, and how that influences the weight of our heads. For example, if your head is chronically tilted because of looking more to one side, even if only a fraction, that weight over time can create tightness in one hip, in the legs, and in your feet. Your eyes are also your brain, and your cognitive process, memories, and emotions are bound up with your vision. So as you do this, pay especially close attention to the eyes.

If you can complete this movement with palms pressing against the ears and the shoulders pressed down, use this position. If not, modify it by putting just the tips of your fingers against the ears. You want a firm grip on the area around and just above your ears either way (see fig. 8.3 on page 112).

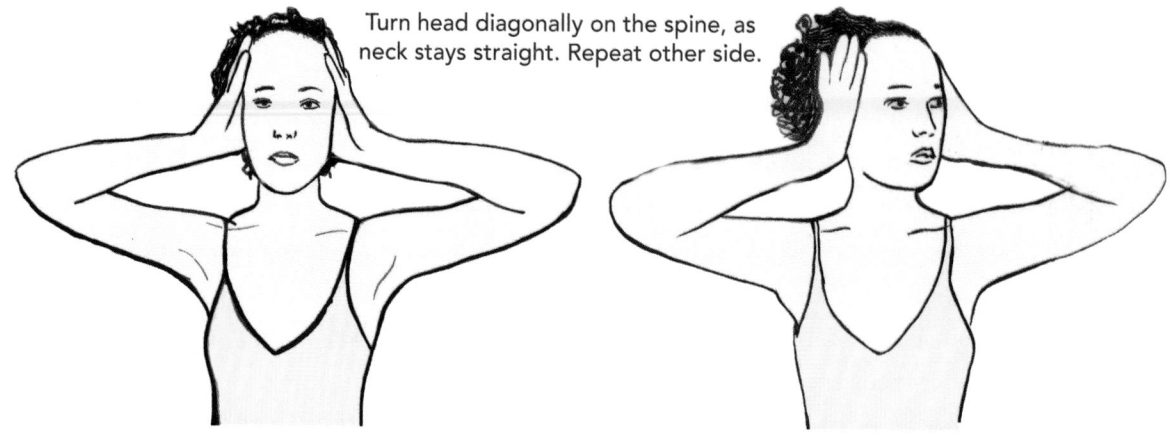

Turn head diagonally on the spine, as neck stays straight. Repeat other side.

Fig. 8.3. Moving Your Skull over Your Neck

1. Keep your neck and chin back, but not tucked in. You want your face on the same plane as the wall in front of you. The underside of your chin needs to be parallel with the floor. You'll probably find that your chin will want to jut forward and so will your neck.

2. Now, keeping your chin and neck back, use your hands to turn the head diagonally on the spine. Keep looking straight ahead—your line of vision will shift, of course. Make sure your neck stays straight, so you are turning the cranium on the spine, opening up some space between the first two vertebrae in the neck, above the level of the skull. Go in both directions, noticing which one is easier.

3. Use your hands to turn your head to the side that is most difficult. Stay there for 90 seconds if you can, pressing *slightly* with the side of your head against your hands toward the more difficult direction. Your head provides a very slight isometric resistance to your hands. Envision sliding the upper hand upward slightly and the lower one downward, pressing your skull and squeezing the cranial bones slightly, as though you were lifting the base of your skull up and very gently turning it in the difficult direction. This will help you feel the separation between the movement of the atlas (C1, the first cervical vertebra) and the axis (C2, the second cervical vertebra), and the space between them and the skull (occiput).

4. Then turn the head in again in each of the two directions, noticing any differences that you feel now.

You can use this exercise for any spiral or bilateral distortions in the spine, scoliosis, eyestrain, and most neck pain.

NECK FLEXORS

Look at the path of the neck flexors (fig. 8.4). You would think that the forward position of the head, unfortunately common in most people, would strengthen the flexors—after all, we are in chronic flexion. However, in this position the flexors shorten and then cannot contract or expand properly (fig. 8.5). Architecturally, the flexors resemble our other troublemaker, the psoas; they support the weight of our heads the same way the psoas supports our torso (see fig. 8.6 on page 114).

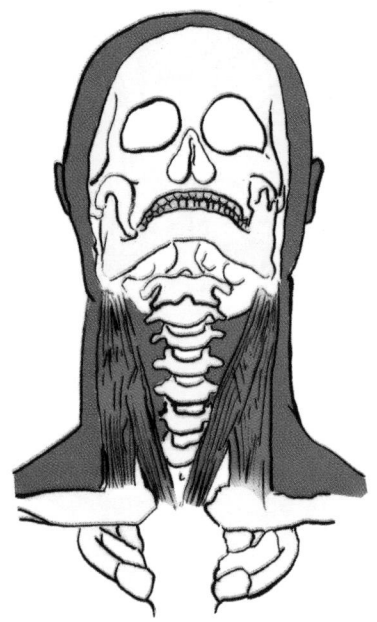

Fig. 8.4. Neck flexors

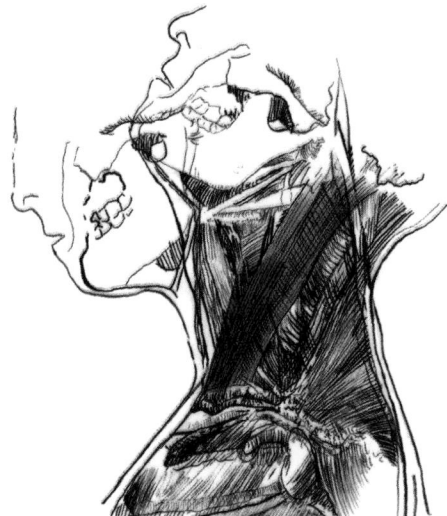

Fig.8.5. Neck flexors in motion

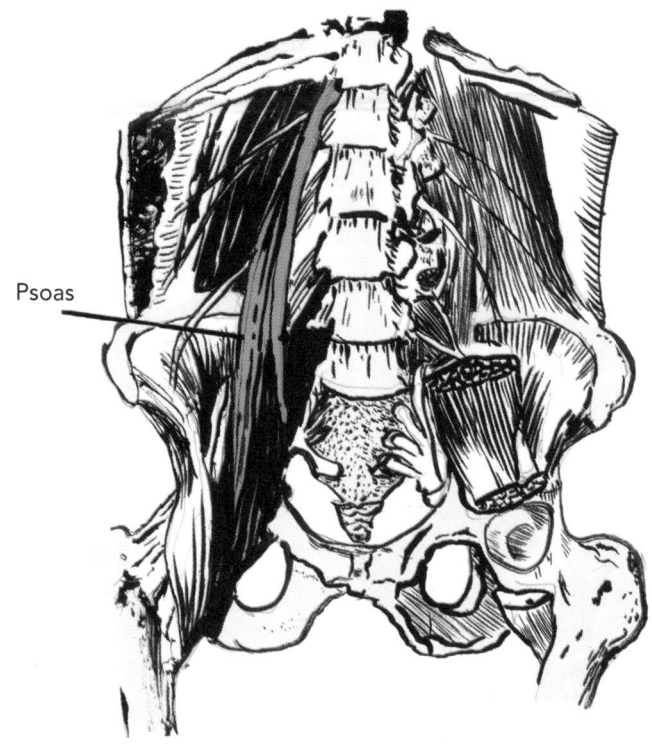

Psoas

Fig. 8.6. Psoas muscle

🌿 Strengthen Your Neck Flexors

Make sure your shoulders stay relaxed. Your chin should be slightly down, but with some space between your chin and your throat. You should feel the work in the front of your neck and in the back next to the base of the skull.

1. Lie on your back, arms by your sides, palms down.
2. Think of stretching your spine long as you bring your head up about 8 inches or so from the floor and look between your feet. The gaze point between your feet should keep the neck in the correct position.
3. Hold for 3 minutes if you can, without shifting position.

This is also a good test to see how strong your neck is. If you can't hold the position for at least a minute, your neck flexors are quite weak and could be responsible for some neck pain. Weak flexors allow the head to fall too far forward, causing pain at the back of the neck.

🍃 Advanced Strengthening Exercise for the Neck

This is a good exercise to deal with neck tension (weak neck flexors and rotators) if:

1. When you do abdominal crunches, your neck hurts unless you support it
2. The position of your head is forward of your body in profile
3. You have had whiplash or another neck injury (but be careful if you have disc herniation or other vertebral issues)
4. You have eyestrain
5. You have neck tension

Try this advanced exercise very carefully. Don't rush it. This is an amazing exercise with fast results if you do it correctly. However, if you practice it with poor alignment, you can easily hurt your delicate neck.

1. Use a bed or table. Lie on your back with your shoulders at the edge and your neck hanging over backward (fig. 8.7). Take a rolled-up bath towel and place it lengthwise on the table directly under the spine of the upper back, so your thoracic spine is supported and the shoulder blades fall down on either side of the towel. The length of the rolled-up towel should run between the seventh cervical and about T12—not up to the neck or down to the waist or lower back. Without this support, you may compress T1, T2, and T3 when you lift your head.

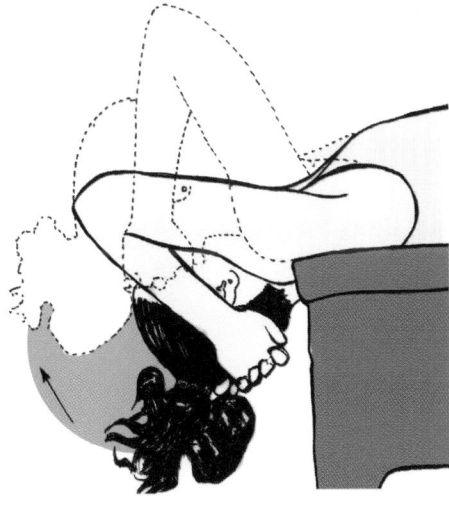

Fig. 8.7. Advanced Strengthening Exercise for the Neck

2. Bring your hands back to a point about a hand's width back from the crown of the head. You will probably feel a ledge of bone there—the edge of one of the cranial plates. Hold it gently with the fingertips of both hands, and lengthen the back of the neck. The neck must stay long throughout the exercise. The chin, with the mouth shut, remains in the same proximity to the throat the whole time—about 3 inches away. Depending on your strength, provide more or less support with your fingertips.

3. Keeping the point you are touching supported, so the head does not fall back and the back of the neck stays long, lift the neck toward the chest. Make sure your chin is right in the center of your shoulders. Keep your gaze directed toward the center of your chest. Come up only as far as you can without lifting your upper back from the towel. You will probably bring the head slightly above shoulder level.

4. Keep your head alignment, and bring the head back down to the starting position. The eccentric (negative) movement is usually a little easier, so relax your fingertips more now and try to feel the movement in the back of the neck, close to the skull. If you feel the movement mostly in the front, you will need to tuck the chin more and lengthen the back of the neck. Adjust your neck position carefully, so you are working primarily in the back, not the front. You may also feel work in the lower back portion of the neck. The contraction of these muscles can feel like a gripping neck tension. This is okay. Gripping and cramping in the throat is not—it's an indication you are compressing your neck.

5. Each movement should be very slow and controlled. Make the upward (concentric) movement of the head to a slow count of five, the downward (eccentric) to a slow count of ten. Five to twelve reps equal one set.

Follow immediately with Jaw Release (page 108).

🌿 Stretch for the Neck

1. Sit on a chair or cross-legged on the floor. Support yourself with one hand on the floor or by holding the chair as you lean away from it (fig. 8.8).

2. If you are sitting on the floor, press your hand into the floor (probably the palm will feel the best, but you can experiment with different hand positions). Bring the opposite ear toward the opposite shoulder. You can support, or gently press,

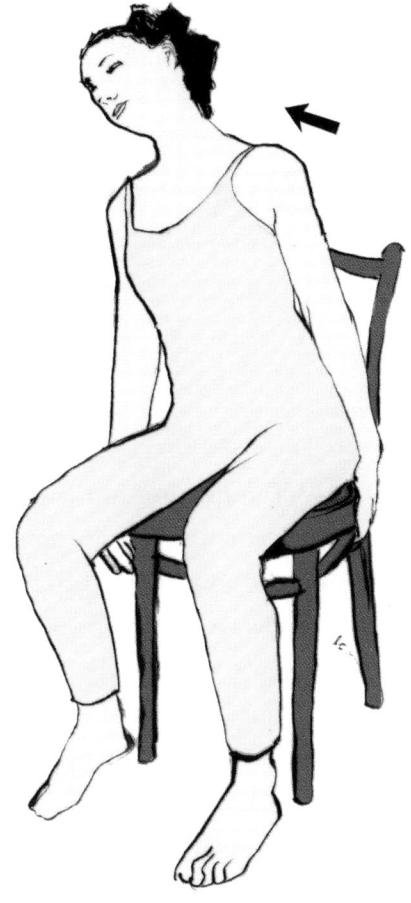

Fig. 8.8. Stretch for the Neck

the head toward the shoulder with the free hand as long as you can relax the shoulder and feel no compression in the neck. If you feel a lot of compression in the neck, you could place a rolled-up towel between the neck and shoulder. Your Neck Roll might also work (page 195). If you don't feel compression, just hold the head in a gently stretched position.

3. Press the collarbones firmly down, while the neck stretches. You can change the angle of your head to find a good stretch between the collarbone and the chin, opening up the fascia in that triangle. Follow your body's guidance and explore different stretches in the front and sides of the neck. Using the dynamic of the collarbone pressing down will open up the lower part of the neck and the upper chest. You may also feel the stretch through the rotator cuff muscles in the shoulder.

9

Breathing

MANY PEOPLE WHO HAVE restriction in their breathing patterns tell me they "forget to breathe." Fortunately, they can't really do that; their bodies will take over, and they will automatically start breathing just to stay alive. In this sense, respiration is an involuntary function we don't have to think about. Breathing is also voluntary—we can restrict it or deepen it as we choose, and we can also train our breathing patterns. Most of us cannot control our heartbeat or our digestion very well (though this is possible and can be learned).

The beginning of all movement patterns is the breath. A change in the rhythm of breathing marks all physical and emotional transitions. If you can identify when the change takes place, you will be able to understand and work with your patterns before they become so entrenched that the connective tissue is involved. Remember that "forgetting to breathe" involves a lot more energy and effort than just breathing.

Most of us, when we are under stress, hold our breath in an effort to control ourselves. If we don't like where we are or whom we are with, we may want to reject our environment by not inhaling deeply. The letting go of the breath in the exhale may threaten our sense of autonomy and control. The diaphragm, structurally, functions as a bridge separating the lower body—the organs and the parts of our bodies we associate with instinct and gut feelings—from the upper body and our conscious emotions and thoughts. It is also one of the first muscles we learn to tighten. Even very young babies, before they are mobile enough to develop structural distortions, can learn to suppress crying by squeezing in their diaphragms. It is one of the first ways we learn to not feel strong feelings and often stays with us all our lives as a shallow, suppressed breathing pattern.

We can also breathe incorrectly because we have the wrong idea about how we should be breathing. There is not a right or wrong way to breathe, but different activities require different uses of the breath, and we can make the mistake of believing that specialized breathing patterns are right for everyday life. These are the most common misconceptions people have about the structural aspect of breathing:

1. The sternum does not move, only the lower abdomen.
2. The shoulders and collarbone initiate the breath.
3. The sternum sticks out, and the lower back shortens.

These ideas come from many different sources. Some yoga teaching emphasizes the lower abdominal breath, and various schools of vocal technique use diaphragmatic breath and work with a hyperextended sternum. To understand normal relaxed breathing, get to know your rib cage.

NORMALIZING YOUR BREATHING

One purpose of training the breath is to shift physical and mental patterns. Yogis discovered that changing breath patterns could quiet the mind as a preliminary to meditation, or wake it up when it was listless. Since we spend so much time attempting to change our mental states through therapies and medications, wouldn't it make sense to explore these possibilities through something as simple as the breath? Maybe it's so simple we don't believe it. The mind seems a very complex thing, and we assume that we need to work on it in painstaking, slow, and difficult ways. Medications have shown us that mental and emotional states can be changed easily by taking a pill, so why not use a completely safe and healthy method that will only serve to benefit us (the breath), rather than turning immediately to more risky interventions such as drugs?

Shape of the Breath

You are already exploring the science of *pranayama*, regulating the life force with the breath, right now, in the sense that the way you are breathing at this moment is influencing your nervous system and your mental state. The way you feel can be changed by the shape of your breath, the parts of your body you use when you inhale and exhale, and whether you use your whole body and lung capacity or restrict yourself to a narrow portion of the torso. You may suppress your emotions by not allowing your chest to move, or your gut feelings by hardening your belly.

It's natural for the flow of air to shift from right to left and back throughout the day. If your breath pattern is stuck in the right nostril your sympathetic nervous system will be overactivated, making you feel stressed and, maybe, interfering with sleep. If the reverse is true, your parasympathetic nervous system will be constantly dominant, making you sluggish.

Or maybe you can only breathe through your mouth. Mouth breathing is emergency breathing, used when the body needs more air quickly, usually when you are exerting yourself. When your heart rate is stable, you should breathe primarily through your nose, which has natural filters in it (the tiny hairs that keep out dust and some germs). You cannot control the airflow as precisely with the mouth.

There is an expression, "mouth breather," that refers to a person easily frightened, without backbone. Mouth breathing when you are not exerting yourself tells your body that there is an emergency and can make you feel anxious or even panicky. The classic way to calm down a person who is hyperventilating (having a panic attack) is to have her breathe into a paper bag, so she inhales her own carbon dioxide, which is a natural relaxant and tranquilizer.

All these forms of breathing are fine sometimes, when in their natural place. What can be harmful is the locking of the body into one fixed breath shape, which blocks our natural flow. Breath shape is the first aspect of the breath that we can work with.

Aerobic Capacity

The second aspect of the breath that we can influence is the aerobic—simply, the health of the lungs. This is so basic that it is overlooked all the time. I've worked with singers who can barely huff and puff their way up a flight of stairs, and then wonder why they can't sing a Wagnerian opera requiring huge amounts of cardiovascular stamina. Without this component, there will be no energy to work with, not much juice.

I want to address this briefly, really, just so we can exclude this as a possible source of difficulty. Certain physical conditions—anemia, asthma, and so on—could affect cardiovascular capacity. But it's usually just lack of fitness.

You can evaluate, and improve, your aerobic capacity easily by exercising on a cardio machine at the gym, like a treadmill, bike, or stair climber. Any kind of sustained exertion that brings your heart rate up for at least twenty minutes will improve your aerobic fitness, but the gym machines also allow you to assess where you are in relation to a norm. You can do lots of exercise of the nonaerobic kind—weights, yoga, Pilates, and so on—and still be weak in the cardiovascular aspect.

The gyms will have training charts that show you what the heart rate "training zone" is for you in your group—remember that this may be different if your resting heart rate is faster or slower than average, and change accordingly. You should be able to stay in your training zone for about twenty minutes without getting winded.

Of course, to do this you need a gym, charts, and a heart rate monitor. But actually you don't need any of this to improve your aerobic fitness—just do something where your heart rate stays up but you don't get so out of breath you cannot talk, for at least twenty minutes. You will need to warm up (your heart rate won't go up right away) and cool down—at least five minutes of light exercise to lower your heart rate gently. Interval training—raising the heart rate to the high end of your training zone, maintaining this for a few minutes, dropping down to the low end for a longer time, rising again, and so on—is actually the fastest way to improve lung capacity.

You can also improve lung capacity by breathing just through your nose, taking your workout to a place where it is difficult but not impossible. Because the air passageways of the nostrils are much smaller than the mouth, it's harder work to breathe nasally, and you will learn to control your breathing and use your full lung capacity. That's pretty straightforward. The other two components of breathing are a bit more complicated.

Breath Control

Breath control is how much you can change and regulate your inhalation and exhalation, how long you can hold in your inhale and exhale (retention of breath), and how long you can practice breathing exercises without becoming lightheaded or dizzy. This is breathing as a skill, something you can learn to manipulate. You can achieve this kind of breathing health through a variety of breathing exercises, the yogic pranayama practice being the prototype. Singing will also increase this particular aspect of breath control.

A good deal of this has to do with your nervous system and how accustomed you are to tolerating the slight fear that comes when we retain breath for a long time or attempt to use the breath in this kind of way.

You may wonder what the purpose of learning and controlling breath patterns is, if you are not a yogi or singer. Most people understand that cardiovascular capacity is an important component of health—after all, doctors give you stress tests to assess this function. But why bother learning fancy, and difficult, breath patterns?

This is where the subject we discussed earlier, the regulation of emotions and states of being through the breath, takes a practical form. The breathing patterns are ways of changing your experience; there are patterns that will calm you, and others that will activate you, reduce stress, and so on. The ability to do this takes for granted that you have adequate lung capacity—you won't get very far if you don't.

BREATHING STRUCTURE

The next component of the breath is the structural aspect of breathing: the health, strength, and flexibility of all the muscles involved in the flow of breath, inhalation, and exhalation, the alignment of the ribs in relation to the rest of the body, the openness of the throat, and the structures of the neck and head (fig. 9.1). You can be perfectly aerobically fit and able to perform long complicated breathing exercises and still be very uncomfortable when you breathe if your structure is distorted and the muscles can't open and release a full breath.

I work with lots of singers who develop vocal injuries as a result of stressing a learned breath that they are using incorrectly, usually because they have the wrong idea about how they should breathe, such as not moving their chest when they breathe, so they then tighten the chest muscles, suppressing the natural breath. That's the most common one based on the idea that when we are relaxed we breathe with our bellies. This is a good example of "a little learning is a dangerous thing." It is sort of true that letting the breath move into the belly is a relaxed and open way to breathe, but not by restricting the movement of the lungs and tightening the chest. You will actually be able to take a deeper "belly breath" by allowing the upper ribs to expand. Try it and see.

I remember teaching a class of singers about bodywork and realizing that none of them even knew where their lungs were. It sounds odd, but do *you* know? Place your hands where you think the top of your lungs are and then where you think the very bottom of your lungs are; now look at fig. 9.2.

About 75 percent of the clients I work with think the top of their lungs is at the level of their nipple line, when they actually reach all the way into the top chest and all the way down to the lowest bottom rib. Of course it is much easier to feel the bottom of the rib cage than the top because the collarbone sits right at the level of the

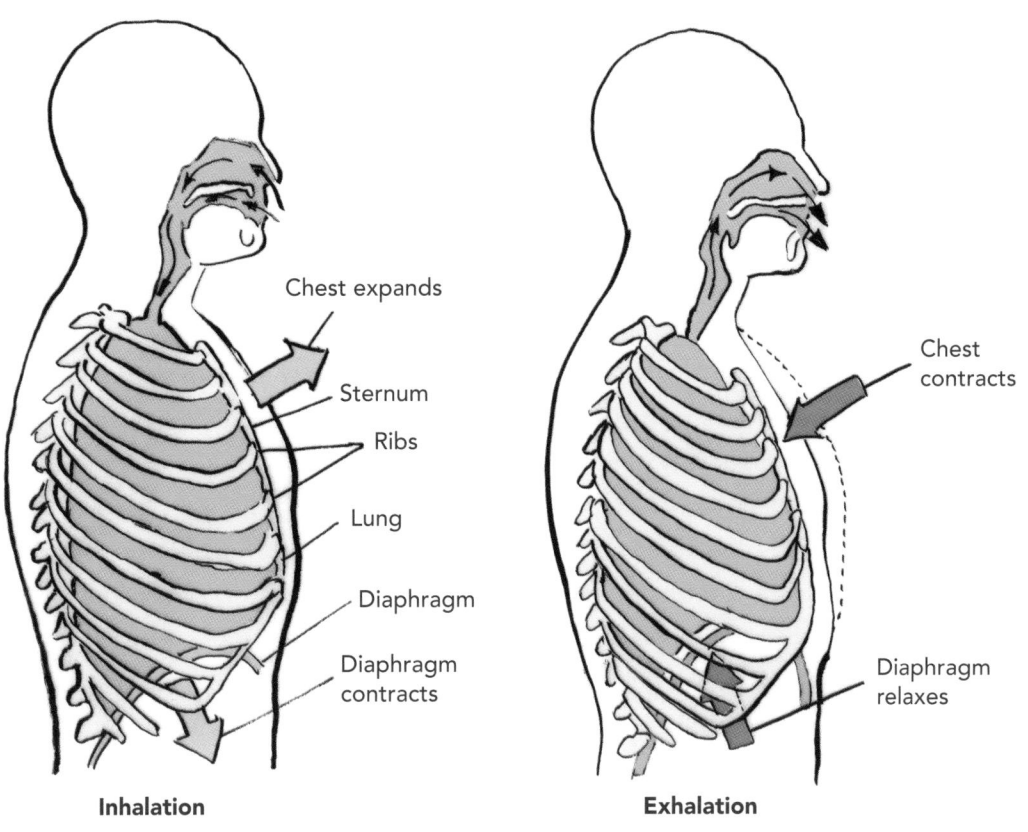

Inhalation

Chest expands

Sternum

Ribs

Lung

Diaphragm

Diaphragm contracts

Exhalation

Chest contracts

Diaphragm relaxes

Fig. 9.1. Breath flow diagram

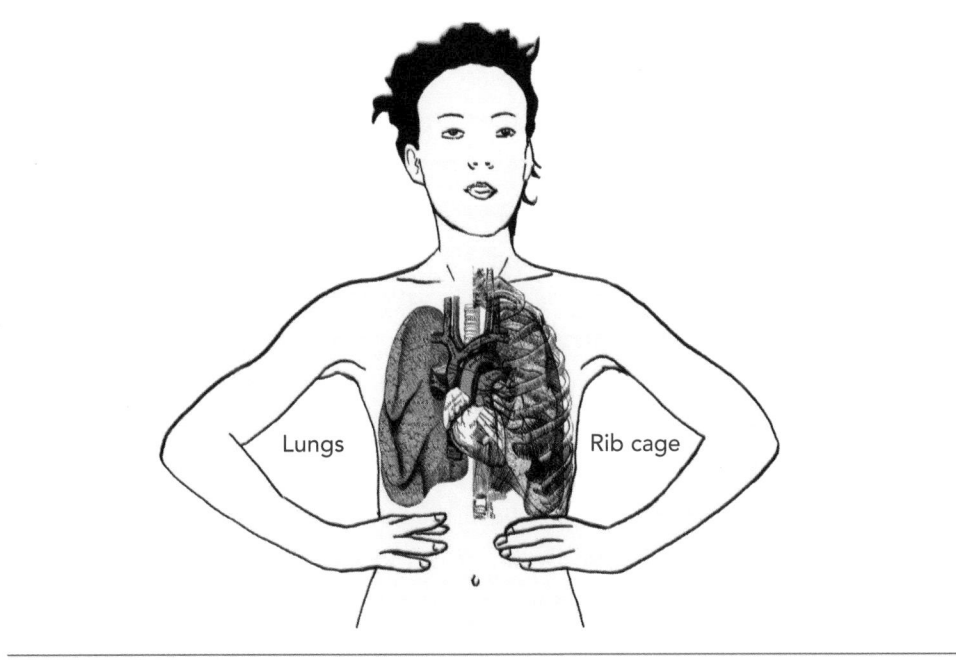

Lungs

Rib cage

Fig. 9.2. Lung placement

top rib and is bigger and thicker. But try out the following experiment to see if you can feel your breath in your top rib.

🍂 *Feeling Your Breath in Your Top Rib*

1. First, touch the collarbone and then move your fingers behind and slightly under it, where there is a sensitive, nervy, triangular hollow. Behind that hollow lies the big and powerful trapezius muscle. Place your fingers on the hollow itself, pressing gently down. The top rib is inside that hollow. Depending on how much tissue you have there, you may be able to feel it.

2. Press down a little harder and breathe naturally. You should feel a small movement there, a slight rise on the inhalation and a gentle release and drop on the exhalation. Keeping your fingers there and maintaining some pressure will stimulate the top rib. Can you feel the movement of the top rib against your fingers and then in front of it the collarbone, which will move slightly outward, widening as you breathe?

3. See if you can activate your top rib a little more and let go of the collarbone completely. The collarbone is a part of the shoulder girdle, which is gently massaged by the breath under it, but it is not a prime mover of respiration.

4. Now notice if your shoulder muscles feel any different. Take your fingers away, and see if you can maintain the activation of the top rib while you continue to let go of the shoulder girdle. We have only explored one side so far, so let's feel the difference. Do your shoulders feel uneven now? How exactly are they working differently? Maybe you have more of a feel now for the relationship between shoulder tension and breathing.

5. Now you can explore the other side in the same way, noticing any differences. All of the muscles in the torso, front, sides, and back, some neck muscles, and muscles that connect with the hips are actively involved in the breath; every tissue in the body is passively involved. So you can understand how muscle imbalances, postural misalignment, and even the condition of the abdominal organs will change your breath.

However aerobically fit you are, however long you can retain your breath in practiced breathing exercises, there will be distortions in the pattern of respiration as long as structural imbalances exist. By far the quickest and, for me as a bodyworker, the easiest way to change the breathing patterns is to work directly on the structures around the lungs and the diaphragm. You can, as you may have experienced when you were exploring your top rib, work on some of these muscles yourself. I'll explain how.

The lungs are big. Everywhere you feel ribs, you basically have lung tissue underneath. Every rib should move away from the center of the body, away from each other, and slightly upward when you inhale and release inward when you exhale (see fig. 9.1 on page 123). The top rib moves up and the bottom rib moves down to allow the rib cage to expand vertically on the inhalation. The rib cage is a cylinder, which moves as much in the back as in the front and sides. Take some time to feel all the ribs, with your fingers from the outside and from the inside of your body. Let your breath go into all the spaces of the rib cage, the armpits, the upper back, the lower back, and especially any parts that feel numb or difficult to feel. Gently tap those places to encourage the breath.

The Intercostal Muscles

Imagine a balloon with soft strings around it, encircling its perimeter. As the balloon is blown up it expands evenly and the strings move farther away from one another. If the balloon were deflated the strings would move toward one another and inward. Now imagine the strings have other small cords like basket weave wrapping between them. If the ribs are strings, the basket weave is the intercostal muscles (fig. 9.3). These muscles allow the ribs to open voluntarily, at least to an extent.

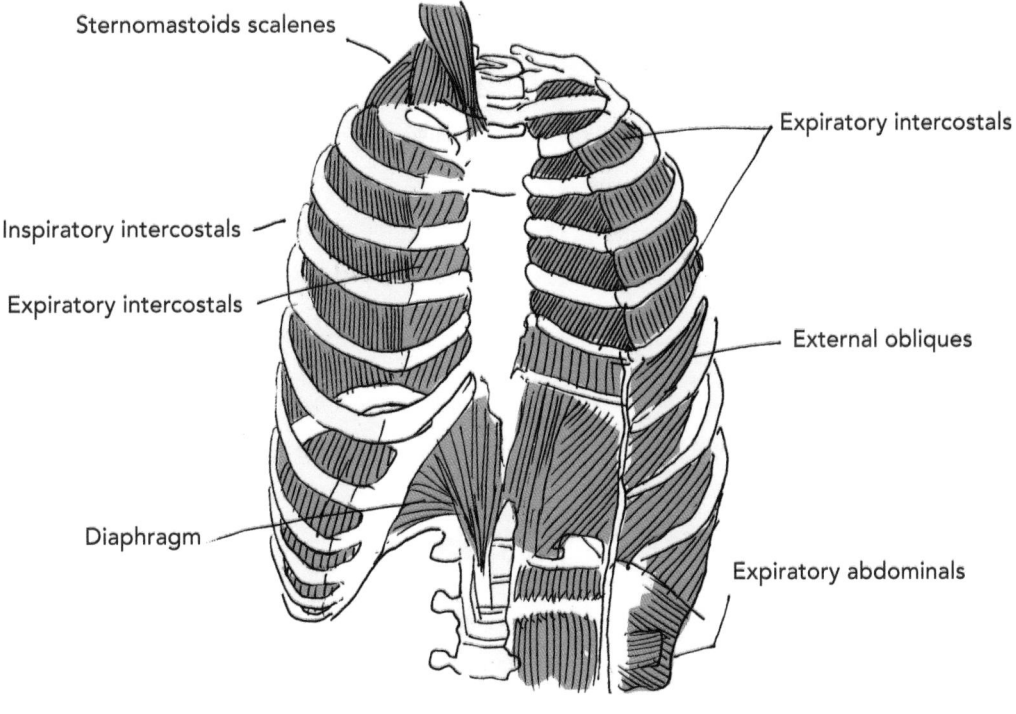

Fig. 9.3. Intercostal muscles

To take our balloon analogy further, imagine that someone dropped glue on the strings and basket weave unevenly, so that some of the strings didn't move properly. The glue is our stuck, glued-up fascia caused by muscle imbalance. When the balloon expands, the pressure from the inside builds up and will only move against the flexible areas, so the glued-up areas don't move at all.

🍃 Releasing Stuck Intercostals

See if you can find the stuck areas on your ribs and start to open them.

1. Start anywhere on your rib cage. Using your thumb and index finger, feel the hard bone of the rib itself. Then move your thumb up or down slightly in the space between that rib and the next one. Even if you have a lot of tissue you can usually feel this area. Press into that space, noticing how much the ribs can move away from each other as you inhale.

2. Then inhale and try to push your fingers away from the center of your body with your breath, consciously moving the ribs apart with your breath. Depending on the area you have chosen, you may feel a free, open movement or not much movement at all, and the space you are pressing into may be more or less sensitive. As you breathe into your fingers and encourage the ribs to move, you are lengthening the intercostal muscles. This will help open the stuck, glued-up places in the muscles.

3. Explore as much as you can of the rib cage this way, lingering at the stuck places in order to open them. The areas that tend to be inflexible and sore are the armpits, the sternum, near the spine if you can reach it, and the lower side back area. Opening the side back ribs this way can alleviate lower back issues too.

Dealing with Lower Back Pain

When you feel what a large area of your back the rib cage covers, you can understand how important the rib cage is, not just to our breathing, but also to any kind of back problem. Each rib expresses the vertebra it is attached to, and you can mobilize the entire thoracic spine by releasing its partner rib. After releasing the appropriate ribs, you may find a new degree of flexibility and maybe less pain, if you had any pain, in your back.

One of the muscles that's often responsible for lower back pain, quadratus lumborum, is also a breathing muscle that shortens on the inhalation, pulling down the lower ribs and increasing lung capacity (fig. 9.4). Quadratus lengthens on the exhalation, allowing the diaphragm to release and the back ribs to soften.

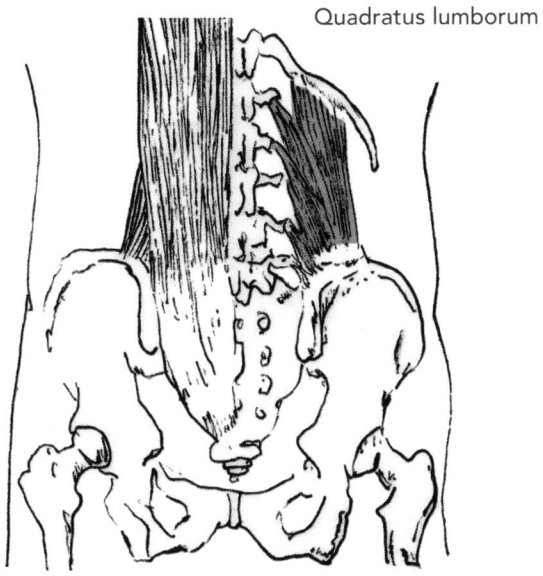

Quadratus lumborum

Fig. 9.4. Quadratus lumborum

Quadratus is worth getting to know in its dual role as breathing muscle and stabilizer of the rib cage and back. Find it by pressing in at the side of the spine just below the lowest rib that is attached to it (fig. 9.5).

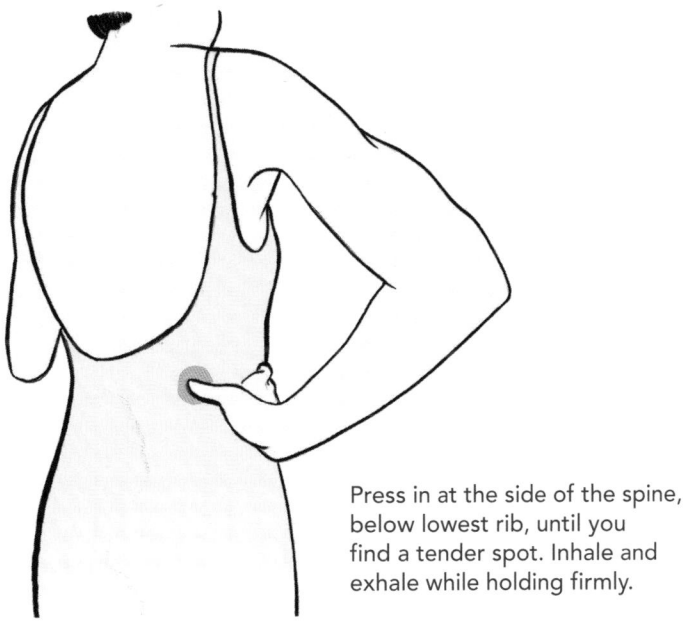

Press in at the side of the spine, below lowest rib, until you find a tender spot. Inhale and exhale while holding firmly.

Fig. 9.5. Finding the Quadratus Lumborum

🍃 *Finding the Quadratus Lumborum*

1. You can work both sides of your spine with your thumbs, or a knuckle. Quite far in to the side and high up under the lowest rib, you'll find a tender spot. If you have lots of surface tissue, it may be harder to find, so bend to the side, stretching that area to make it more accessible. You'll find it!

2. Now, hold your hand in that area and see if you can feel the movement of the back ribs away from where you are holding. You may not feel much—this tends to be one of the laziest areas of the rib cage. Breathe into the back ribs consciously, inflating both sides equally to the side, as you hold the tender spot firmly. This may help relieve lower back pain.

You can work this way with any tight or painful area in your back. Locate the ribs that run through that area and work the spaces between them as we described, all the way round the body. Usually you will find tender or stuck places in the ribs, often more sensitive on the opposite side of the painful places in the back. See if the pain is relieved at all this way.

This is how I work with scoliosis—I've found that working the ribs thoroughly enough to reposition them opens up the spine in a way that working directly into the spine itself cannot accomplish.

See if you can work into chronic back problems this way also. When you get more practice at it you'll know your trouble zones and just work there. If you want a stronger pressure, you can use a very small hard rubber ball, about the size of a plum, and lie on a mat with the ball between you and the mat so that it presses into the spaces between the ribs. This will be a much stronger pressure if you want that intensity. Soft small balls don't seem to fit properly in the intercostal spaces, but you could try lying on a thicker mat if you find the pressure too strong. The advantage of using a ball this way is that you don't have to work at the same time. Once you have found the right places, you can relax on top of the ball and focus on the breathing.

Correcting Breath Imbalance

Now you can check the sides of the rib cage with your hand to see which side, left or right, you are breathing more on. Usually we breathe more deeply into one lung than the other, quite unconsciously, but you can see how that might affect your structure, opening up and strengthening the back and chest on the dominant side, and shortening and tightening the same areas on the weaker side. There's one common reason for this you can check now, which is if the nostril on the weak side is closed, either from muscular weakness or congestion. So see if that's the case.

If you find one nostril not able to breathe fully, check this by blocking off the other nostril. There is a natural switch over every few minutes from one nostril to the other. If a nostril is chronically blocked you won't be able to shift your breath into it easily. Don't be surprised to find you can't breathe through one nostril at all.

You may be familiar with alternate nostril breathing, a yoga exercise that balances the brain hemispheres. The left nostril stimulates the right brain, the more creative intuitive side, and the parasympathetic nervous system, which controls involuntary systems in our body, such as digestion, and allows us to relax. The right nostril stimulates the left brain, which controls logical thinking and the sympathetic; that is, the more activating part of the autonomic nervous system. So of course we need a balance or we'll have trouble either mobilizing ourselves or going to sleep. For most right-handed people the left nostril is more chronically blocked or weaker.

🍃 Balance Yourself

You can experiment with this very simply by finding the nostril you have most difficulty breathing through. Then block the opposite one, making sure you don't push your head into an uneven position.

Just sit however you're comfortable and breathe through the weak nostril. You may need to use your other hand to open the nostril. You can breathe slowly and deeply or try a yoga breath of fire: that's a short, fast, sniffing breath with equal emphasis on the inhale and exhale. I feel a shift in my energy after doing this for about five minutes and a lot more change after fifteen minutes or so. Try it and see how and when you feel the subtle changes of your energy as different brain centers open up.

For most people the left nostril breath is calming and centering, the right nostril more stimulating. Slow deep breathing is relaxing; breath of fire, energizing. So you can combine these factors, as you like, to create the effect you want. If you have a headache on one side, try breathing on the other side. This works on the kyo/jitsu principle (see page 11) of shifting excessive energy, the pain, to the depleted location, the other side.

After balancing yourself this way, sit for a while and notice the flow of breath in and out of both nostrils. We hold a lot of tension in our noses. That's the first place your breath will shut down. Mostly you don't feel tension in the nose; most nasal tension is unconscious and related to holding in the eyes and jaw. This is one way you can tell if you are tight; a relaxed breath will be felt more in the septum area, the inside channel of the nostrils, than the outer edges of the nose. Direct your breath there, and relax the muscles under the nose, the triangular area beneath the nose. Think of this area widening as you inhale, and lifting slightly. That will relax the muscles around the nostrils. Then keep the widened feeling, and let go of the lift as you breathe out.

Muscles Involved in Breathing

The various muscles involved in breathing are shown in fig. 9.6.

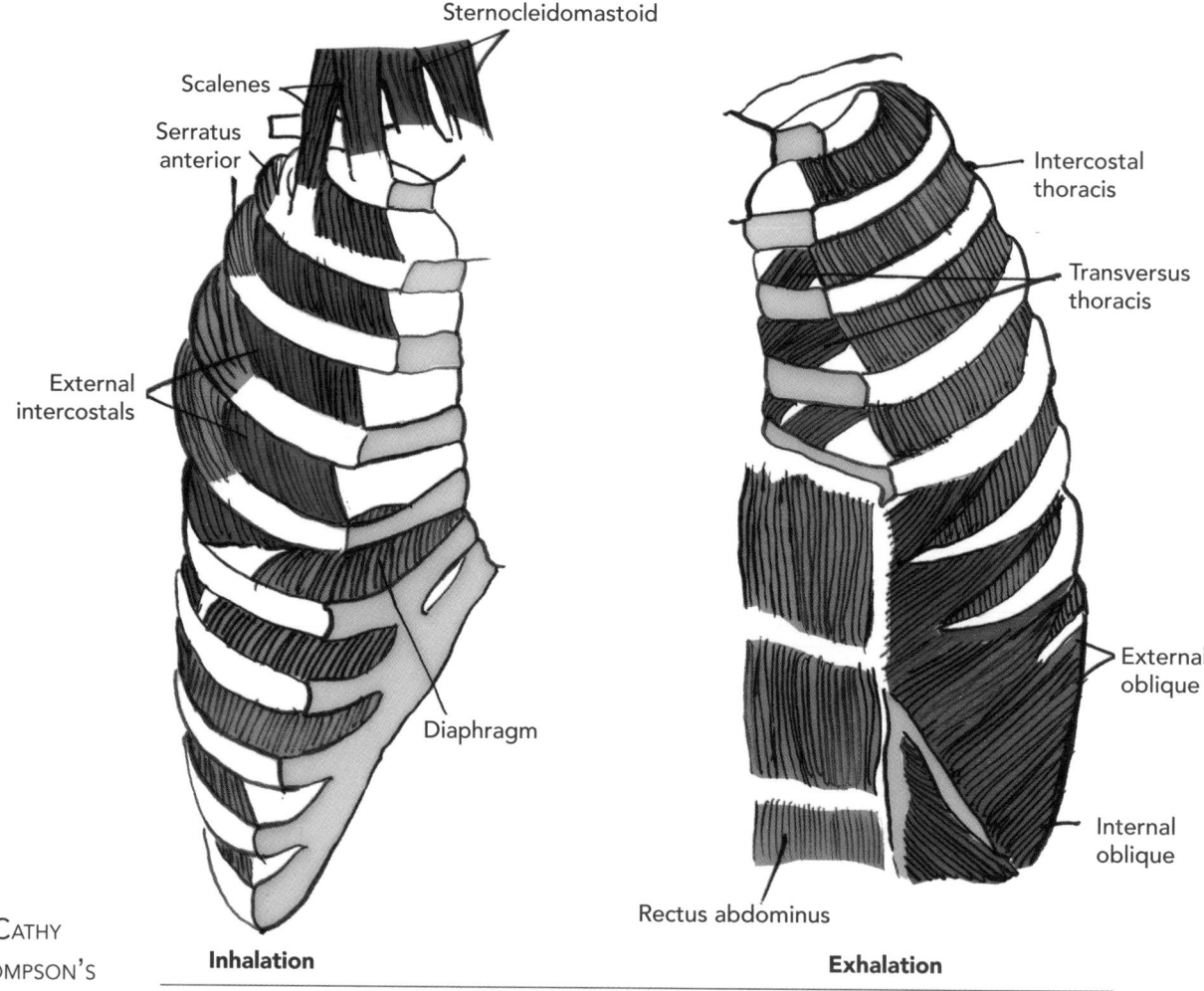

Fig. 9.6. Muscles involved in breathing

Running from the top rib to the inside of the cervical vertebrae you'll see the scalenes. They shorten on the inhalation to allow the lungs to expand upward and then release down on the exhalation. These are the muscles that control the slight movements you felt when you explored the top rib area. You can see now how neck tension influences the breath and vice versa.

As the top rib is pulled up, the collarbones widen and slightly separate, deepening the well in the throat, the sternal notch. They do not lift upward with the top rib but move only to allow space for the expanded lung area. The upper area of the sternum, the manubrium sterni, lifts up toward the chin and slightly rises as it moves away from the body. All the upper ribs open gently up and away from the body, the middle part of the sternum moves outward away from the body, and the lower part, the xiphoid process, mostly stays still to stabilize the rib cage.

You'll notice that most people, maybe you, move the lower part of the sternum much more than the upper. Think of a piece of string attaching the lowest part of the rib cage right under the xiphoid process to the spine, so it can't move at all and the ribs separate from each other as you inhale. Notice how that forces you to expand the side and upper areas of the rib cage; it is more muscular effort but ultimately more relaxing.

The spine expands along its whole length, and the back ribs move upward and outward. The shoulder blades move very slightly away from each other to allow for the expansion of the upper ribs. The stabilization of the xiphoid process creates a framework for the diaphragm to move freely, expanding the lungs.

To feel the breath moving into the upper parts of the lung, first run your fingers between the ribs in that area including the sternum, the armpits, and as much of your upper back as you can reach. Then lie on your back with your arms raised and crossed behind your head. This is the easiest position to feel the upper ribs.

Even Chest Breathing

The top part of the chest and the upper back hold the emotional breath, and when this opens we can start to feel deeply held grief and longing. Symbolically and energetically it is the movement from the heart, the center of feeling, to the throat, expression. Due to some misunderstandings about the nature of the breath and the role of the diaphragm, many people deliberately block off this part of their breathing, clamping down on their emotional energy and creating tension in the chest and shoulders.

One misunderstanding involves the role of the shoulder girdle in breathing: it should be passively moved by the ribs beneath it, not actively engaged. In an effort to not involve the shoulders in breathing, many people tighten the whole upper rib cage. Unfortunately, many singers and vocal practitioners have been trained to avoid shoulder breathing, by cutting off the breath in the upper chest. This leads to emotional constriction, neck and shoulder pain, and vocal strain. You should be able to breathe easily while keeping the abdomen tight and the rib cage lifted. Chest breathing is an even movement in all directions of the upper chest, including the upper back.

CORRECT DIAPHRAGMATIC BREATHING

Diaphragmatic breathing comes from widening the lower rib cage and opening the back lower ribs without much movement of the front lower rib cage or the solar plexus. For most people this is counterintuitive, and they restrict the breath to the in-out movement of the solar plexus. This comes from and creates anxiety. The adrenal glands are on top of the kidneys at approximately the location of the lower back ribs. When we are shocked, frightened, or very stressed, they pump out stress hormones into the blood.

It seems as though this fight-or-flight reaction causes us to contract our side ribs, narrowing our vulnerable and sensitive solar plexus area. Think about what happens when someone is punched in the gut; he contracts his ribs inward, making the space of the solar plexus smaller and tighter. This is the adrenal reflex; it's as though the many shocks we experience cause chronic, self-protecting, curling over and narrowing in the gut. But long term it doesn't protect us; it only restricts our diaphragm so we can't breathe freely.

✿ Freeing the Diaphragm: Freeing the Breath
Experiment with this.

1. Put your hands on your side ribs and breathe into them, so your hands move farther away from each other. The ribcages are pulled away from each other on the inhalation. You should feel a significant (at least 2 inches) movement sideways. To do this you will have to suppress the opening of the front lower ribs to some degree, not entirely; there will maybe be a half an inch outward of movement.

2. Notice how this diaphragmatic breath makes you feel, and breathe as you naturally do. Is that different? Maybe there is less movement or none in the side ribs, more in the solar plexus. How is that; does it feel different? Without a good diaphragmatic side breath you will not be able to obtain much stamina, in exercise or vocal work, and you will probably feel pulled in and anxious as the adrenal glands are overstimulated. It's like putting yourself in a tight, confining box.

3. Now lie on your back and press your hands gently onto the front ribs, suppressing the outward movement slightly and the upward movement slightly. Imagine you have a band expanding from the bottom front of one side of your rib cage to the other. The solar plexus area does not change much as you breathe, only the side back and upper ribs expand.

4. Imagine little balloons inflating under your side ribs as you inhale. Let the back ribs drop to the ground; it's a relaxed easy breath with no tension. If the deeper muscles are not strong enough to create significant movement, work the side ribs and visualize the balloons moving. See if you can feel the spaces between the ribs moving outward and upward as you inhale.

5. As you exhale, keep the rib cage lifted and bring in the lower abdomen, about 2 inches below the navel, not the upper part.

6. The solar plexus stays soft and relaxed through the breathing cycle. You'll probably find, if you have the breathing habits of most people, that at a certain point in the exhalation your solar plexus will want to tighten. If that happens, raise the rib cage even more and think of pulling the pubic bone up toward the navel, slightly firming the lower abdominal area, just slightly, and you should feel a deep contraction under the navel, pulling in and squeezing together laterally (this is engagement of the transverse abdominis to support exhalation).

🍂 Diaphragm Opening

The diaphragm is not a muscle that can be strengthened, nor would you want to. The effort of breathing comes not from the diaphragm, but the auxiliary muscles of inhalation and exhalation. The diaphragm needs to be relaxed and released so that it is free to move properly, allowing the auxiliary muscles to do their job.

1. To relax the diaphragm, lie on your stomach with a 5- or 4-inch ball under your solar plexus, below your rib cage. Breathe into the rib cage and relax. It may be

slightly painful at first, but that should lessen after a minute or so. The smaller the ball, the less the sensation.

2. You can also stretch and open the area by lying on your back, with a 7-inch ball under your back at the level of the solar plexus or slightly above it. Stay in that position for a while, breathing in the rib cage. Turn to your side to get off the ball.

3. If you have a large physio ball, you can lie back over it and stretch the diaphragm that way.

4. You can also do the Psoas Stretches (page 202) because of the position of the psoas and the diaphragm attachments to the spine. The psoas must be released for the diaphragm to move properly.

🍂 *Advanced Diaphragm Technique*

You can also try this more advanced technique.

1. Sit any way you are comfortable, and bring your fingertips to slightly above your navel, pressing in hard. Of course, make sure your stomach is empty. You should feel the navel pulse, which is the pulse of the main artery (the aorta). Is this pulse on the navel, or to the side, above or below? For you to feel strong and steady, it should be most clear and powerful just below your navel.

2. Now lean forward, and press the fingertips hard below the navel. Breathe long and deep, pushing in farther as you exhale. You may feel a lot of tightness in the solar plexus, where the diaphragm meets the spine. It will release as you breathe in the sides, back, and chest. Continue for at least a minute, longer if you want.

3. Then bring your fingertips out slowly. Now feel the navel pulse and notice any changes. When the diaphragm is relaxed and moving freely, the pulse will probably drop lower, to be felt most strongly just below the navel.

Don't do this at all if you are pregnant or menstruating.

INHALATION

Inhalation, anatomically, involves the synergistic action of many muscles in the torso, mostly in the rib cage. The assessment of how many muscles are involved varies between forty and fifty-five—anyway, lots. It involves freedom in pectoralis minor (fig. 9.7) and between the ribs.

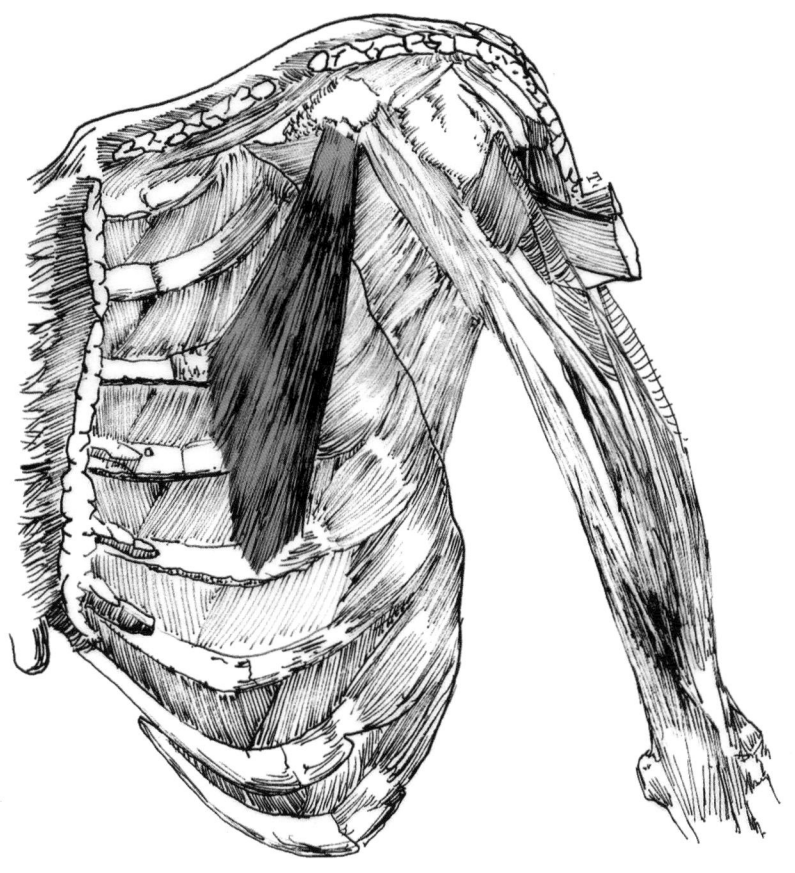

Fig.9.7. Pectoralis minor

Traditionally, ease on the inhalation (in other words, being able to inhale a long, deep breath easily and comfortably) is associated with self-assertion, the ability to start things, and to create prosperity. Ease in maintaining the inhalation is connected to keeping things going, to holding on to what you have, and to containing feeling.

Exhalation is supposed to represent the ability to deal with anxiety, and to tolerate the idea of death. Do you think this is true?

🍃 Equalizing Breathing Pattern

Try a breathing pattern with an even count—four counts for the inhale, four for the retention of the inhale, four for the exhale, and four for the holding of the exhale—then repeat over and over with no pause for at least three minutes. You can use any count you want; the point is to keep each portion of the breath pattern equal. You will find out which is hardest and which is easiest for you. For most people, holding out the breath is the most difficult and unpleasant. But not for everyone.

Let's look at how you might use the information you get if you do this exercise.

Tight, hunched shoulders that rotate inward and a collapsed chest—a slumped posture—will inhibit inhalation. I associate this type of posture with depression. In Core Energetics Theory (a method developed by John Pierrakos, M.D., which brings consciousness to how we block our energy and recreate defense patterns adapted in childhood that keep us limited and disempowered), the body type that expresses itself this way is called the oral type and is considered to have been deprived of nurturance at an early developmental stage, causing repressed oral desires and a kind of unsatisfied neediness. Whether this is true or not, we do associate the posture resulting from lack of strength and flexibility with an inability to assert oneself and take in what we need.

For women, this kind of slumping often comes from having large breasts that they don't want to stick out. They may have attracted a lot of unwelcome attention when they were growing up, so they got into a habit of slumping to disguise their chest. I see this in a lot of opera singers, who usually have large ribcages, if not big breasts. The feeling of shame and self-consciousness, and whatever negative sexual experiences they might have had, became locked into the posture. When we change posture through bodywork, those repressed feelings surface. As they feel the greater comfort and ease in being able to breathe more freely, the nervous system will process the negativity held in their bodies, which (hopefully) is no longer relevant to them as an adult.

The weight of the breasts themselves can also lead to rounded shoulders—it does require more muscle strength to maintain an erect posture. In this case, the person has a choice: strengthen the muscles that support the breasts or get surgery.

🍃 Releasing the Shoulders

The ability to separate the rib cage from the shoulders is needed to inhale fully. The shoulders can easily get welded to the sides of the chest. I'd associate this pattern with tight pectoralis minor and serratus anterior and weak rhomboids (the "winged" shoulders we see when there is this muscle imbalance). I work serratus anterior and the intercostal muscles in the armpit to release this pattern. You can do this for yourself, as long as you can get your hand up into your armpit. I think it's easiest and feels best to use the thumb of the hand on the same side.

1. As you worked in the other parts of your rib cage, press the spaces in between the armpit ribs with a firm pressure.
2. When you find a good sore spot, keep your thumb pressure firm and focus on sending the breath up and out, pushing your thumb away. Keep your shoulders relaxed!

These points—the Chinese call them the "fire points," and they are associated with the heart meridian—can be extraordinarily sore and sensitive. Releasing them can begin to open up the part of the chest that holds in grief, longing, and emotions that have to do with connection and relationship. The muscle around the armpit and the roots of the shoulders reach out, push away, and pull things toward us.

Even if none of these things are issues for you, notice the change in your shoulders and neck after you work into the ribs of one armpit. It's usually much more successful to work shoulder tension this way than to massage the top of the shoulders.

Think of the shoulders as they exist functionally, a girdle of bones, sitting on top of the rib cage and moved by the breath as it ebbs and flows under and around this girdle. Activate the breath in the ribs around and under the shoulders, and notice how this energy focus allows the shoulder girdle to give up some of its excess work and tension. I think of the shoulders being massaged from the inside by the rhythmic movement of the lungs.

EXHALATION AND THE DEEPER ABDOMINALS

The key to letting go of all the air in your lungs in a relaxed way is to keep the rib cage somewhat lifted and open on the exhalation, just as we learned to do when we inhale. The work of expelling the breath comes from the squeezing and pulling in action of the lower and deeper abdominal muscles, specifically transverse abdominis. To find this movement, inhale and exhale fully, not letting the rib cage drop down. Then, with the breath held out, pull your navel in as sharply as you can toward your spine. Focus on the area about two inches below the navel. The purpose of keeping the rib cage lifted is to suppress the action of the upper/outer abdominals, which will close in and squash the natural movement of the diaphragm, if they engage.

Look at fig. 9.8 on page 138 to see the relationship between the surface, usually much stronger, rectus abdominis, and the underlying transverse. Transverse abdominis is a deep abdominal muscle that functions as an inner girdle, shaping and holding in our organs, supporting the spine, and controlling the position of our diaphragm and the depth of exhalation. Think of its function in breathing as being similar to the handles of an old-fashioned bellows. As you squeeze the handles in (by contracting transverse abdominis), the membrane of the bellows (diaphragm) pushes up to expel air.

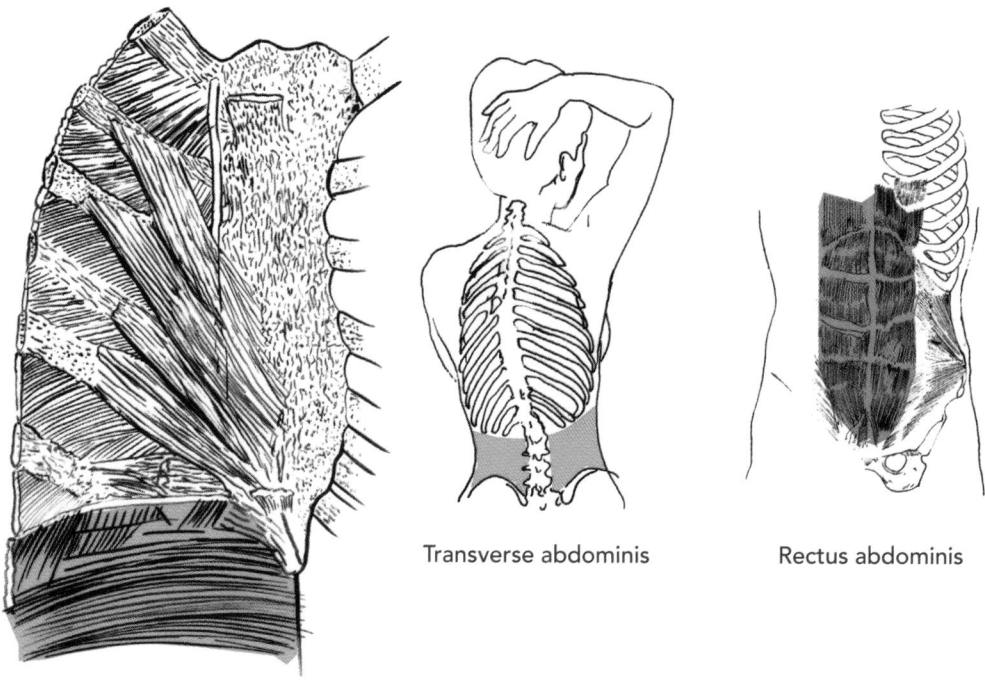

Transverse abdominis   Rectus abdominis

Fig. 9.8. Transverse abdominis and rectus abdominis

The outer muscle, rectus abdominis, creates those "six-pack abs" when it is developed and can bulge outward when built up. Its main function is to flex the abdomen forward as in a sit-up. When we pull the belly in toward the spine, moving the abdominal wall straight back, not up or down, we are using the lower fibers of transversus. When we tighten the abdomen, pushing the central area out slightly and hardening the belly, as though protecting ourselves from an anticipated blow, we are flexing rectus abdominis.

It is important for our purposes to understand the difference between the two muscles. For example, if we engage rectus instead of transversus on a deep exhalation, over a period of time we will develop the flexion of the muscle to such a degree that the rib cage will be held down and the diaphragm restricted. To engage transverse abdominis on the exhalation, keep the rib cage lifted, create even more length in the abdomen, and contract the muscles under the navel, squeezing in and back, while keeping the solar plexus as wide as possible.

Transverse abdominis will automatically contract slightly if you squeeze your "Kegel" muscles (the pelvic floor area, which you use consciously in bladder and bowel control). You may feel a slight but deep pulling, deep in the abdomen under the navel. When you need to inhale, keep the contraction of the abdomen and with the rib cage lifted, breathe in the chest.

Deep abdominal work, as in Pilates and other deep core strengthening, will help develop transverse abdominis, but the muscles must be worked in conjunction with exhalation to be strengthened for breath work.

This is where the belly breathing controversy can finally be cleared up, I hope. The bad habits some kinds of belly breathing can lead to have to do with a misunderstanding of the differences between rectus and transverse abdominis.

Rectus is an easily accessed, phasic muscle. If you employ rectus to power the breath, as you will if you push out your belly and lower your rib cage, whether on inhalation or exhalation, you will shorten the distance between the rib cage and the pelvis, and between the two sides of the rib cage. Over time, this will compress the tendons of the diaphragm, restricting rather than freeing your breath.

You have probably seen bodybuilders who have built up rectus at the expense of the deeper muscles to such an extent that they hunch over. This can even cause back problems over time as the lower back becomes overstretched. Now, most of us are in no danger of that, and abdominal flexion is an important function in back health. But using rectus and not transverse abdominis in breath work is easy, and since the upper fibers of rectus tend to develop more easily than the lower, diaphragmatic compression is a real issue.

There's a simple way to avoid this happening, which doesn't depend on the strength of transverse abdominis. On exhalation, just keep the rib cage lifted, front, sides, and back, or try to—it will depress somewhat. You cannot use rectus then; it is stretched too far. To exhale you must squeeze your belly and part of your back in, like squeezing a tube of toothpaste.

Don't let the sternum depress, either. That may be difficult since there is often a lot of internal tension, and contracted fascia, between the sternum and the abdomen. Rub into your sternum with your knuckles to release some of this. You can also focus more on the squeeze below the navel—that will help.

🍃 *Finding the Action of Transverse Abdominis in Exhalation*

1. Exhale with the rib cage lifted. Keep it lifted, and exhale fully.
2. Hold out your breath, and pull your navel in hard toward your spine. Think of squeezing in from your back toward your belly also, as though compressing an interior place slightly below the navel and right in the center of your body. Hold this contraction, and release all the other places that have probably tightened up!
3. If you can't find this movement at all, engage your pelvic floor muscles (the Kegel exercise) used in bladder and bowel control. This will automatically engage transversus. You may feel a slight, deep pulling in the abdomen.
4. Now, when you need to inhale, keep the contraction and breathe into the upper body. Lift your rib cage even higher, relax the shoulders, and repeat.

If there is a lot of tension in the rib cage and the chest, inhalation can be difficult and feel forced. Exhalation can be hampered by tensions in the gut and fascia pulling around the lower abdomen.

All breathing will feel like hard work if the central tendons of the diaphragm that attach to the inside of the spine are restricted by tensions in the surrounding muscles. Then the auxiliary muscles of breathing have to work extra hard to compensate for the lack of freedom of the diaphragm and may even tighten up, restricting the breath further. The Transverse Abdominis Exercises I and II (pages 173 and 175) will strengthen the middle to upper part of transversus, providing a natural shelf for those tendons, allowing the auxiliary muscles to release. This is one of the areas that provide support for the voice for singers—and for the rest of us too—the speaking voice needs as much support as the singing voice.

🍃 *Breathing Exercise for Diaphragmatic Problems*

Diaphragmatic problems include tightness in the tendons of the diaphragm; inability to open the side ribs; pushing the breath; hypertension of the sternum; lifting the chin up in an effort to breathe; lower back shortening and lower back rib area weakness.

The pattern in this exercise will make serratus posterior and anterior work together in a way that will open the ribs to the side, forcing the intercostals to engage, and the various muscles involved in stabilization of the rib cage (quadratus lumborum, the serratus group, obliques, lats, and so on), have to coordinate to use this pattern.

You'll have to do the exercise for at least 5 minutes, preferably longer—up to 15 minutes—to feel the effects kick in. Keep your back straight, lift the back ribs, and support as you need. You may feel a "stitch"-like pain in the sides as the diaphragm releases and the correct muscles engage. Slow down if you need to, but try to work through the sensation—it's usually just a sign that the muscles involved are starting to strengthen.

1. Sit with your back straight, any way you are comfortable. Lengthen your spine, close your eyes if you can, but keep looking straight ahead, even with closed eyes. Press your palms together by your chest until you feel the bottom tips of the shoulder blades engage and slightly pull down and toward each other.

2. Keep that straight pressure, and with palms together, breathe in and out quite fast through an O-shaped mouth (pursed lips) (fig. 9.9). The cheeks will suck in a little. The lips are engaged and the O-shape is about the size of the circumference of your thumb. Keep your lower back ribs lifted, side ribs engaged, and the bottom of your shoulder blades engaged.

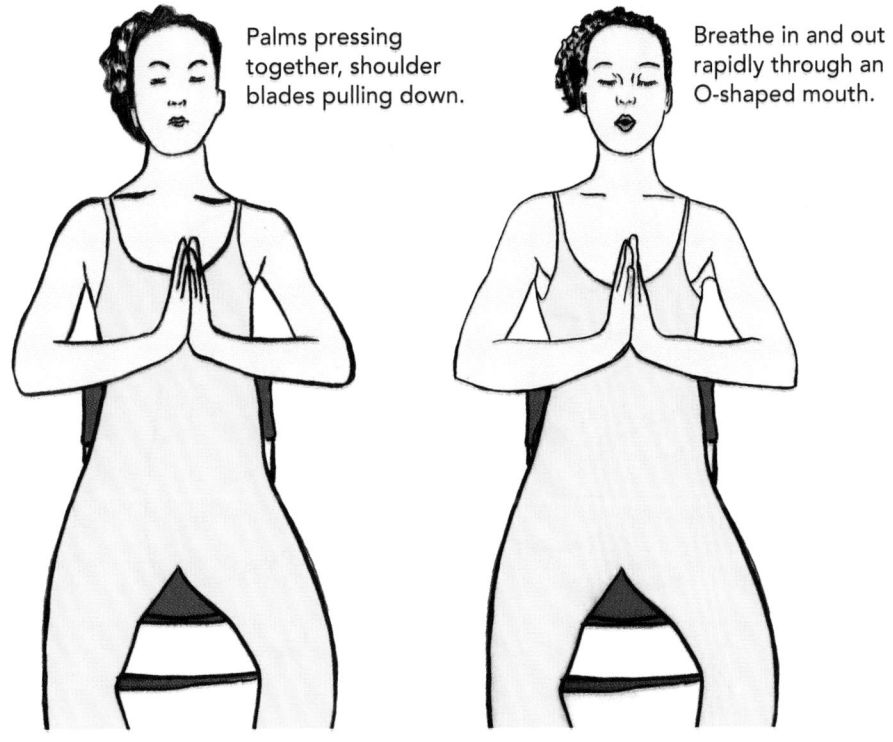

Palms pressing together, shoulder blades pulling down.

Breathe in and out rapidly through an O-shaped mouth.

Fig. 9.9. Breathing exercise for the diaphragm

3. Keep breathing, with equal time for inhale and exhale (about 1 second each). All breath is through the mouth. Breathe as vigorously as you can, for at least 5 minutes.

4. Release, with slow nose breathing, for a minute or so after.

🍃 *Breathing through Water*

This simple exercise can help asthma. It will also increase cardiovascular strength faster than any other exercise. To do it, simply inhale through your nose, and then exhale slowly through a straw into water (fig. 9.10). The bubbling will tell you if you stop exhaling. Your exhale should be slow and even. Build up to 60 seconds for the exhale.

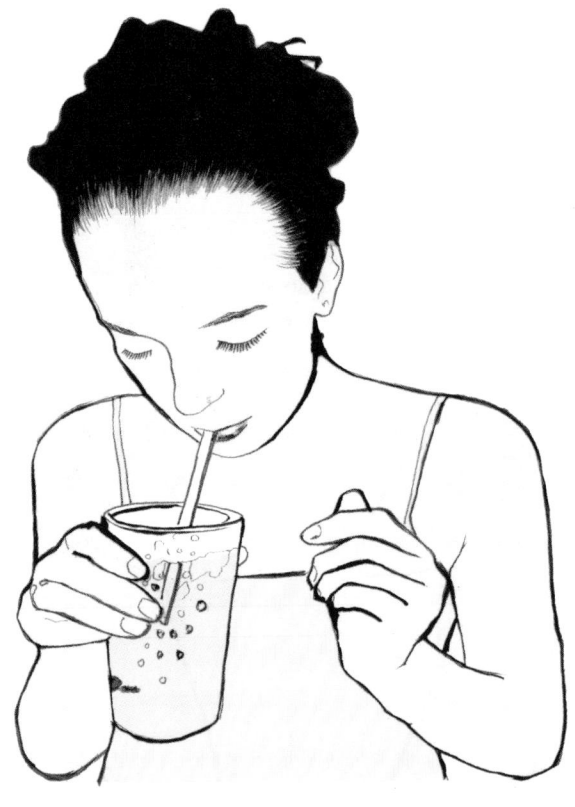

Fig. 9.10. Breathing through Water

10

The Voice

FOR MOST OF MY CAREER, I've worked primarily with singers—maybe 70 percent of my practice—because of my connection with Joan Lader and other body-oriented voice teachers and my general interest in the voice. Since most of what is required for the vocal structures, and thus the voice, to be free and avoid injury is simply for the rest of the body to be free and open, singing has proved to be a useful arena for me to develop some of my ideas. This chapter is written specifically with singers in mind. However, the material is useful for nonsingers as well, because the body affects the voice, and the voice is an expression of the whole body.

Anyone who uses his voice a lot will notice that even slightly poor posture and alignment will be reflected in his voice. It is like being an athlete in that you need to be in top physical condition to use your voice excessively and not damage it. If the muscles of expression such as the throat, jaw, tongue, and diaphragm, mostly in the front of the body, are being asked to take on the role of support, there will be excess vocal tension and strain. Most of what we do with our bodies in everyday life reinforces these habits, so it takes conscious awareness and engagement of the muscles of support—mostly the deep core muscles attaching to the spine, transverse abdominis, multifidis, the back of the body, and the pelvic floor—to support the spine, throat, diaphragm, jaw, and head so they can be free for expression.

Just as everyone can benefit from this chapter, singers and speakers can benefit from the other chapters in this book, particularly those dealing with the exercises for the deep core muscles, most of which are applicable to singing. The postural muscles can be difficult to feel, so it may take time to learn to use them correctly. With patience you can gain support for free vocal expression.

Any tension in the body, any fixity or distortion, is going to show up somewhere in the voice. When a singer, or anyone else for that matter, calls me for an appointment, my first diagnosis is usually based on the sound of her voice on the phone. The telephone can be deceptive, of course, and I wouldn't diagnose whole-body issues that way. But initially, at least, it can give me a lot of valuable information. All of us should listen to our voices on a recording and evaluate our physical and emotional state through the speaking voice. Since the speaking voice, which of course is an issue for all of us, is the basis of the singing voice, let's look at, or rather listen to, how the sounds we make can be an expression of ourselves.

Good vocal production requires proper support in the lower body, and a relaxed upper body, specifically the rib cage, jaw, tongue, and muscles connected to the larynx. The structure of the torso and throat repeat each other. The larynx, ultimately responsible for all our sound, is dependent on the alignment, strength, and flexibility of the surrounding musculature, just as the organs of the torso depend on the strength of our core abdominal muscles. Support needs to come from the back; the entire back of the body from the heels to the top of the head, and from the pelvic floor, which supports the spine and the breath. The latissimus dorsi and serratus anterior muscles must be strong to support the rib cage and breathing properly. These muscles strengthen the sides of the body and anchor the shoulder blades.

🍃 Strengthen the Latissimus Dorsi and Serratus Anterior Muscles

To strengthen and identify these muscles, stand facing a wall, two or three feet away.

1. Place your palms flat against the wall, as though you were pushing it away from you. Make sure your shoulders stay down throughout the exercise.
2. Gently push into the wall with your palms, being aware of the sides of your rib cage, especially around the armpit. Do not push so hard you lose the sensation there.
3. Hold for 10 to 15 seconds, repeat 4 times.

VOCAL SUPPRESSION

All of us, singers or not, have vocal tension—lots of it—and we're usually unaware of it. Vocal control, as in learning the muscular patterns that shape language, is a part of education and should not create any tension. However, at around age five or six at the latest, when children go to school and are expected to be "teachable," vocal tension and eventually suppression begin. Of course, we can't have little Johnny yelling his lungs out so none of the other kids can be heard. Temporary suppression of the desire to yell is simply learning self-control. However, there is an internal suppression that, I believe, has more to do with emotional expression. It's usually crying and tears that are held in by contracting the tongue and the throat (soft palate), and when a client gets bodywork, often the first expression that comes out is tears.

I remember my son coming back from school, telling me, "Why aren't boys allowed to cry and girls are? It's so unfair." I was shocked, because he was right. Nobody told him directly, but he picked up from his peers and teachers that he should suppress his crying. From then on, he did, despite my telling him that boys need to cry. And of course, girls aren't really that lucky, as we know; they are expected to suppress their feelings, too.

The voice has the interesting characteristic, like breathing, of being half unconscious, half conscious. We should be able to yell and scream powerfully without getting hoarse and running out of air. Yet most of us, singers or not, have a significant degree of vocal suppression. These habits, which are mostly detrimental, become unconscious. The habits become part of us and cause strain. When I work on people, they quite often release emotions through sound—yelling and screaming—and usually they do not get hoarse afterward, as the efficient, natural sound of the voice is released in tandem with the physical release.

The physical areas that hold tension and reflect vocal suppression are, principally, the diaphragm, the soft palate, the tongue, and the TMJ (temporomandibular joint). You can experiment with these places yourself by manipulating and massaging them, which we will discuss throughout this chapter. In terms of kyo/jitsu (see page 11), the line of energy between the pelvic floor and the soft palate and the deep core and back muscles are kyo, and the diaphragm, jaw, and laryngeal elevators are usually jitsu. That central channel can be blocked because of tightness, weakness, and imbalance anywhere in the body. The more you can energize and connect the pelvic floor and the soft palate, aligning the soft palate over the center of your pelvic floor, the more the other areas holding tension can let go.

It is important to be able to manually release the muscles that most directly affect the voice because the same muscles are used in daily life for mostly unconscious processes such as swallowing and breathing. For example, normally in swallowing, the larynx raises as the soft palate depresses, and this is also part of the "gag reflex." We train singers to manually learn to release and lift the soft palate, through direct manipulation, so that the soft palate can raise as the larynx stays released, which is what is needed for optimal use of the singing voice.*

The throat and jaw are areas that can be difficult to consciously release, and physical manipulation of the musculature can help to bring them into awareness. It is much easier to release using vocal exercises, visualizations, and so on once the body knows what it feels like to be free of tension. Tensions held for decades feel "normal" and often it is not until they release through bodywork, or by another means, that they are even felt. It is beneficial if you can find a bodywork practitioner to work with who understands the vocal structures; however, there is a lot you can do on your own.

Retraining the Breath

The number one problem most singers have is that they breathe incorrectly, usually tightening their ribcages and obstructing the natural movement of the diaphragm and the lungs, creating unnecessary tension and actually limiting the airflow. To release the breath, and effect change in the power of the voice, preventing "pushing" and overuse of the more delicate small muscles of the mouth and larynx, we must free and strengthen the intercostal muscles first, then release tension that obstructs the movement of the diaphragm. This technique is described on pages 125–26 in the previous chapter on Breathing.

You'd think that after undergoing a great deal of training singers would breathe wonderfully. But it's the training that is the problem. Often, singers are taught to belly breathe, because the exhalation is of such primary importance in singing; a good, powerful usage of the lower abdomen to control the outward flow is crucial. But most of us don't have the requisite strength and awareness in the deeper layers of abdominal musculature, especially in the transverse abdominis, to accomplish this without overuse of the superficial layers and lots of tightening in the rib cage. So my first task with a singer who has vocal issues is usually to open the ribs, encourage the client to widen the rib cage on the inhalation, and free up the whole thoracic structure. Since the emotional breath is contained in the chest, it is interesting that those in the performing arts, who need to feel and express in order to perform, are often taught a breathing style that constricts the sternum and thus the heart center.

*For more in depth discussion of this please see Scott McCoy, *Your Voice: An Inside View* (Gahanna, Ohio: Inside View Press, 2012).

All the relevant breathing material is covered in the chapter on Breathing, but to reiterate—

1. Inhale away from the diaphragm, relax and soften the solar plexus, widen the side and back ribs and stabilize the xiphoid process, expand the rib cage in all dimensions, widen and lower the collarbone, lift the top ribs, widen and relax the jaw and larynx.

2. Exhale by contracting the area between the navel and pubic bone, particularly just above the pubic bone, contracting it upward, with a very slight contraction of the pelvic floor. Keep the rib cage soft and lifted during the exhalation. In other words, the ribs stay roughly in the same position during exhalation as during inhalation; they do not collapse forward. Think of air releasing from the lower abdomen, then the back ribs lift to allow the air to pass out from the spine and into the larynx.

When the breathing is corrected, about half the time the vocal issue is too.

Easing the Throat and Tongue Muscles

Notice your tongue and larynx. You can probably feel a holding and tension all the time, which you can't let go of. Your throat and tongue muscles are deep muscles; you won't be able to consciously release them unless you have extraordinary control. They connect into the hyoid cartilage (see fig. 8.1 on page 104) and affect its ability to move freely. The hyoid, which houses the larynx, is connected entirely by muscle; it does not connect directly to another bone. The only other bone in the human body that shares this situation is the patella, the kneecap. From this, you can understand: first, how much the larynx requires free movement, space, and blood flow; and second, how distortions in any of the numerous small muscles can distort the sound.

🍃 Relax the Larynx, Jaw, and Tongue

The larynx, jaw, and tongue must be relaxed to sing properly without stressing the vocal cords. What you experience as tightness in the larynx is tightness in the strap muscles, which tighten and pull the larynx toward the chin.

1. You can push the larynx down directly by placing the heels of the hands against the sides of the throat and pushing gently down toward the collarbone.

2. To release the base of the tongue, place the tips of the fingers of both hands on the larynx and find the ridge in the middle. If you find several ridges, it is the one nearest the chin. Place your fingertips right above that ridge, in the hollow.
3. Press the fingertips gently toward each other, squeezing the larynx slightly. Let the tongue relax, stretching it slightly out of the mouth.

Releasing the Cranium

After releasing the breath, usually the next place we work with singers is the whole cranium, paying special attention to the muscles around the occipital ridge. In terms of kyo and jitsu, the jaw is generally jitsu, consciously tight and overworking, while the other cranial bones and the cranial fascia are devoid of movement and blood flow, holding the cranium in a fixed, inflexible position on the body rather than having very slight movement in the cranial bones, particularly the inner ones such as the sphenoid. We can release the cranial bones through bodywork and release the tight fascia of the scalp. We can also influence the position of the sphenoid bone by working in the hard and soft palate, despite not being able to palpate it directly.

When the muscles attaching to the occiput at the back of the skull are too tight, as though the head is glued onto the neck, the jaw has to compensate muscularly because it cannot release from the skull; the chin (which is the jaw, of course) will point up and out instead of releasing downward with gravity. It is then held in a state of constant tension, which results in an inability to release the larynx and lift the palate. In other words, the muscles of the jaw must be released, which means that the whole cranium must be released and positioned well on the top vertebra inside the skull in order for the laryngeal elevators to be able to relax enough while the palate lifts and the larynx maintains freedom of movement.

FREEING THE TONGUE

The most flexible and changeable structure in the mouth is the tongue, which also has a significant effect on releasing vocal tension. A well-known yogi once said that all the words we tell ourselves are formed by our tongues, soundlessly. You can feel a slight vibration in the tongue all the time. It cannot be stopped and goes on even during sleep. That is harder to prove, of course, but I've watched people's tongues as they sleep, and I believe it to be true.

The tremendous ability of the tongue to change shapes also creates the sounds of speech and singing. It needs to be mobile and free in order for the muscles to have full range and create the many possibilities of positions the tongue is capable of. Stiffness and immobility of the tongue cause strangled sound, sore throat, and so on.

🍃 Exercise for Tongue Tension

To understand where the ideal resting position of your tongue is, try this five-part exercise.

1. First, stretch the tongue by pulling it out of your mouth with your fingers—you can use a paper towel or a piece of gauze so that your fingers don't slip. Pull it gently up, down, left, and right.

2. Now push your tongue against the back of your lower teeth as far to the right of your inner gumline as you can, and then push your tongue as far to the left as you can, as though you were pushing your teeth outward from the inside, running back and forth along the teeth with moderate pressure, not to the point of creating tension. Repeat 10 times on the upper gums and 10 times on the lower gums.

3. Push your tongue hard against the roof of your mouth, and then push the floor of your mouth down with your tongue; open the mouth using the strength of your tongue, without tightening the jaw. Repeat both the up and down 10 times.

4. Now stick your tongue out of your mouth as far as you can. In this outstretched position, move it as far as you can to the right, turning the head with the tongue. Allow the tongue to lead the head. Repeat this moving to the left. Repeat both 10 times.

5. Next, very gently turn the head from side to side with the tongue relaxed outside the mouth and the mouth slightly open, not moving the tongue separately this time. Allow the movement of the relaxed tongue to follow the movement of the turning head, as exactly as you can. You should feel a widening and relaxation at the base of the tongue. Repeat this movement 10 times.

When you have completed the exercise, notice the position of your tongue relative to the teeth and the roof of your mouth. Is it touching the upper or lower teeth? There is not a right or wrong way. Believe it or not, much of it has to do with the length of the tongue. See if you can figure out why this might be.

Manual Release of the Tongue and Jaw

Because the tongue and muscles that tighten the throat are so difficult to release consciously, it can be a great help to release them manually. The jaw needs to be able to release open without the larynx rising, which is physically impossible if the muscles of the tongue and jaw are overly tight. If the jaw muscles, such as the masseter, are too tight to allow the jaw to release open, the digastrics has to work to open the jaw. The digastrics is a muscle that engages to open the jaw, but it also raises the larynx because of its connections with the hyoid. If the jaw is relaxed enough to release open, then the digastrics doesn't have to work to open the jaw and the larynx can also stay released. This is just one example of the type of tension that this manual work can help. This work will help most vocal problems—I'm not going to specify too much because any tensions can affect all vocal problems.

Working in the Mouth to Release Vocal Tension

Although we cannot work directly on the entire vocal structure, we can help most vocal problems and general vocal tension to improve the singing and speaking voice by working inside and outside the mouth to release many of the muscles of the tongue, jaw, and palate that affect the voice. You can explore and loosen them yourself.

First loosen the outer cranium, including the forehead and temporal area, as well as the occiput, by rubbing your entire scalp with your knuckles. Then go to the mouth. The cranial structures are usually stuck, which leads to excessive jaw tension. The jaw is the jitsu, and overworking because of misalignment of the skull and lack of subtle movement in the other cranial bones is kyo.

You may choose to wear gloves to work inside your mouth, as the oils in your hand can be irritating to the tissues. You absolutely must have clean hands and short nails to do this work.

1. First, go back between the outer back teeth and the inner cheek. You will feel a ridge—part of the inner structure of the mandible. The movements you use are scooping and widening, as you move the flesh away from the center of the head. Start inside the ridge, moving up toward the top of the head first, and then scooping down. There may be no space to go far back. Do not force. Work the rest of the mouth first and come back.

2. Next, go to the upper part of the jaw where it abuts the inner cheek. Scoop out the flesh gently.

3. Repeat on the lower jaw and inner cheek surface of that side. Pay attention to the chin area, where occipital tensions are reflected.

4. Repeat on the other side.

5. Next, go to the pterygoid muscle and the hard and soft palate (fig. 10.1), which influence the sphenoid (fig. 10.2). Start at the hard palate in the centerline with both index fingers or thumbs, and move them to the outer edge to widen. Go back into the soft palate with one index finger if you can. But don't force it!

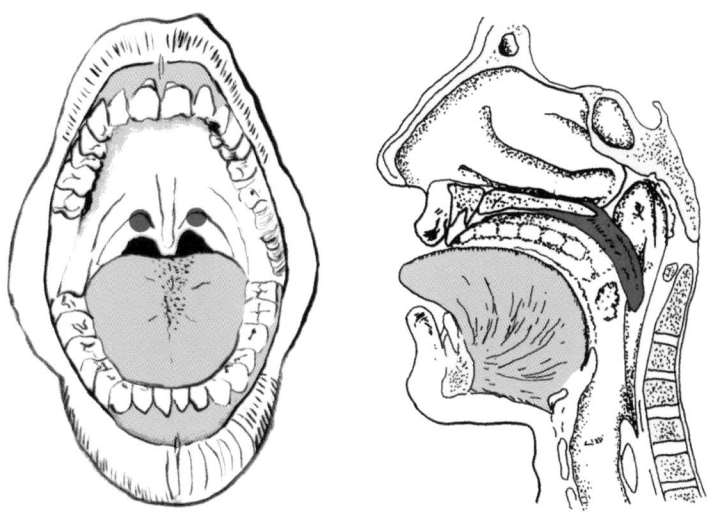

Fig. 10.1. Soft palate

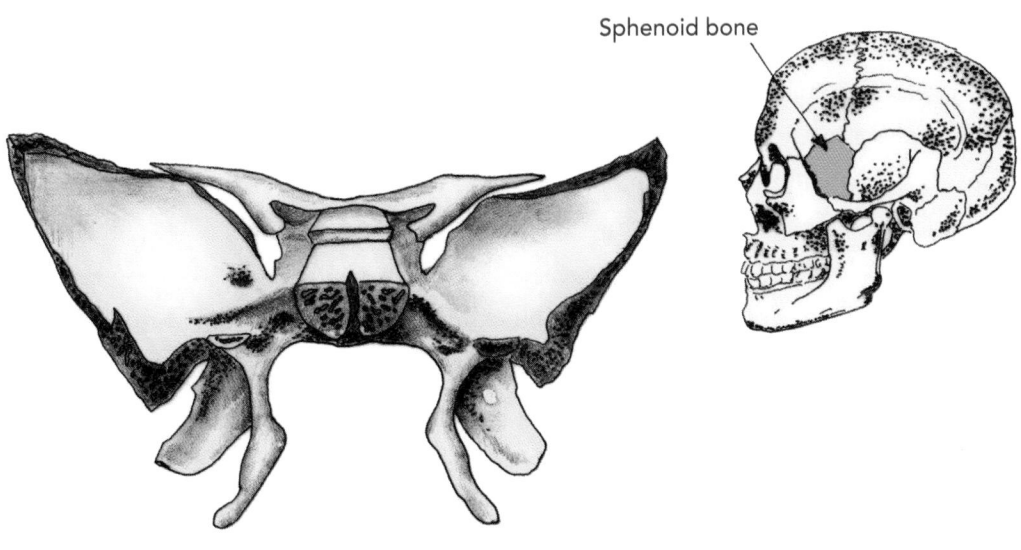

Sphenoid bone

Fig. 10.2. Sphenoid bone

6. Now, one side at a time, go to the upper part of the pterygoid (between your upper and lower jaw on the inside) and the soft palate. Scoop and lengthen down. Repeat on the other side.
7. Now come back to the first position, way back inside the TMJ (temporomandibular joint), the outside of the upper teeth. Use both fingers, one on either side of the mouth, if there is enough space. If not, don't force. The space will open over time.

🌱 Soft Palate Release: Advanced

The soft palate and base of the tongue are the second place we learn vocal suppression; the first is the diaphragm. After the general mouth release outlined above, the soft palate can be traced back in the mouth using a clean, gloved index finger. If you practice this in a standing or sitting position, you'll be much less likely to gag. Practice widening and going as far back as you can.

Lift up gently toward the ceiling as though your thumb or finger were a little hook. Then allow the TMJ to drop and the lower and upper parts of the jaw to separate without forcing. Eventually with practice you may be able to feel the very beginning of the atlas vertebra (C1, see fig. 8.2 on page 105). You may feel changes at the base of the tongue.

🌱 Breath Pattern for Breaks
in the Voice (at any place)

This pattern establishes control of the transitions through different parts of the voice. This exercise actually has more to do with the nervous system than the muscles and has to do with the ability to tolerate blood chemistry changes, flexibility in coordination of different structures, and the ability to use weaker muscles when needed, without strain.

First, find the dominant nostril by blocking one off and breathing through the other. Which nostril is easier to breathe through? If you are not sure, pick the left nostril to work with—that is, assume the right one is dominant. In this exercise you will block the nondominant nostril with your thumb (the left one for our purposes), inhale through the right. Then you will block the right and exhale through the left in the following pattern:

Exhale for 4 seconds.

Hold the exhale for 4 seconds (don't breathe in at all).

Exhale for 4 seconds.

Hold that exhale for 4, and so on, until you have to inhale.

So this will be the total pattern:

1. Breathe in through the right nostril, blocking the left.
2. Then unblock the left and block the right.
3. Exhale slowly through the left nostril only, *not inhaling at all* as you exhale for 4, hold exhale for 4, exhale for 4, hold for 4, exhale for 4, hold for 4.
4. Then block the left nostril and inhale through the right.
5. Repeat the cycle for at least 5 minutes.

You'll discover something very important when you attempt to lengthen the exhalations, or 20 more cycles of 4/4. If you let out all your air at once, you won't get very far. You must exhale so lightly that the passage outward through the nostrils is almost imperceptible. This is how you develop strength and power in the breath, not through vigorous breathing. To allow this slow, controlled exhalation, release your muscles as much as possible, even if your nervous system panics.

One of the biggest mistakes both singers and public speakers make (it's actually much more important in speaking than in singing) is to pull air as though starving for oxygen, as fast and hard as possible, and then push it out way too fast, with the result that not much control develops, and a great deal of tension builds up in the body. It is actually a panic reaction—we gasp air in suddenly when we are shocked or startled. Continuing a chronic panic reaction creates huge stress in the nervous system. Remember how breath controls the mind? This way of breathing disturbs and panics the mind.

When you are under stress, breathe very, very slowly, in a crescendo pattern, starting with pulling in almost no air, and building with continuity until the peak of expansion is reached. That peak is the place where there is a small effort, but no tension. Then exhale slowly the same way, letting out the air as though not even a flower petal under your nose would be disturbed. The interrupted exhalation pattern in the exercise will force you to exhale this way. Otherwise, you'll just run out of air.

COMBINING STRUCTURAL WORK
AND TECHNIQUE

The many singers I have worked with over the years found the exercises I have presented to you here beneficial for their voices. I hope they prove helpful to you too. We have only addressed structure in this chapter, not usage. This work is most helpful for singers when used in conjunction with improving usage and technique with a talented voice teacher or therapist. Nonsingers can also benefit tremendously from working with a voice teacher, as singing can be a tool for accessing and releasing physical and emotional blocks as well as improving your speaking voice. You need a good voice therapist or teacher to train you in the correct speech patterns. That's not my province. However, working with the vocal structure can assist greatly in the work you do with your voice teacher.

11

The Shoulders

THE DESIGN OF THE SHOULDER JOINT makes it vulnerable to injury unless we strengthen the internal muscles, primarily the rotators, but also some parts of the larger muscles. Since the joint is designed to move through such a wide range of motion, it is held together by soft tissues: ligaments, tendons, and muscles. The joints are shallow and not tightly connected. So the design that makes it possible for us to do all those amazing things with our arms also makes the shoulder susceptible to tension (overworked muscles) and injury.

The most important aspect of shoulder health is the relationship between the head of the arm bone and the joints (see fig. 11.1 on page 156). For a well-functioning shoulder and also to correct a lot of neck problems, you need to be able to keep the head of the humerus (the upper arm bone) within the confines of the shoulder joint, especially when you lift and carry things. The sequence in the chain of movement of any shoulder action should be small internal muscles engage first, then the back. If you are lifting anything, learn to pull in the head of the bone first and then engage whatever other muscles you need.

I would say most shoulder problems and a lot of neck tensions would be prevented completely if this were the case. So if you don't do anything else for your upper body, do the following exercises, which not only help to support the head of the humerus, but also increase your ability to sense when the bone slips out, so you can consciously pull it back in.

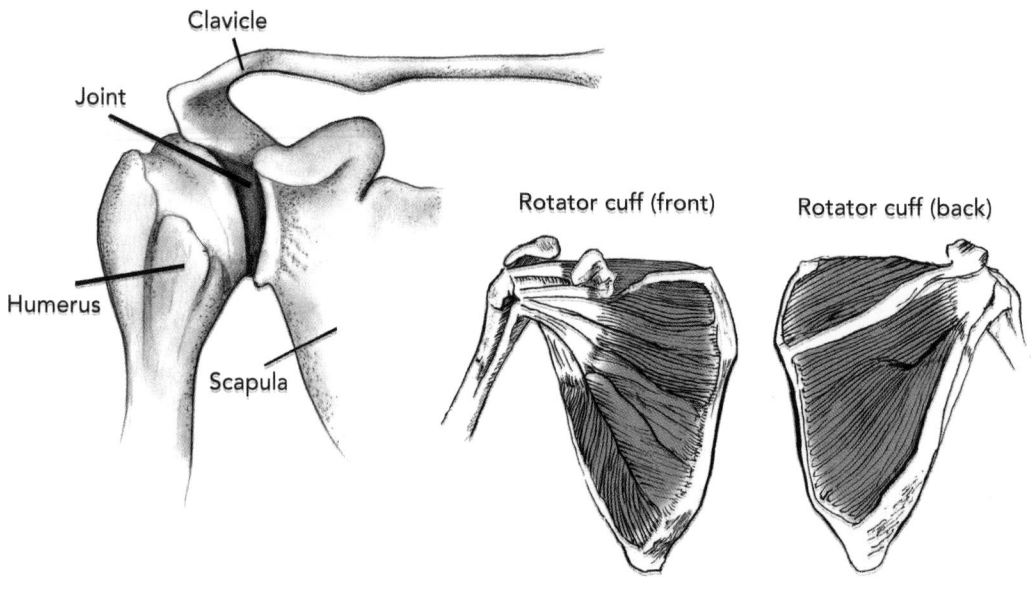

Fig. 11.1. Shoulder and rotator cuff muscles

🍃 Shoulder Joint Exercise

Look at the structure of the shoulder first, and then try this movement.

1. Keeping your arms straight in front of you, lift them up to a 60-degree angle, as though lifting something light (fig. 11.2). Notice what happens to the shoulder

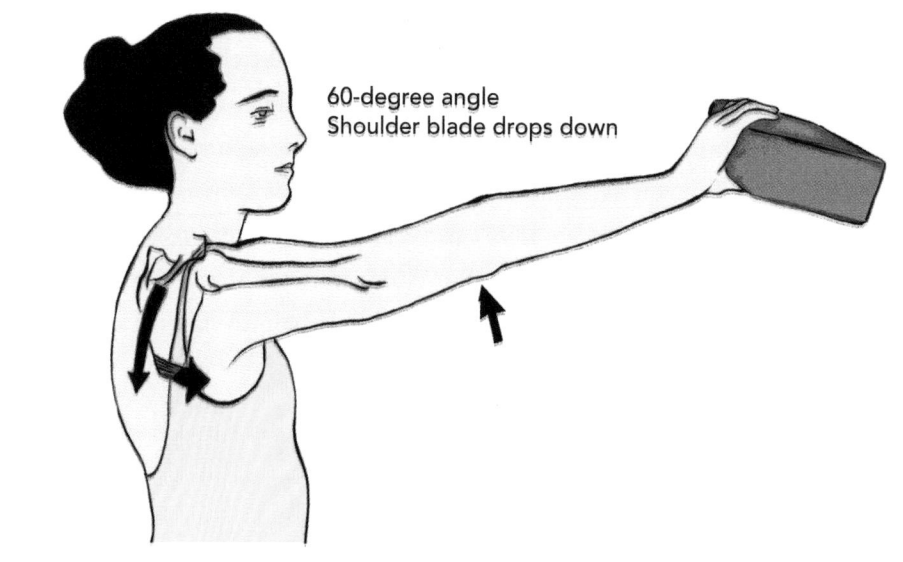

60-degree angle
Shoulder blade drops down

Fig. 11.2. Shoulder Joint Exercise

blade in the back, especially at the bottom tip. Does it lift up with the arm or drop down?

If the whole shoulder blade lifts up with the arm, bringing your shoulder closer to your ear, you are using your upper trapezius to lift. You can see this pattern of development: the upper back looks somewhat collapsed and weak, or rounded and overstretched, and the upper shoulder muscles feel hard and tight. This way of lifting can be useful if you must lift a heavy weight; otherwise it's an inefficient and counterproductive action. It's a habit people get into when they have a shoulder injury, since it saves pressure on the joint, but when the arm bone is no longer moving separately from the scapula, the small muscles that control that movement weaken.

2. Now swing the arms loosely up and down, using momentum. Swing them one at a time, then together. Can you feel the movement of the bone in its socket? Imagine it, looking at fig. 11.1, so you can visualize where that movement should occur. As the arm lifts, the scapula drops in the back, without the back ribs shifting at all. Notice any difference in the two sides, and see if you can let the arm that moves less easily learn from the more differentiated one.

3. Now raise the arms up to 90 degrees. Keep them completely straight and rigid; don't let your elbows bend, but also do not hyperextend your elbows. Move the arms straight back behind you. Keep them in their sockets, and experiment with raising them as though you are lifting something. Make sure your neck stays back and is relaxed, that your jaw hangs loose, and your front ribs stay back.

4. Swing the arms now. Probably you won't have to think much about keeping the head of the arm bone in, so let the movement be loose and free. Notice the difference. When you lift objects, envision your shoulders as a girdle, equal front and back, supported by your rib cage, with the mobile arm/shoulder joint as the focus of movement. This will prevent that ubiquitous shoulder tension. Keeping the awareness of the bottom tip of the shoulder blade and its position on the rib cage may help center your focus.

✻ Exercise for Shoulder Alignment

This exercise will help to correct rounded, internally rotated shoulders; tight chest; "winged" shoulders that do not lie flush on the back. It corrects muscle imbalance in the rhomboids (weak and loose), serratus anterior (tight, weak, or strong), and pectoralis minor (tight, probably weak).

1. Bring your palms over your ears at a right angle to your forearm (fig. 11.3). Engage the bottom of the shoulder blades to pull both shoulders down, and keep them dropped (you will have to keep thinking about this). Make sure both shoulders are even and your head is in line with the spine. Gaze straight ahead or slightly upward.
2. Now keep the alignment and draw the elbows back as far as you can. Make sure the upper arm comes back with them.

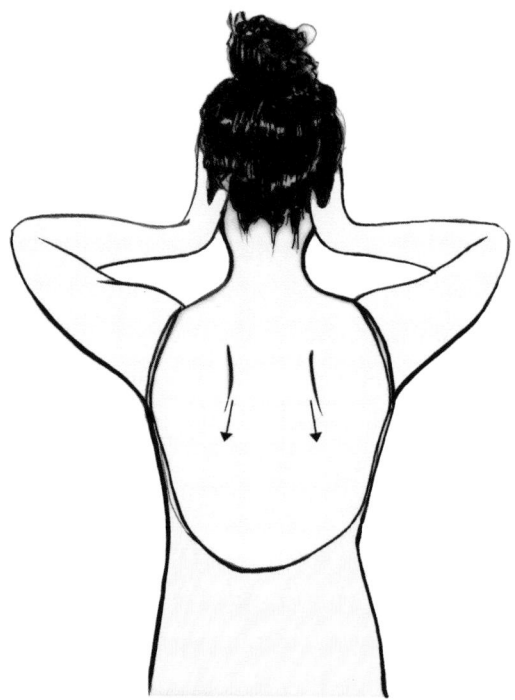

Fig. 11.3. Exercise for Shoulder Alignment

3. Engage the muscles between the shoulder blades (rhomboids) tightly; squeeze hard. Use these muscles to press the shoulders down farther.
4. Hold this, and check your position—head in line, palms pressed into ears, shoulders even and down, chest open, back straight. Try to bring the inner wrists to the ears.

To modify: Take the same position, but this time bring the wrists away from the ears as far as you need to, keeping the fingertips on the sides of your head. Hold as long as you can.

EXTERNAL ROTATION OF THE SHOULDER

Most of us greatly overuse the internally rotating (forward) muscles of the shoulder, because almost all the activities we do are forward facing. Driving, writing, manual labor, and even exercise all involve forward movements of our shoulders. Any activity that takes place in front of us and demands that we use our hands will require forward rotation, because our eyes are in the front of our bodies. Jumping rope is the only everyday activity I can think of that uses external rotation.

The hunched-over look most of us acquire as we get older comes from this chronic forward rotation and leads to shoulder tension as the large muscles of the shoulder and upper back get overextended and weak and struggle to pull back the shoulder joints. Massage and stretching will help temporarily, but to effect a permanent change we need to strengthen our external rotator cuff muscles and rhomboids.

🌿 Reposition the Shoulder Joint

To reposition the shoulder joint, experiment with externally rotating your arms. Internal rotation means turning the arm from the thumbs up to the shoulder in toward the center; external rotation is turning them outward in the opposite direction. In the first part of the exercise you can work with one arm at a time or with both at once, spiraling from the fingertips into internal and external rotation.

1. Standing or sitting, let the arms dangle at your sides. Then rotate the arms externally, away from the body, as though the thumb of each hand was drawing a small circle on the floor. If there were a clock on the floor, just below your hands and facing up to the ceiling, the right hand would make a clockwise movement and the left hand would move counterclockwise. Make sure your arms move equally from the thumb up, and the back and neck stay still. Go as far as you can with the external rotation. Now, turn the arms the other way, in toward the body. Feel how the shoulder joint rotates outward when the arm makes an internal rotation. Make sure your back and neck stay still and your collarbones face straight ahead.

2. Externally rotate your right arm as far as you can; then bend at the elbow, keeping the rotation. The hand will be about nipple level.

3. Keeping the rest of your body still—no arching of the back, which is what you will probably want to do—bring the right elbow forward toward the front of the

room. Then take that elbow in your left hand and pull it forward and up and as far as you can. Experiment with the angle of the forearm and the distance of the elbow from the body for a good stretch.

4. Very slightly bend your body forward for a deeper stretch. You want to feel all the movement and sensation in the shoulder joint. It is quite possible for the elbow to rotate all the way up and over to your back—this advanced stretch is a part of some yoga positions. Most of us can't do that (and don't force it), but use the image and possibility of that amount of freedom in the joint to open the area up fully. You may find that changing the distances between the upper arm and the body and the angle of the forearm gives you a better stretch.

5. Repeat with the left arm.

🌿 Rotator Cuff Muscle Exercise

This one is great, worth all the trouble, because it stretches and strengthens the whole rotator cuff with the shoulder girdle in correct alignment. But it does take some setting up.

1. You'll need a mirror initially, or someone to spot you. Stand with your back to a wall, a mirror (or your spotter) in front of you. Bring your legs away from the wall so only your hips, shoulders, and spine and the back of your head touch the wall—if something doesn't touch, or is uncomfortable, use padding.

2. Then bring your arms up to shoulder height, palms down, pressing as much of the back of your upper arm into the wall as you can (fig. 11.4). Your wrists, elbows, and shoulders are in one line. Gaze straight ahead.

3. Then bend your elbows so the wrists and forearms form a right angle with the upper arms, palms facing downward. Your wrists and hands stay in line with your elbows, the knuckles in line with the wrists. You can hold a one- to three-pound weight if you want or you can strengthen and align with this exercise without using any weights. You should start without any weights to get the hang of the alignment.

4. Keep your wrists in line with your elbows, and the elbows the same distance from the head, as you bring your hands very slowly down, keeping a perfect right angle—that's the hard part. Watch for the elbows dropping down (press back into the wall with your upper arms the whole time); the hands moving closer in or farther away from the right angle; and your shoulders or head moving away from the wall.

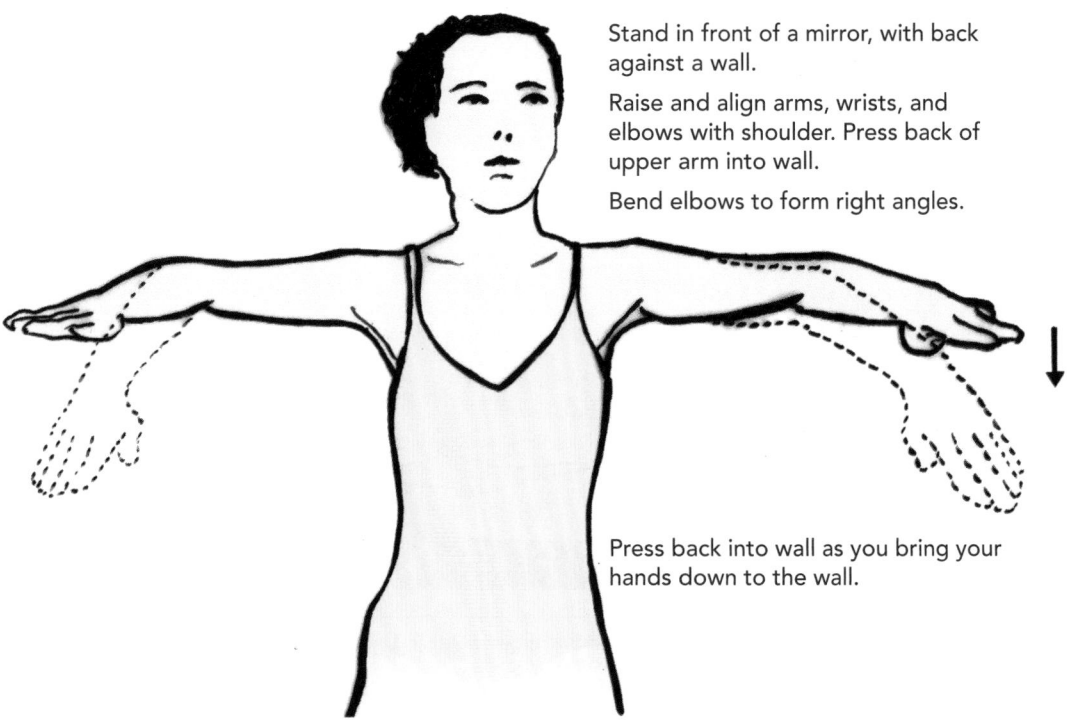

Stand in front of a mirror, with back against a wall.

Raise and align arms, wrists, and elbows with shoulder. Press back of upper arm into wall.

Bend elbows to form right angles.

Press back into wall as you bring your hands down to the wall.

Fig. 11.4. Rotator cuff muscle exercise

5. Press back into the wall as you bring your hands down, watching the wrist/knuckle alignment (keep wrists straight) at the bottom. Feel a good stretch at the bottom of the move, hold a few seconds, and then come up to your starting position slowly. Each repetition should take about 30 seconds. Repeat 3 to 5 times.

🍃 Shoulder Stretch Series

◈ Shoulder Stretch I

1. Lie on your stomach, head toward a wall. Bring your elbows to the wall, directly in line with your shoulders, hands up the wall (see fig. 11.5 on page 162). Your wrists should line up with your shoulders—they may not do this easily, so make sure both wrists are even in relation to the elbows and shoulders—and press down hard into the wall at the inside of the wrist, thumb, and index finger; the forearms will rotate slightly internally. The upper arms and shoulders will then rotate externally, opening the armpits toward the floor.

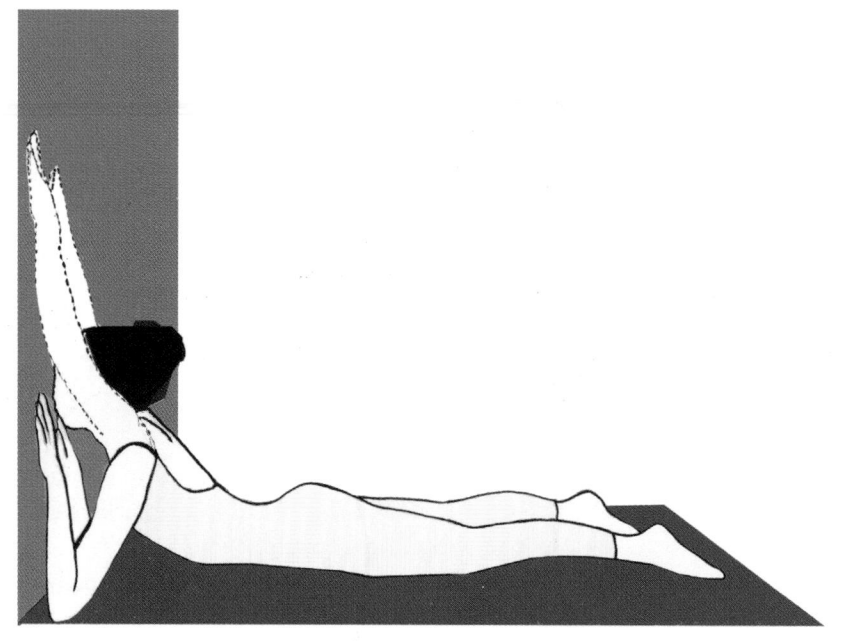

Fig. 11.5. Shoulder Stretch I

To intensify this stretch, keep your elbows on the wall, press the forearms and hands against the wall, and scoot the rest of your body away from the wall. Rest your head wherever it feels comfortable. If you get someone to press gently on your upper back in this position, you will feel even more of a shoulder stretch.

2. Now, from the same starting position (more or less, depending on the length of your neck and where you want your head in the stretch), bring your arms straight up the wall, chest off the floor slightly. Elbows and wrists must be in line, collarbone straight so shoulders are even. The unmodified version has the elbows on the wall, forearms pressing in, and head dropped. To modify, use yoga blocks to support your elbows, at any height, leaving a gap, so your head can drop in between (fig. 11.6). You can rest your head on the wall if this is uncomfortable. Make sure you keep your wrists, thumbs, and index fingers pressing into the wall.

Let the upper spine drop in between the shoulders, relaxing and softening it into the stretch as deeply as you can. You will probably feel the stretch in the shoulder joint, deep inside the structure. It will intensify as gravity pulls your head and torso toward the ground, so start from a position that you can hold for

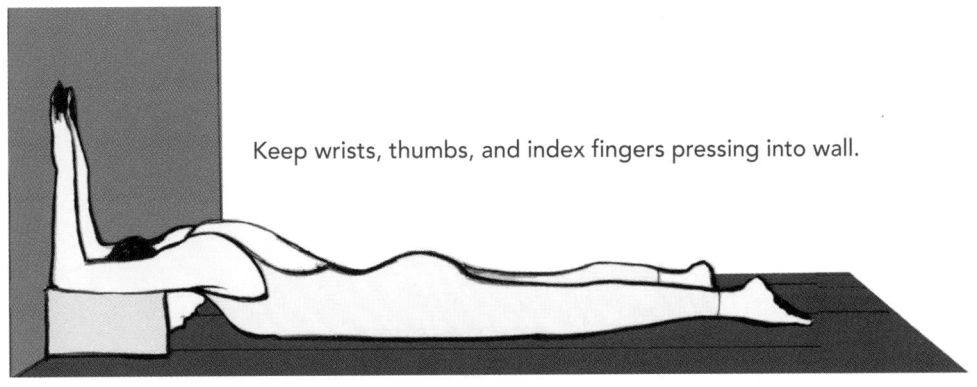

Keep wrists, thumbs, and index fingers pressing into wall.

Fig. 11.6. Shoulder Stretch I Modification A

at least a minute without tensing your body. Allow the stretch to open the chest and diaphragm, breathing throughout the entire rib cage.

3. Make sure your lower back is relaxed, unclench your buttocks, and pull the tailbone toward your feet. If your lower back will not disengage, you can do the same stretch kneeling, facing the wall and working with your psoas until you can relax the pelvis in this position (fig. 11.7).

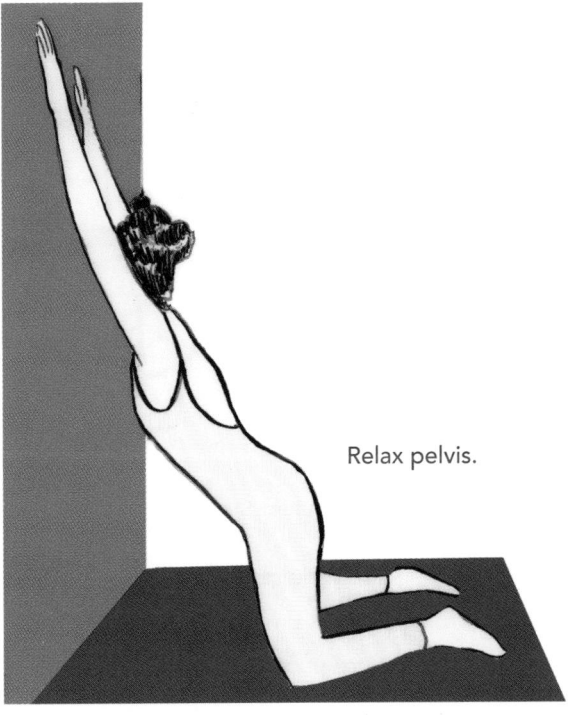

Relax pelvis.

Fig. 11.7. Shoulder Stretch I Modification B

Follow with any forward bend—the Wall Hang Stretch (pages 190–92) is ideal.

◈ Shoulder Stretch II

1. Stand two to three feet away from the wall, back to the wall, arms above your head, wrists on the wall, palms flat on the wall, and fingers pointing straight down to the floor (fig. 11.8).

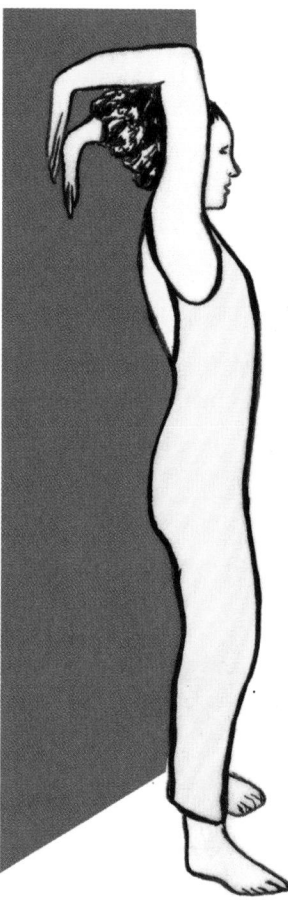

Keep hands even, and press palms into wall. Squeeze elbows in toward one another.

Fig. 11.8. Shoulder Stretch II

If you can't do this, you can use a shelf behind you, if you can find one the right height. Place the inside wrist and palm under the shelf and press against the shelf for leverage. It's hard to see if your hands are even. You can look at your elbows, aligning their positions, and bring them toward your body. This will tend to even up the hand position. The elbows will want to splay out away from you, and the success of this stretch will depend on how far you can engage your triceps to bring them in. You could tie your upper arm muscles in this way with a yoga strap.

2. Now push your palms hard against the wall or the bottom of the shelf, keeping elbows pressed in and lifting your sternum. Don't—very important—arch your lower back at all. This is not a backbend, and you could hurt the back this way. Your head should stay forward. Think of the collarbones lifting up and toward the ceiling and away from the wall, elbows squeezing in tightly, and shoulder blades pulling in toward each other, supporting and lifting your chest and shoulders.

◈ Shoulders and Upper Chest Stretch

1. Bring the front of your right shoulder to the wall, arm straight out along the wall behind your body, elbows bent a little or a lot, whatever feels best to you. Turn your body away from the arm and shoulder, trying to keep the shoulder on the wall, or as close to it as possible (fig. 11.9). Repeat with the left shoulder. You will feel a stretch in the chest and shoulder, maybe in the arm.

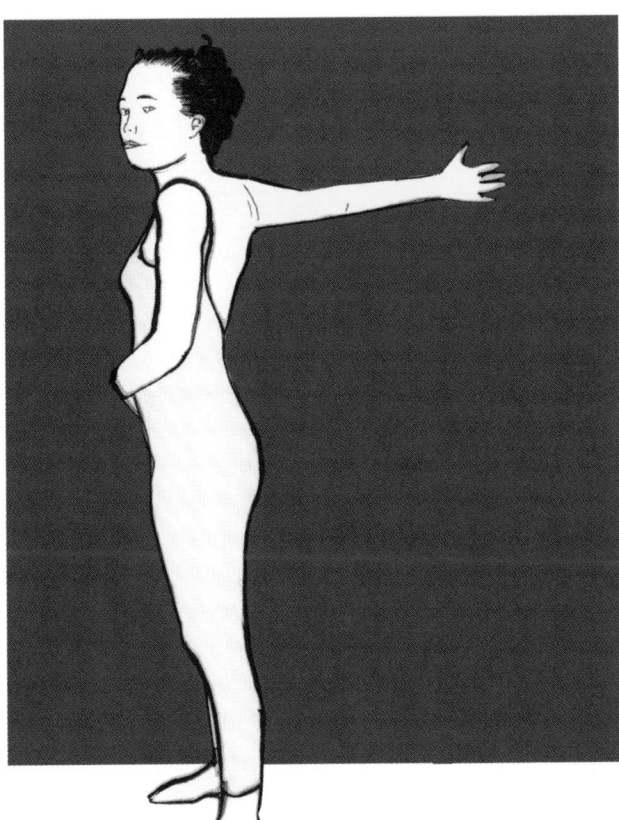

Fig. 11.9. Shoulders and Upper Chest Stretch

2. Use the hand that's not on the wall to gently pull the other side of your rib cage away from the shoulder. This is a free-form stretch, so experiment with the elbow position—more or less bent, higher or lower on the wall—and the body position—hips turned farther, chest turned farther—for a variety of sensations.

To modify: Use a corner or a doorjamb or put padding between your shoulder and the wall. If the shoulder or elbow hurts, it is best to modify this exercise by bringing that shoulder toward the ear. This will isolate the stretch in pectoralis minor. Breathe in the upper outer portion of the lungs.

12

The Spine and
Deep Core Muscles

MOST BACK PROBLEMS come from an imbalance in the spirallic lines of movement in the spine. Scoliosis, where the spine has a visible S curve from right to left, is an obvious example and probably the cause of much undiagnosed chronic back pain. The spirallic movements can also be distorted when the spine appears straight right to left but is actually rotated incorrectly along its axis—in other words, when the left or right side of the vertebrae are in front or back of each other. The spine will attempt to balance itself by curving more and more in different directions, so eventually the condition becomes chronic and results in "traveling" pain—one day the upper back hurts, the next day it's the lower.

Spiral line distortions originate in genetics, and they can be congenital. (There is a theory that pressures against the uterus from the mother's own spinal distortion can create uneven formations in the connective tissues of the fetus.) Mostly, however, these distortions are acquired by injury or habit.

SPIRAL DISTORTIONS

Look at fig. 7.4 on page 91 to get an idea of the complexities of spiral distortion. The other issue that we must understand to change this condition is that some parts of the spine are naturally very mobile and will compensate more—and usually hurt more—than the rest of the back. As you can see from the illustration in fig. 8.2 on page 105, the atlas and axis, under the skull, have an interesting and limited mobility. You can see how easily they might "stick" in one position and how difficult it would then be to free

167

them up. The entire thoracic spine has a similar formation; because of the rib joints attaching, it can't rotate much without lengthening. Otherwise, our ribs would snap off or grind into each other. The lumbar and cervical spine are much more flexible.

C3 and T12 (which is half lumbar and half thoracic in its formation), are usually the most mobile vertebrae in the spine—and those are the locations where many people have pain (see fig. 2.17 on page 39). These areas will take on the extra work that the stuck parts of the spine can't do, so the overworked muscles around them go into spasm. These areas may feel as though they need loosening—and it's true the muscles do—but the best and more long-term solution is to free the thoracic spine by learning to lengthen and then rotate it and to free up atlas and axis by mobilizing the cranium, addressing the underlying kyo.

C3 and T12 seldom herniate because of their mobility. The likelihood of injury is highest at the stress points of the spine, where there is much wear on the discs. C5 and C6, adjoining the thoracic spine, and L4 and L5, connecting the flexible lumbar spine to the less mobile and heavy pelvic structure, are particularly vulnerable to herniations.

THE ROLE OF THE DEEP BACK MUSCLES IN BACK PAIN

A good deal of back pain, whether it's caused by weak muscles or not, can be helped by strengthening certain muscles. You can have disc herniations, osteoporosis, and even more severe spinal injury without having any back pain. One interesting study showed that 64 percent of people with no back pain, who said they had never had back pain, have some disc herniations that show up on an MRI. Different conclusions have been drawn from this study, of course.

John Sarno, M.D., believes that studies like this show that almost all back pain is psychological in origin.[*] Jim Johnston, P.T., draws the conclusion that the difference between the pain-free and pain-full group is the strength of the back muscles, specifically the multifidus.[†] Since there also appears to be a correlation between psychological difficulties and weak back muscles, they could both be right.

John Sarno has his own stress reduction program outlined in his book, and it has

---

[*]John E. Sarno, *Healing Back Pain* (New York: Warner Books, 1991).

[†]Jim Johnson, *The Multifidus Back Pain Solution* (Oakland, Calif.: New Harbinger Publications, 2002). His book includes some excellent practical exercises and his website (www.BodyMending.com) is a good resource for more good information about this important muscle.

helped many people. However, I naturally tend to see those people for whom his program has not been successful, and they are usually helped by the back strengthening exercise approach and by my work, so let's look at the role of the deep back muscles in the correction of back pain.

The Multifidus Muscle

There are a lot of deep back muscles that run by the spine. The one that we'll look at is multifidus, which physical therapist Jim Johnson credits as being responsible for almost all back pain. I have found his approach invaluable and have drawn a great deal from his writing. You will see that I have included many exercises for both multifidus and transverse abdominis. These two muscles work together: the action of transverse abdominis stimulates the lumbar fascia, which in turn activates multifidus (fig. 12.1). The transverse abdominis is supposed to fire to support the spine whenever we move. However, this pathway is turned off if there has been back pain, any

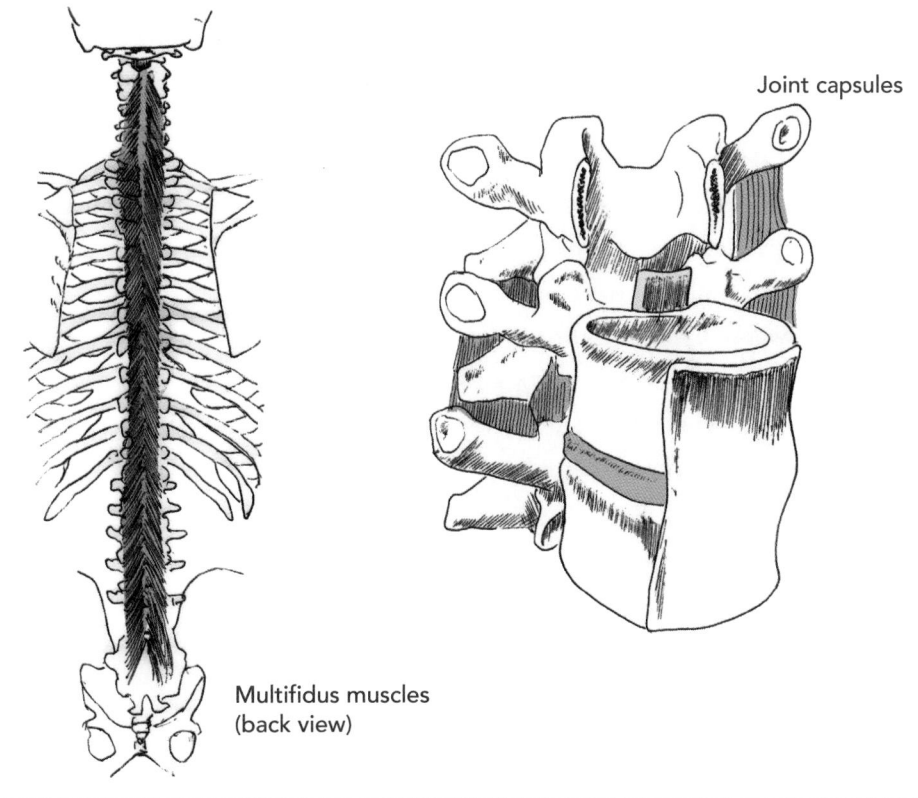

Joint capsules

Multifidus muscles
(back view)

Fig. 12.1. Multifidus and joint capsule

spinal or abdominal surgery, including caesarean, often after childbirth, and so on. In order to regain the support of these muscles, they must be consciously and patiently retrained.

Multifidus differs from the other deep back muscles in two important ways:

1. It is attached to the joint capsule of the spine, rather than to the joints themselves.
2. It connects only with the nerve that innervates that section of the spine to which it attaches, unlike all the other deep back muscles.

Now, why is this important enough that I'm including it? Look at our joint capsules (see fig. 12.1 on page 169). They are just tissue that surrounds and protects the facet joints of the spine, sort of like the bursa of the elbow or the shoulder. We know how painful bursitis is. Well, if the multifidus is weak, or not synchronized with the other muscles, it may not fulfill its function of pulling the joint capsule tissue away from the joint itself when you move, especially in sudden movement, which can result in nipping the facets—ouch! The result: the back goes into spasm. This accounts for about 80 percent of seemingly inexplicable back spasm attacks—I was just vacuuming the floor, lifting my child, and so on.

The multifidus is vulnerable, since it can only use one spinal nerve, at the level of the spine to which it is attached. Other back muscles can pick from a variety of spinal nerves. Why? We don't really know the evolutionary reason for this—maybe it strengthens the multifidus/neural pathway somehow. What we do know is that if one vital nerve is compressed for any reason, the multifidus muscles at that part of the spine will suffer.

That is why most of my back exercises also include strong multifidus work. Here's one that isolates multifidus.

🍃 Exercise for Multifidus in the Back, Especially the Lower Back

1. Rest your weight evenly on your hands and knees (fig 12.2). Make sure wrists are over shoulders and hips over knees. Press all four stabilizing points into the floor (hands and shins) equally.
2. Now, simultaneously lift the right hand and left knee up off the floor just 2 inches, no more, without changing your torso position. If you lift your hand or knee too high, you won't be able to do this.

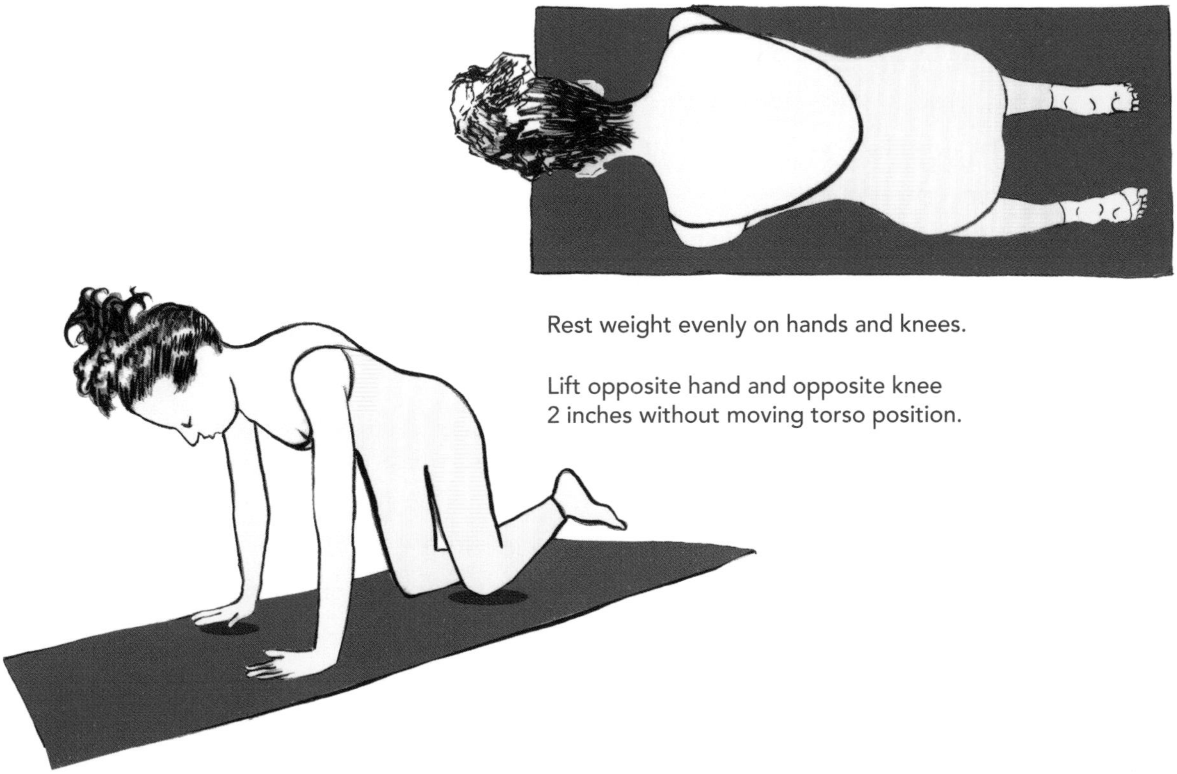

Top View

Rest weight evenly on hands and knees.

Lift opposite hand and opposite knee
2 inches without moving torso position.

Fig. 12.2. Multifidus Exercise

3. Hold for 90 seconds. Repeat on the other side.
4. One side is probably easier than the other. Hold the weak side twice as long as the strong side, same number of repetitions on each side—probably 3 or so before muscle fatigue. Build up to 10 repetitions on each side.

ALIGNING THE SPIRAL PATHWAY

Any imbalances in the core spiral shape and the rotational movement of the spine will reflect in various right/left distortions in the rest of the body. And any inequalities in the right/left alignment of the pelvis, torso, shoulder girdle, and head will show up in distortions of the rotational pattern of the vertebrae, somewhere in the spine.

There are grids you can stand against that will show you which shoulder and hip are higher, as well as other postural deviations that become apparent when you look at the body from one plane without movement. You can see these imbalances yourself if you look carefully, facing forward in a mirror. The spiral distortions are subtler and may only show up in movement. Even if they appear structurally, they're harder to catch. One shoulder may be in front of the other without being higher or lower. That condition won't be very easy to see, but it means that more muscles are imbalanced than in a high/low distortion, because the spine is involved more directly.

Adjusting bone or massaging muscle offers only temporary fixes for back pain because neither muscle nor bone forms the shape of the spine—connective tissue creates the shape of our physical structure. However, muscle, strengthened and stretched appropriately, can change the shape of the fascia over time. Permanent pain relief happens when fascia is changed through bodywork, concentrated and deliberate exercises, and changes in the nervous system that correct long-term habits.

The series of spiral pathway exercises included here involve the whole spine because of the nature of compensation and balance in the rotational movements. You will find these four exercises useful if:

- Any part of your body hurts more on one side than the other
- You have traveling pains, pain and tightness that move around the body
- You spend, or have spent, time in an asymmetrical position habitually (e.g., working on a computer with the head slightly turned or playing a violin)
- You have loose joints

These are alignment exercises. This means that the purpose of the movement is not fulfilled if you make the shape of the movement or posture but don't use the correct muscles. This is the hard part, because every other body part will want to work, except the weak stabilizing muscles we are trying to get to! So resist the temptation to do it wrong. You're much better off holding the position correctly in a modified form. That way your body will learn a new way of being that is more comfortable. New neurological pathways will be created, but you must hold each position for at least ninety seconds *minimum* for the muscle memory to be created in the brain.

I suggest you start with a modification that you think will be too easy for you and hold it, paying attention only to your form (and the clock) for at least ninety seconds. Focus on the areas you want to use as well as the compensations that are happening, and let your attention scan your whole body every ten seconds or so. Stay aware and alert; make sure your breath stays open and continuous. As soon as you lose concentration, old habits will creep back in.

For all the exercises except the fourth one, the hips and shoulder are square and level. Pay a lot of attention to this. Don't let the head or torso move to the right or left. You are strengthening the central line of your body so that the spinal movements can free up and equalize. There should be a lot of sensation in the inner core of the body, inner legs, abdomen, and spine.

Scoliosis is an obvious spiral line distortion; there are lots of others that show up in movement patterns in which you twist more easily in one direction than the other. You may not even be aware of these patterns.

Whatever your problems are, start with the first exercise; initially don't add more than one exercise each day, holding the postures once or twice, no more. So on day one you'll do exercise No. 1; day two will be exercises No. 1 and No. 2; day three will be No. 1, No. 2, and No. 3; and day four, No. 1 through No. 4. Then you'll do either all four every day or every other day, as you choose, and leave out anything unsuitable.

The exercises are very mentally challenging—you can't do them successfully while watching TV. You're better off visualizing and thinking correctly while messing up the exercise—well, at least, not being able to do much of it—than not thinking and mechanically completing a correct movement. It's actually in the effort that the change happens. So if you can do the unmodified exercise without any effort, there's a 90 percent chance you're doing it incorrectly and a 10 percent possibility that you just don't need it, in which case, go to the next one.

✑ Spiral Pathway Exercise No. 1: Transverse Abdominis Exercise I

You can refer back to fig. 9.8 to have a clear picture of the muscle being worked.

1. Stand by a doorjamb so you can hold on to a corner of it. Facing forward, place the outer edge of the right foot, the side of the hip, and the side of the rib cage on the doorjamb, your right hand and arm on the other side of the wall slightly behind you, holding on to the molding or the wall (see fig. 12.3 on page 174). If you can't touch your rib cage to the doorjamb without twisting your body, place some padding between your rib cage and the edge so you can face front

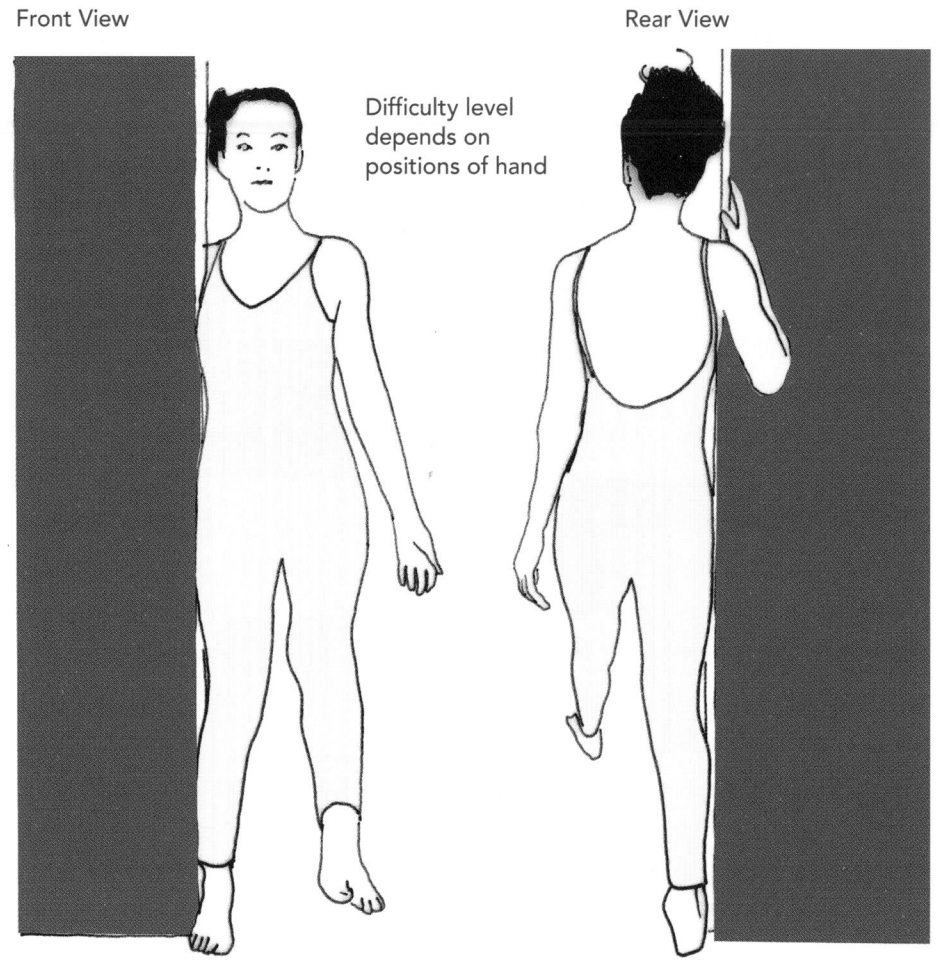

Front View

Rear View

Difficulty level
depends on
positions of hand

Fig. 12.3. Transverse Abdominis Exercise I

squarely, without any distortion. The hips should be square and level, both feet parallel at hip distance.

2. Make sure the shoulder at the edge of the doorjamb is comfortable; all doors are different and you may need to experiment a little to find the right one. The distance your hand is from the edge will make this movement more or less difficult—the farther away, the harder it will be to balance.

The hipbone, where it contacts the edge of the doorjamb, must be straight and not tilted up or down. You want to feel as much distance as you can between the crest of the bone and the bottom of the pelvis, as though someone were squeezing your hips together and they were elongating. The rib cage also should not tip forward or back, so let the lower back part of the rib cage widen and lift up toward the ceiling while the shoulders relax. You want to feel as much length as possible in the torso before you start the movement, so concentrate on drawing the rib cage away from the pelvis and lengthening the spine.

3. Keep the length and the alignment against the doorjamb, hold on firmly, and check alignment pointers again—connections to doorjamb, foot position, hips square and level, relaxed shoulders. Hold on with your arm muscles rather than the shoulders. Then lift the leg farthest from the doorjamb about 45 degrees, very slowly. You should feel a strong contraction, like a belt, around your navel, pulling in. That's the upper part of transverse abdominis working. If you don't feel this, start again, and check all your alignment. Don't lose any length as you lift the leg. There will be an optimum place where you can lift the leg and feel the "belt" action—it may be lower or higher than 45 degrees.

   As you lift the leg slowly, think of the ankle rising easily and the head of the thigh bone softening back into the socket, engaging your abs rather than leg muscles, without losing hip placement. If you can't lift your leg, raise the foot slightly on a block and just think of lifting to find the same muscles.

4. Stay in the optimum leg lift position for at least 90 seconds, continuing to lengthen the torso like a snake sliding up the wall. If you can find a lift in the back of the head, let that help you too. You are feeling the support of transverse abdominis under the stomach and diaphragm.

5. Do the exercise on both sides, holding for 90 seconds, with one repetition on each side.

After you release the position, your breathing may feel easier and more relaxed. If you had tightness in the solar plexus, it may release. The spine will also feel more supported. Enjoy the sensation; ultimately it can lead to a core strength that will allow your movements to feel less effortful and more graceful.

You can use this lengthening feeling in the back between your rib cage and pelvis when you are sitting. Imagine your rib cage in the back floating up and away from the pelvis and, when you can maintain that, feel the whole torso lift up away from the pubic bone and the structure of the pelvis in the back.

🌿 Spiral Pathway Exercise No. 2: Transverse Abdominis Exercise II
This exercise strengthens side, abdominal, and some leg muscles. This pathway corrects imbalances in the back, which you can feel as lower and midback pain, inability

to sit and stand up straight, and lower back pain that is primarily on one side of the body. The exercise will also help scoliosis.

1. Kneel parallel to a wall, with the space between your knee and the wall as long as a yoga block. Kneel upright with padding under your knees, if you want, and the block touching the side of your knee and the wall. Your hips are up, directly over the knees. You may (you will!) need a chair in front of you to hold on to.

2. Now bring the yoga block between your hip and the wall, so the distance is the same between the hip and the wall as it was between the knee and wall (fig. 12.4). Keep the block there to support your hip. Hold on to the chair in front of you, however you feel comfortable. Keep the hips square and level and straighten the leg that is farthest from the wall, so that the toes of that leg and the knee of the leg closest to the wall are in a straight line. Try to lift the straight leg only 2 inches from the floor, keeping the hips square. Hold for 90 seconds, one repetition.

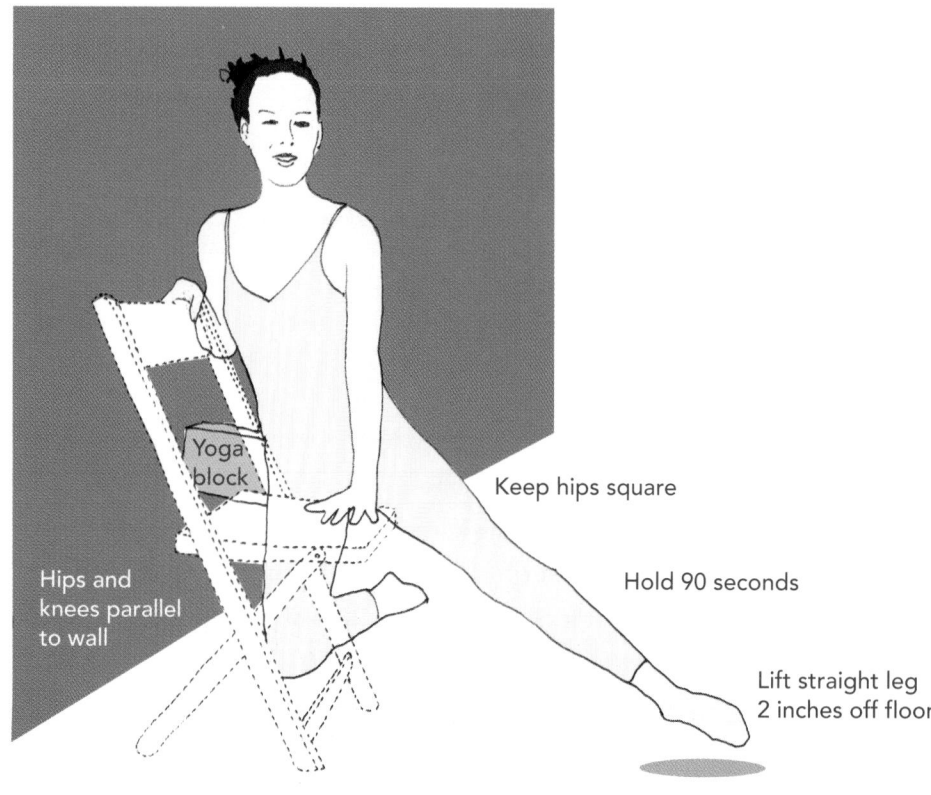

Yoga block

Keep hips square

Hips and knees parallel to wall

Hold 90 seconds

Lift straight leg 2 inches off floor

Fig. 12.4. Transverse Abdominis Exercise II

3. Repeat on the other side. One side will probably be stronger. Work the weak side first, and then the strong side, and then the weak side again.

To modify: Bend the leg slightly, and lean forward onto the chair. You can cheat just a little by bringing the knee closest to the wall a little farther away. If it is not possible for you to lift the leg at all, you can simply hold the position and envision lifting it until you get stronger.

This is a very hard exercise for most of us. You must be able to do it while keeping the hips square and level, tailbone *slightly* dropped, so the lower back is straight and your shoulders are *over* your hips. Don't let the shoulder nearest the wall veer in toward it or rise up.

To make this easier, you can use your arm strength, lean forward, and use some isometric pressure of the hip against the block to push against.

◈ An Easier Version of Transverse Abdominis Exercise II
If you can't get this one at all, here's an easier version.

Adopt the same position, but this time position yourself next to a doorjamb so you can hold on (fig. 12.5). The outer leg, hip, and rib cage (use padding if necessary) touch the edge of the doorjamb. Same alignment.

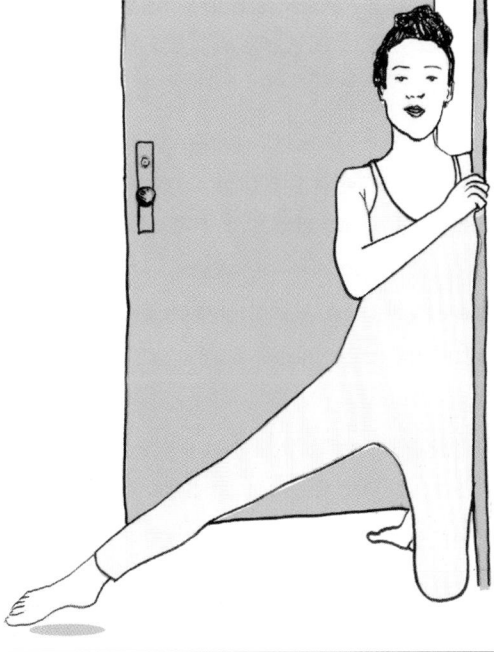

Fig. 12.5. Transverse Abdominis Exercise II Modification

🌿 *Spiral Pathway Exercise No. 3: Outer Spiral Exercise*

Just as the Transverse Abdominis Exercise works the deep inner muscles that help the inner part of our spiral movement pathway, so this one engages the deep outer muscles that support the outer part.

◈ Outer Spiral Exercise Level I

1. Lie on a mat or any comfortable surface that has a straight edge (but not one you can fall off). Position yourself on your left side, with your left arm straight and under your head. Bring your left side into a straight line by using the edge of the mat, so the side of your hip, your rib cage, your shoulder girdle, your left arm, and your head line up.

2. Then position your legs so they line up too. You can use your right hand to stabilize as you move, but then move your right arm on top of your right side, palm on the side of your right thigh (fig. 12.6).

Extend   Stretch Spine   Reach Out

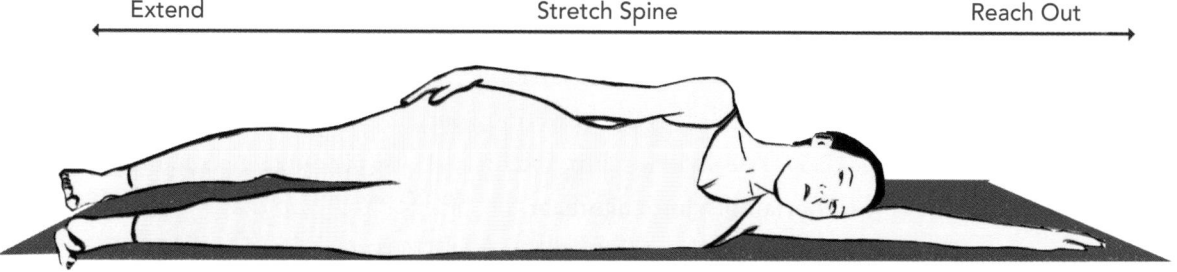

Fig. 12.6. Outer Spiral Exercise Level I

3. Stack your hips so they are square and level. The right hip will probably want to roll back a lot, so feel the side of the pelvic bone to allow you to roll it into the correct position. It should be square with the ceiling, as should your shoulders. Feet are flexed and active. The outside of your left foot should press against the floor, at a right angle to your leg. Your head must be in line with your spine—not forward—so the weight of your head will rest in the middle of your left arm.

4. Gaze ahead, and check that the top of your head is in line with your pelvic floor. It will want to roll forward on its own. If that happens, don't go farther; press the outer left side of your body down into the mat, and think of lengthening your spine.

5. Hold this position for 90 seconds, and then repeat on the other side. Work the weaker side first for one 90-second repetition, and then the stronger side for the same time, and then the weaker side again.

6. The degree of difficulty you'll discover does not depend on strength exactly, but on

the amount of torsion in your lumbar vertebrae. If the position as I've just described it is not challenging, keep the alignment in your hips, shoulders, and head the same, but move your legs an inch or so back, using the right hand for balance.

7. Now realign as we did initially—spine straight, hips and shoulders square, head in line with spine, gaze in front, and bring back the right arm to the starting position, palm down on the side of your right thigh. Roll the right hip forward again.

8. Keep moving the legs back until you feel a challenge—if you are doing this correctly, you won't need to move more than a few inches. The position should be possible to maintain, but will take some work. Then lift the right leg up a few inches, keeping it in line with the left leg exactly. There will be an optimum distance for you to position the leg so that the challenge is right.

   The left leg must be able to keep its starting position. It is very important here that only the distance between the right and left leg change, not the angle, and the hips stay stacked. Hold this position for 90 seconds, and then repeat on the other side.

9. Work the weaker side first for one 90-second repetition, and then the stronger side for the same time, and then the weaker side again.

◈ Outer Spiral Exercise Level II

1. For the next level of challenge, make sure the hip point on top stays rolled forward so you are in line. Then bring the top leg forward, keeping the hip stable. Keep the foot flexed and straight. Make sure your gaze stays straight ahead. Keeping the outer edge of the foot and the leg itself straight, bring the leg to the place of maximum challenge (fig. 12.7).

Start parallel with other leg and then roll forward

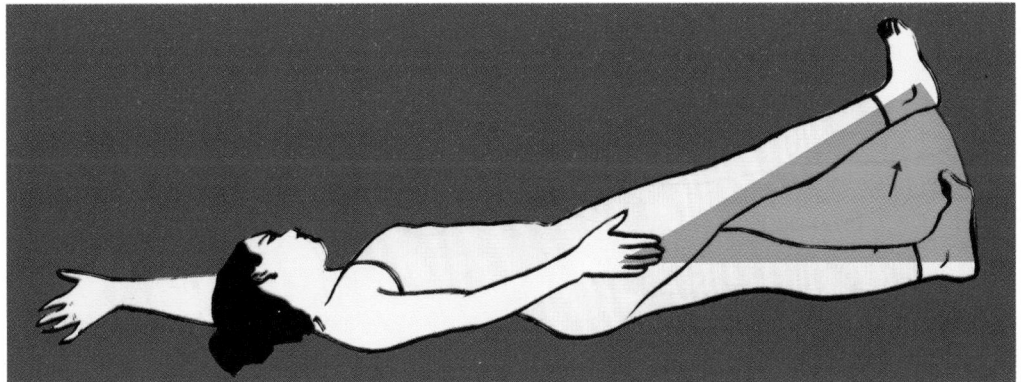

Right arm palm down side of right thigh

Fig. 12.7. Outer Spiral Exercise Level IIa

2. Then, keeping alignment, rotate your leg in by bringing your heel toward the ceiling as you think of lengthening the leg. The leg and hip do not change position (fig. 12.8).

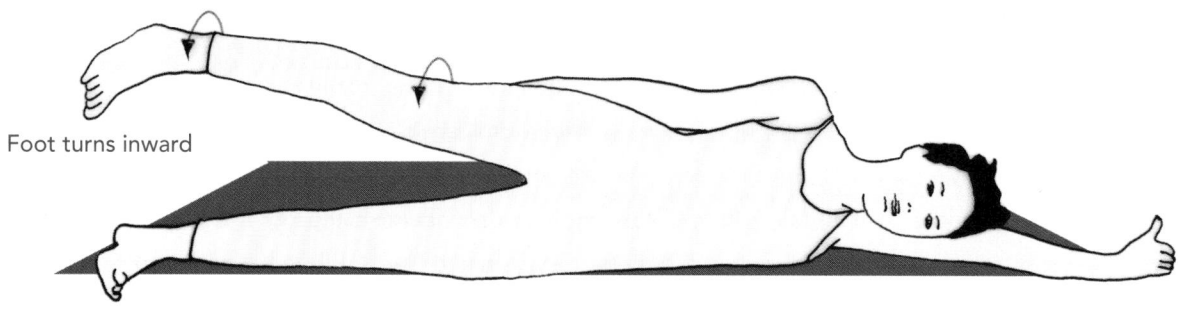

Foot turns inward

Fig. 12.8. Outer Spiral Exercise Level IIb

3. You can then externally rotate the leg by turning the foot outward, so the toes move toward the ceiling (fig. 12.9).

Top View

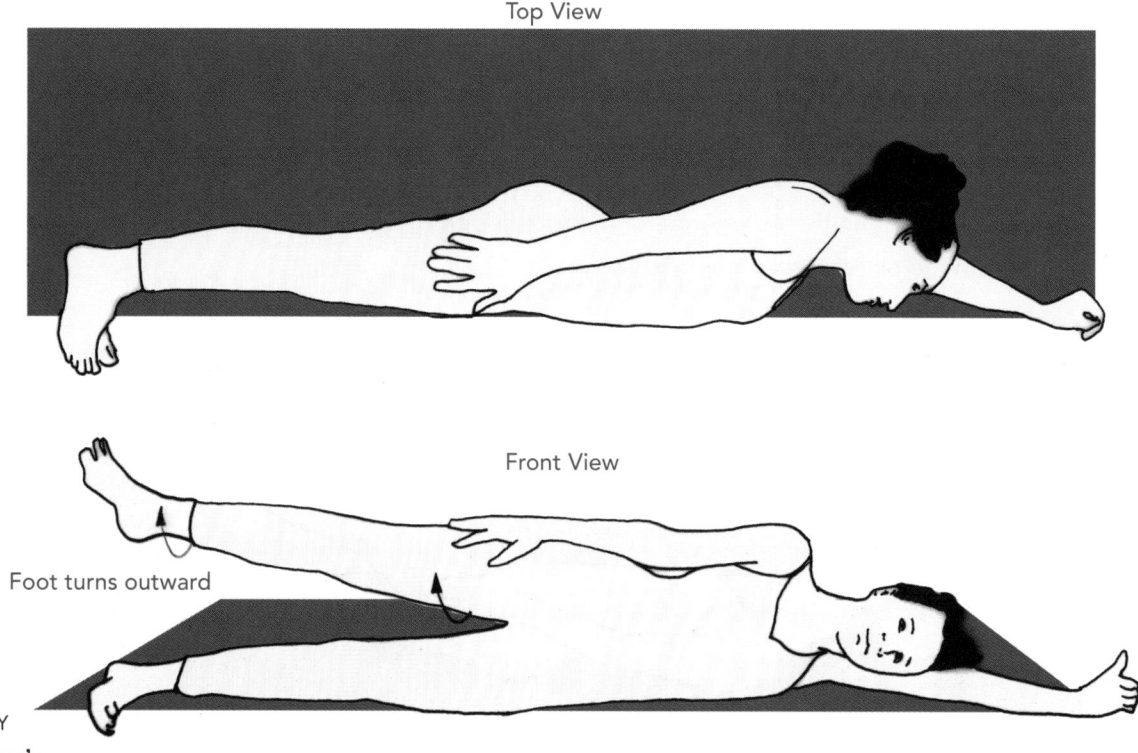

Front View

Foot turns outward

Fig. 12.9. Outer Spiral Exercise Level IIc

4. Notice which is more difficult. Hold the leg with the foot straight for 90 seconds, and then repeat the more difficult movement for about 10 seconds.

5. Repeat the sequence on the other side.

🍃 Spiral Pathway Exercise No. 4: Lower Back Exercise with Physio Ball

This exercise works to stretch and strengthen obliques, quadratus, and sides of the back. This move is very safe and works for most lower back pain, both short and long term. You will need to use a physio ball of the appropriate size for your height. If you are not sure of your balance you can use a wall to steady yourself. You can even use a corner of the room, so you can prop the side of the ball against both walls. However, you should not use the wall unless you absolutely need it, because you want to strengthen your stabilizing muscles—the ones you use to balance on the ball. Although this is a tricky exercise, it is well worth the effort for the magic effect it has on the lower back.

1. Position yourself *exactly* on the ball (as shown in fig. 12.10) in order to work the side of the body. You should feel the movement on the side between the

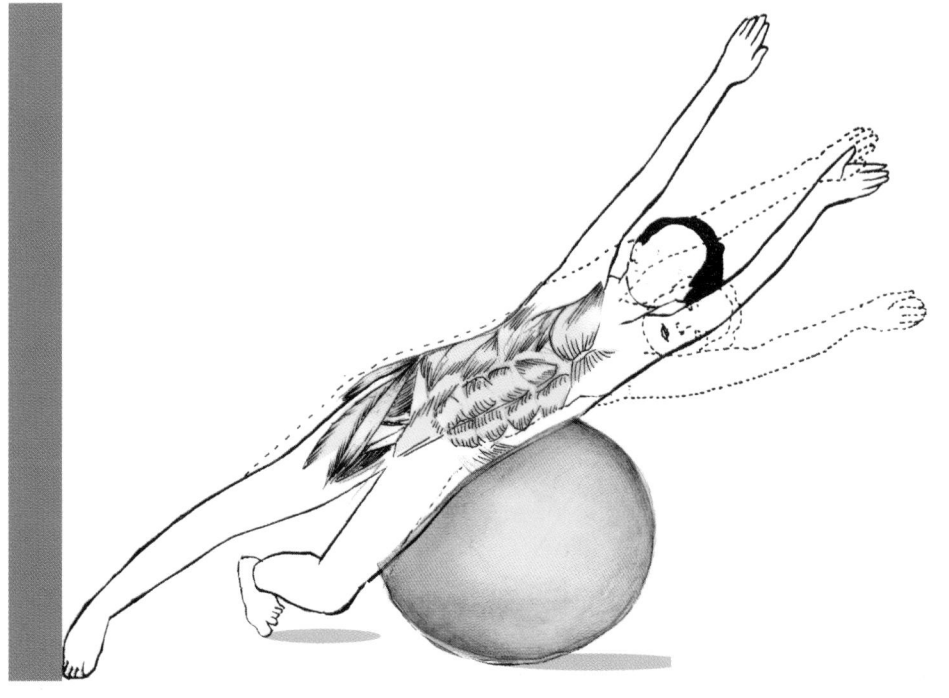

Fig. 12.10. Lower Back Exercise with Physio Ball

hipbone and the rib cage and maybe up the rib cage and down into the side of the hip. Place your feet on the wall with the top foot behind the bottom or with one foot on the floor and one against the wall as shown. Knees can be bent as much as needed. The exercise is easier when your knees are very bent, so you can use your feet against the wall to stabilize your body. Your hips are square and stacked, one on top of the other.

2. Your body lies in a straight line, as though following an imaginary line drawn on top of the ball, and your hips are directly over each other, shoulders stacked in the same way, as though both the front and back body are pressed between two panes of glass. You can bring your hand behind your back to make sure you are not leaning forward or back. Your head should be in line with your tailbone (it will want to jut forward, especially when you move). Check that the side of your rib cage faces the ceiling. Your gaze should be straight ahead.

3. Bring the bottom hand down on the floor to align yourself, and stretch over the ball as far as you can. Start the movement from the most stretched-out position you can obtain. This allows you to stretch the outer muscles of the side body so you have to access the weaker deep muscles and to engage the postural aspects of the lower back—the parts of the muscles that support your spine.

4. Bring the elbows by the ears, arms straight, or bring the hands to the top of the head for an easier move. You could even keep the bottom hand on the floor to modify, or the top arm on the body.

5. Keeping 100 percent aligned, as described, slowly and evenly raise your side body, using a controlled movement. Do not use the weight of your head to lift up. Look straight ahead, and relax your neck—the effort should come only from the side body. Push your feet or foot into the wall to stabilize yourself. Do not come up above the angle where your body forms a line (as shown), in order not to contract the outer muscles too deeply. You want to keep a slight stretch in the side body.

6. You can repeat the movement up to 6 times, for a count of 10 seconds for each repetition—10 up and 10 down. If you can do this without tiring, your alignment is almost certainly not correct. Check it, and try again. One repetition may be enough.

7. Repeat on the other side. Start on the weaker side, and then work the stronger one, and then the weaker again.

❖ Lower Back Exercise with Wall and Physio Ball

This exercise can be modified in a few ways to make it easier. One is to use a firm ball and prop the ball against a corner. You can also use a stool to raise your hands, so your starting position is less extreme. Or you can lean with your back against a wall, feet a comfortable distance away, so your back is flat on the wall and your head touches the wall. It's best if your shoulders touch the wall too—if they don't, work at bringing them back without losing the contact of your back against the wall.

1. With your back flat against the wall, raise your right arm, elbow at right ear, palm facing out. Then slowly bend to the left side, keeping the hips still and the back flat. Here's the more difficult part—you must keep both sides equally long, so the left side of your body keeps quite straight and does not collapse at all.

2. Go as far as you can without losing the straight edge of the left rib cage. Keep the right shoulder and arm against the wall. You probably won't get very far without losing alignment. Go to where you can keep form, and then bring up your left arm to your left ear. Hold for 90 seconds, and repeat on the other side.

BALANCING THE MIDBACK (12TH THORACIC VERTEBRA)

The 12th thoracic vertebra is a common "problem" area, located at a junction point between the upper back and lower back. This area is an especially complex meeting place, because the vertebra itself is formed as a thoracic vertebra at the top and a lumbar vertebra at the bottom. This allows more movement, yet because of the greater ease of twisting in the lumbar, it often gets stuck rotated to one side or the other, causing back pain.

As the neck and the lower back are the most naturally flexible parts of the spine, they compensate for tightness and immobility in the thoracic spine. They go "out of line" when they are pulled beyond their limits, and then the muscles around the overstretched parts of the spine can go into spasm for protection.

We can solve this problem by (a) strengthening the neck and lower back and (b) stretching and opening the spaces between the thoracic vertebrae.

🍂 *Arm Raise Twist*

This twisting exercise will correct the rotation by aligning the muscles around this part of the spine, gently persuading the vertebrae to line up.

1. Sit cross-legged on the floor. If you can't sit cross-legged, sit on a chair with your feet flat on the ground. Bring your right elbow to your left knee, and use the leverage of the knee to twist as far as you can away from the knee. You will probably notice the left hip move back to facilitate your twist. Press the left hip forward as you turn, so the hips stay level. This will prevent the lumbar vertebrae from turning too much.

2. Allow the midback to open. Make sure your neck stays in line with the rest of your spine by aligning your chin with your sternum. You don't want to drop your head, though; think of slightly bending back rather than forward, which will help to straighten the spine. You will feel the twist deep in the lower, mid-, and upper spine.

    If any part of the back feels tight or sore when you twist, check that:

    • You are not leaning back or forward; your spine should be straight
    • Your shoulders are turning with your body and are level with each other
    • Your lower ribs are level and not tipping unevenly right or left

3. Your shoulders should be slightly back over the ribs, so there is just a little back bend in the upper spine—think of widening your collar bones and pulling the shoulders away from each other. That will contract the muscles between the shoulder blades slightly. Relax your hands!

4. Think of lifting the crown of your head up toward the ceiling, and feel each vertebra lengthen and open.

5. Now go back to your hips and make sure the right hip is square with the left—not moving back. Bring it forward, keep it there, and go through the steps again!

6. Then raise your left arm, and twist farther if possible, looking up at the left hand (fig. 12.11). Ideally, there will be a straight line from the left hand through the left shoulder and the chest to the right elbow and left knee. Hold for about 30 seconds.

7. Repeat on the other side. Then reverse the cross of the legs and repeat the two movements. You have a sequence of four movements: left arm up, twisting right,

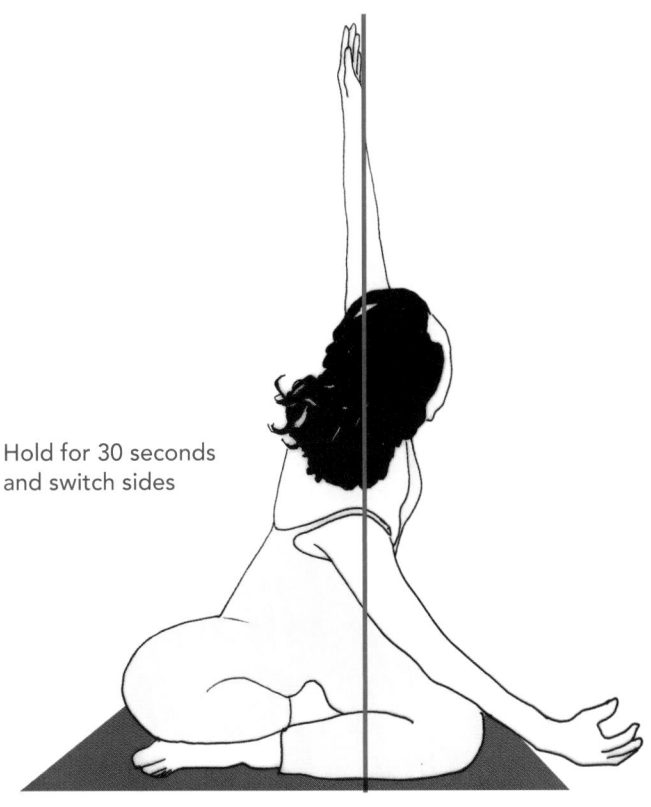

Hold for 30 seconds and switch sides

Fig. 12.11. Arm Raise Twist

and the same two with the legs crossed the opposite way. If you are sitting in a chair, you will have only two movements.

8. If the 12th thoracic area is "stuck," one or two of the movements will be more difficult. Go back to the difficult movement(s), and stay with it until you can perform all four movements with equal ease (or as close to this goal as you can accomplish).

Do this exercise regularly for chronic back issues, scoliosis, and other ailments, and occasionally if you want temporary relief from midback pain.

USING THE HORSE STANCE TO STRENGTHEN AND ALIGN THE BACK

The Horse Stance is used by qi gong and tai chi practitioners as a meditation posture. They'll stand in it for much longer than suggested in this variation, sometimes for an hour or more. The complete straightness of the spine that the posture demands allows them to channel energy up the core of the spine with various breathing techniques.

For our purposes, the straight spine forces us to use the lower abdomen as the center of gravity. At the same time the exercise strengthens the back muscles and realigns the "collars" of the body. These horizontal bands of fascia can distort spiral movements. Because the spirals run across the body, they will be interrupted by a tight band that prevents the open flow of movement—this will become obvious when you do Horse Stance. Since you will be preventing all spirallic movement while doing this posture, any tight horizontal fascia will be pulled and stretched by the bones. It may feel as though your muscles are tight, but the difference is that you can't consciously release the fascia. Just let the bones hang into the fascia, let the back muscles strengthen, and eventually, the fascia will soften.

The most important part of the Horse Stance exercise, for the purpose of relieving back pain, is the engagement of the lower back and abdominal muscles in the pelvic tuck. The stance itself prevents the utilization of the wrong muscles.

🍃 Variation on the Horse Stance

1. Stand with your feet parallel, shoulder width apart. Position yourself close to a mirror so you can see yourself from one side. Weight is even on both feet to start. Lower your hips about 6 inches, making sure your knees do not come past your toes as you look down. You'll have to keep checking this, as your knees will want to creep forward as you progress, so make sure you check by just glancing down, not by moving your whole body (fig. 12.12).

2. Now curl your tailbone under and pull up your pubic bone, feeling engagement in the lower abdomen. Keep the area between the navel and the rib cage long—don't lean forward.

3. Bring the back directly over the tailbone in one straight line with your arms making a circle in front of you, palms facing you, as though you are holding a large, light ball. Your spine will be completely straight, with no curves except for the neck. Make sure your shoulders come back too, and don't let your arms pull forward. They should feel relaxed.

4. At this point, you are likely to experience some difficulty. Your feet may want to come up off the floor in front if the tibia (shin bone) is normally positioned too far forward. To help this long term, you can stretch the front and back of your calves and feet (see pages 258–62). If you are really in danger of falling over, position yourself so your toes go under a door, or put something heavy on your feet. For

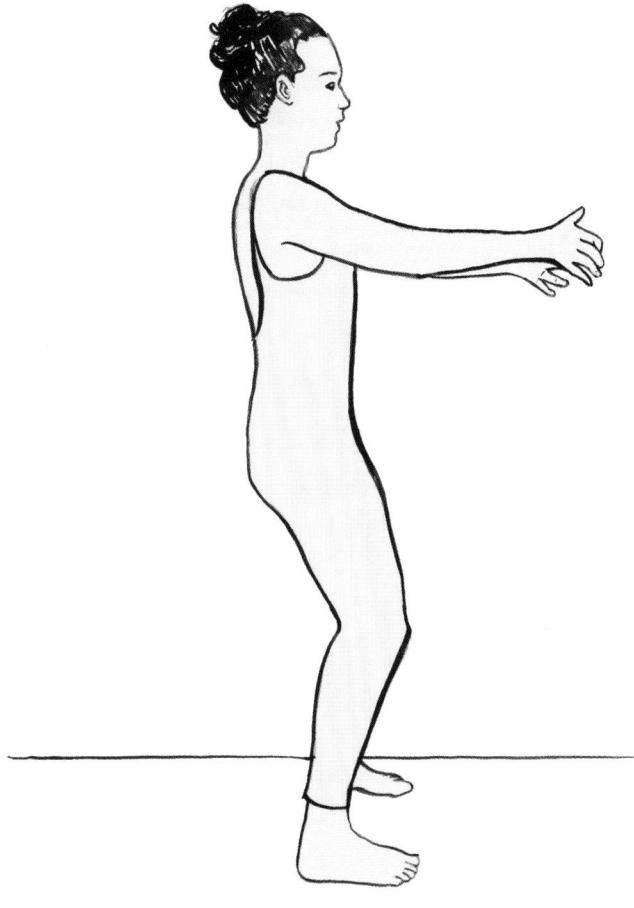

Fig. 12.12. Variation on Horse Stance

now it's okay if your weight falls mainly on your heels. Just keep pressing the balls of your toes into the floor until the alignment changes.

5. Your knees may creep forward. Keep pressing them back and then retucking the pelvis. Your back must be completely straight. For most of us, who are chronically forward flexed, this will feel like we are falling backward.

6. Now fine-tune the position of the head and shoulders: Gaze straight ahead, and position your head over your new center of gravity, the crown of your head over the middle of your pelvic floor, your chin parallel with the ground. Your shoulders must be back, down, and as relaxed as you can get them. To release the shoulders and chest, bring the hands in front of you, palms facing you, and touch them together lightly, just to the roots of the fingers, to give a very minimal support to the arms. Now release the hands completely. Feel the collarbone and shoulder blades drop.

THE SPINE AND
DEEP CORE
MUSCLES

187

Bring the head up toward the ceiling about ¼ inch, feeling that connection between ceiling, crown of head, and all the way down the spine. Imagine that your spine is as thick as your neck, and stretch it up slightly with the crown of your head. You may be able to feel a very slight stretch inside your sacrum. Let the entire shoulder girdle relax. Relax your tongue and jaw.

7. Now check that you have your:

   - Feet parallel, weight evenly distributed between your left and right foot
   - Knees behind your toes
   - Pelvis tucked, engaged in lower abs
   - Arms in front, shoulders back, not pulling forward
   - Spine completely straight, no forward lean at all
   - Head back, chin parallel to floor, and crown in line with middle of pelvic floor
   - Shoulders, neck, hands, and jaw relaxed
   - Breathing focused into lower abdomen in a relaxed way
   - Focus on lower abdomen, legs, hips, and back

8. Ideally you should feel a nice strong contraction in the lumbar spine (multifidus) and the lower abdominals (transverse abdominis). Put your hands there to check—try to engage front and back equally, if you can. Feel a pleasant stretch in the lower back; it shouldn't hurt.

9. You'll notice that, as the lower back and abdominal muscles tire, you'll feel other muscle groups chime in. That's natural—they're just helping out—but for our purposes, we want to keep the back/abdominal tension. So just as though you were meditating, draw the focus back to that area as the muscles drift, until you no longer can, and then stop.

To modify: The obvious way to make this easier, you might think, would be to support the back. I thought that too and tried it, and it took me a while to figure out why it didn't work. You've probably guessed already. The back of the head sticks out behind you if your head is aligned. You would need to use either a good six inches of padding between your shoulders and hips on a wall, or else use a wall that has a hole where your head sticks out. Both these ways present some logistical problems.

You could support your hands on a shelf, making sure the shoulders relax back and down. Or if you need just a slight modification, come down only an inch or so. You can do this sitting, if standing is difficult. Just sit with your feet parallel, knees over ankles, sit bones even on the chair. Then line up your torso, shoulders directly over hips, just as though you were standing. Everything will be the same from the hips up. You can't really tuck the pelvis successfully while sitting on a chair—you'll slide your sit bones forward too much—so pull the pubic bone up toward the navel by tightening your abdominals and draw your navel up and in. You will still keep the lumbar curve that way.

SPECIFIC TARGETS AND OVERALL STRETCHES FOR THE BACK

In this section, there are two exercises that each have a specific target and then two that stretch the entire back.

🍃 Exercise for the Paraspinals

You may have a very strong back, but weak postural muscles. This exercise will challenge the paraspinals, which are part of the postural muscles.

1. Make your body into a perfect L-shape. Make sure your hips don't pull back too far (keep them as far forward as your body will allow—it is hard) and that your head and arms are in line with your straight spine. Your arms should be straight and close by your ears (fig. 12.13).

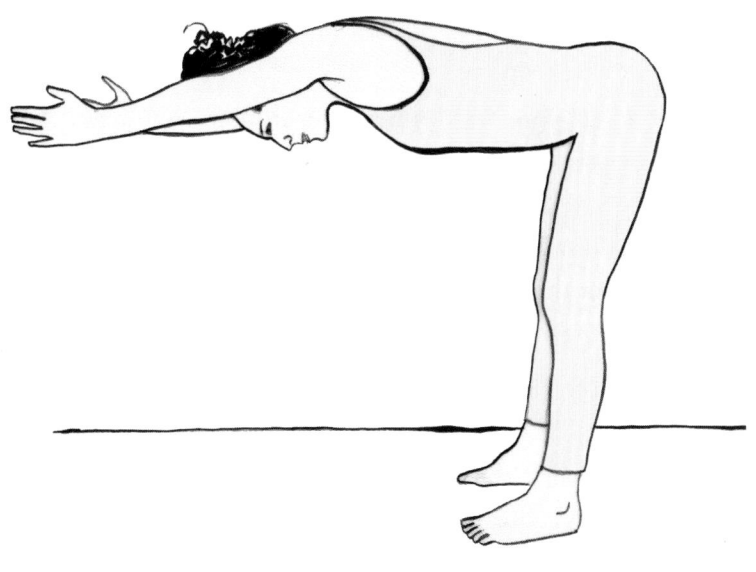

Fig. 12.13. Exercise for the Paraspinals

2. Bring the bottom tips of the shoulder blades down the back, and reach forward with the fingertips. (If you can't straighten your arms without pulling the shoulder blades up your back, it's actually shoulder tension that's the problem, so try the Shoulder Stretches (page 161). Hold this position as long as you can. This exercise can be sobering if your back is strong in other areas. It will help to strengthen the muscles that prevent back pain, so persist.

To modify: You can support your hips against a wall; you can even touch a wall with your fingertips.

🌿 Exercise for the Sacroiliac Joint

1. Lie on your stomach, preferably on a thick mat or with some padding under your pelvis (but don't let the pelvis rise up very far). Bring the legs together, making sure the knees are connecting. Then bend at the knees. Make sure your thighs are parallel.
2. Then raise the knees off the floor (if you can), pressing the pubic bone evenly into the floor. You probably won't get very far. Hold as long as you can. A person with a moderate degree of back strength could hold this position with the knees a few inches off the floor. It would be wonderful if you have a friend who could gently press the tailbone down toward your knees, lengthening the lower back. But if you don't, just think of dropping the tailbone down between your legs—or just imagine your friend is there, pressing the bone down gently.

If this position hurts, you may be uneven—tilting to one side or the other—or you may have too weak a lower back to practice this successfully. Avoid it until the other exercises have strengthened the supporting muscles sufficiently.

🌿 Wall Hang Stretch

If you do only one thing, do this stretch. It opens up the entire back of the body, from heels to the neck, and uses gravity to gently traction your lower back.

1. Stand facing a wall, with your legs apart. The farther apart your legs are and the farther from the wall you are, the easier the stretch will be. You need to be able to lean forward and lean your upper back on the wall comfortably (fig. 12.14).

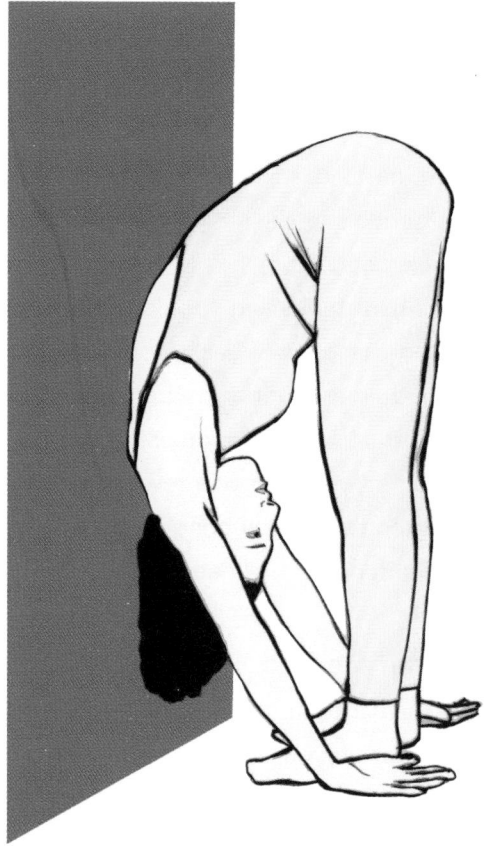

Fig. 12.14. Wall Hang Stretch

2. After you do this, relax and give your weight to the wall so it is supporting you completely. Bend your knees if you need to, and change your position so that the stretch is felt in the backs of your legs and your back.

3. Shuffle around until you find your optimum position. Then align yourself. If your hamstrings are so tight that you cannot bring your heels to the ground, put padding under the heels. Look at your feet and ankles, especially the inner bones of the ankles. Make sure they are not dropping inward or turning outward. The ankles should be straight and even.

4. Then check your hips. You will want to lean toward the most flexible side, so move your hips to get a good stretch, even if it makes you a little uneven. But stay in the stretch for a longer period with correct alignment; that is, with the hips straight and your body hanging evenly between the hips. If you don't have a mirror behind you, or a friend who can spot you, run your hand up the outside of

your legs and torso, and you can probably feel where your hips and torso are in relation to each other. Most people have a chronic twist to one side or the other, and this exercise can help correct it.

5. This is also a good position to check how your neck is aligned between your shoulders, and give it a gentle stretch with your hands. You can turn the neck to the right and left, if it feels good.

6. This stretch involves your hamstrings and your lower back. Tight hamstrings will pull on the pelvis and can cause lower back problems. You want to make sure you are stretching the middle and upper part of the muscle, not just the area behind your knees. So start out with your knees slightly bent, even if you don't need to bend them. Then lift your tailbone toward the ceiling and toward the wall at your back. Straighten the legs by bringing the upper thighs back behind you, rather than just straightening your knees.

🌱 Stretching the Back and the Neck

It's important to stretch all the back muscles together, because they tend to shorten together. Imagine a line that starts at your heels and goes all the way up your body to the base of the skull. Any shortening or tightening along that line will result in some degree of shortening everywhere along its length. That's why stretching the neck on its own usually doesn't do much to loosen it up. This sequence of back stretches lengthens the muscles that usually tighten in the course of daily life. Using it just five minutes a day will help to prevent back problems.

1. Start by sitting on the floor with your legs extended and your heels touching the wall. Your feet should be hip width and straight (not rotated out or in). For some people, this position alone is uncomfortable. If you are one of them, find the degree of bearable discomfort you can maintain and stay there until you gain more flexibility. You can put padding under your knees if you can't straighten them on the floor.

2. If you can sit this way easily, let your head drop slowly toward your knees, arms relaxed, and hold for 2 minutes. Then stretch toward the toes with your hands on the floor, head still dropped (fig. 12.15). Stretch from the lower back; don't pull with the arms. This is a lower back stretch. Hold.

3. Now, maintaining this position, push the balls of the feet into the wall and push the heels away. This stretches your shins. Hold.

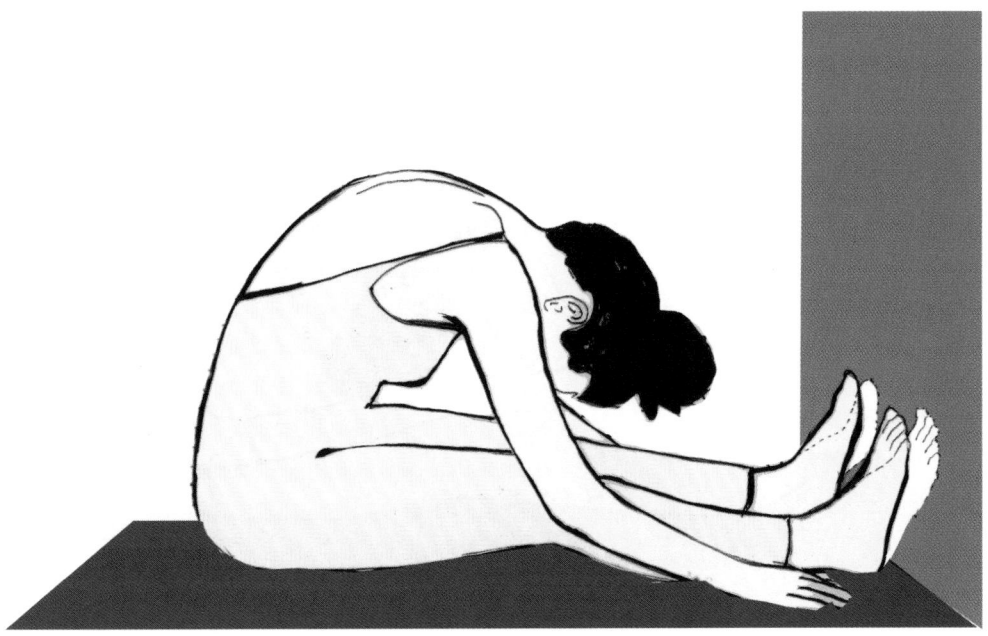

Fig. 12.15. Lower back and hamstring stretch

4. Then reverse this posture by flexing the feet and pushing the heels into the wall, toes away from the wall. You should feel the stretch in your hamstrings at first. Wait a minute or so to feel the stretch in the deep calf muscles and the Achilles tendon.

5. Go back to the "slumped" sitting position, head dropped toward the knees. Interlock your hands behind your head, keeping your shoulders relaxed. Don't push at first. Feel the stretch in the upper back, and then gently, if you want to, increase the pressure, making sure your shoulders stay relaxed. Turn your nose to the left for a stretch to the right side of the trapezius, keeping your arms in the same position, and then turn to the right. Go back again to the starting position.

6. Now bend your right arm, extend the elbow up to the ceiling, and slide your palm down your neck and upper back as far as you can. Bend forward to feel a stretch in the shoulder (see fig. 12.16 on page 194). Now repeat on the left side.

7. Go back to that starting position again, and now try to touch your head to the floor on the right side of your legs at about knee level. (Unless you are very flexible, you won't get very far.) Stretch your arms out diagonally in front of you, so that both arms and your head are in parallel lines (see fig. 12.17 on page 194). Make sure both hips stay on the ground for a stretch in the lower back. Repeat on the opposite side.

Interlock hands behind head, keep shoulders relaxed.
Turn nose to the left to stretch right side. Switch sides.

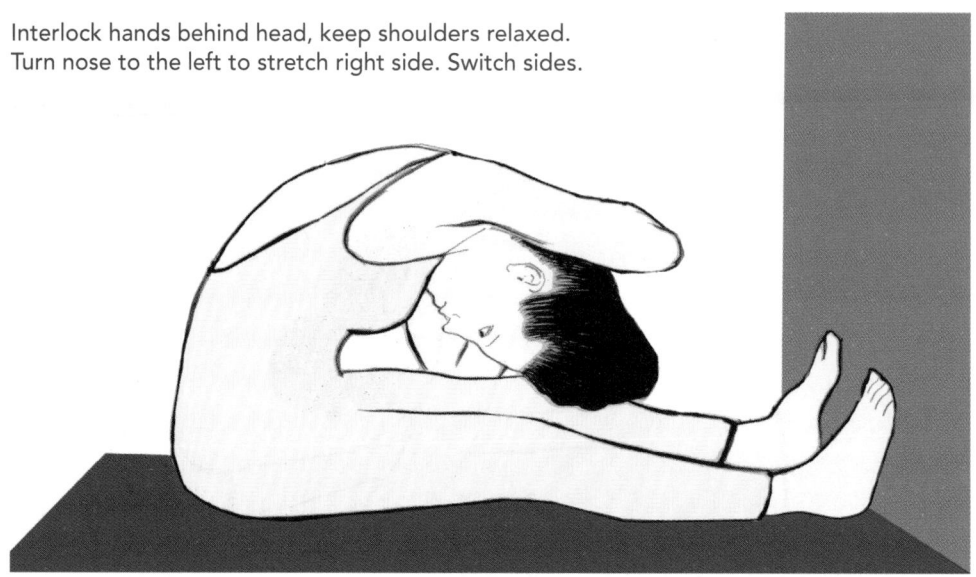

Fig. 12.16. Upper back and neck stretch

Stretch arms diagonally in front, keeping arms and head in parallel lines.
Keep hips on ground.

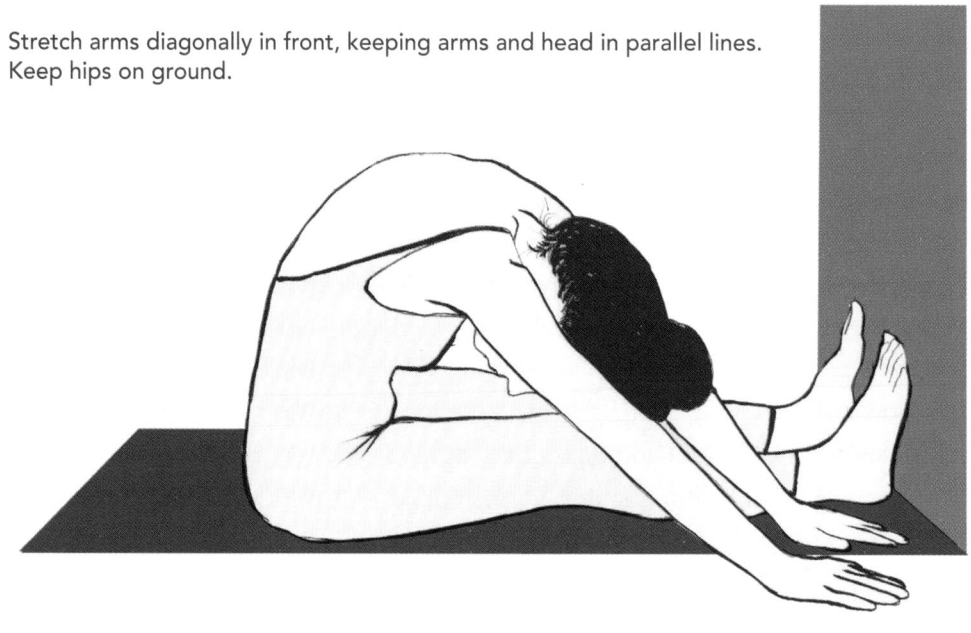

Fig. 12.17. Upper and lower back stretch

SPINAL ALIGNMENT WITH ROLL, BLOCKS, AND BALLS

You can change the shape of your spine simply by practicing small movements while lying on different kinds of props, using the forces of gravity and the combination of passive shaping and movement that has such a powerful effect on structure.

Using props may seem like a lazy person's way to do his own bodywork (and one reason I've had a chance to develop this system is that I can get almost any client to do these exercises on his own), but the body learns in a powerful way when it is able to be completely relaxed and passive. The props give the system new information about the shapes that it can incorporate, which might be more efficient for its movements.

Most of the positions I describe here should be held for about five minutes. You will feel very little as you lie there initially. Then, as the body stretches and starts to reform around the props, you will feel stretching and maybe some discomfort. Then these sensations will pass, and the props will start to feel comfortable and minimally present. This shows that your body has integrated the information. You can then remove the props, and relax for a minute lying down. This last step is important—don't skip it—it helps the brain process the change. You'll feel an immediate and often dramatic change in your body after you take the props away and lie back down.

You need to be able to relax on the props and breathe consciously and slowly. Modify if you can't relax into the sensation or your breathing tightens to a place where you cannot consciously release it. Intensify if you can't feel any sensation at all, or use the props for longer—a half hour or so. That will intensify the exercise also.

Then move around as you normally would—or just go to sleep if you do the exercises in bed at night.

Neck Roll

The first prop—you might as well make this one yourself if you are going to use it—is the neck roll. You will find this useful if you have an overstraightened (reverse curve) neck. About 75 percent of people with neck problems have this configuration of the cervical spine, and the neck roll will be useful to them. The other 25 percent have the opposite problem—too much curve in the neck—and the neck roll will be of no value to them.

How can you tell which alignment you have in your neck? If you tend to look downward and tuck your chin in, if you have pain at the base of your skull, tension in your throat, or if you have had whiplash injuries to the neck, you probably have a reverse curve in the cervical spine. This usually happens because the scalene muscles, deep neck muscles that attach to the inside of the cervical spine and run through to the top rib, tighten up or are damaged in some way (you can see from fig. 8.5 on page 113 how a whiplash injury might cause tearing and scar tissue here). These diagonal muscles provide the architectural support for the head, as the psoas does for the torso. If you imagine them shortening, you can see how that might either straighten the back of the neck and pull the chin toward the chest or compress the head down while tilting the chin up, like a swayback in the neck. The shape the scalene shortening gives the neck depends on where in the scalenes the damage has occurred.

Both types of reverse curve will benefit from using the neck roll. To make a neck roll for yourself, you can either roll up a bath towel very tightly until the circumference is about the same as your fist, then secure it with rubber bands, or do the same with a yoga mat (you could cut the mat if it's too big). The size (thickness) of the roll will depend on the natural length of your neck.

Using the Neck Roll

Lie on your back with the neck roll under your neck, not your head. Your head should lightly touch the floor or bed (fig. 12.18). The neck roll should be firm enough that your neck doesn't compress it at all; you will feel each vertebra move away from the ones next to it, even though the spine is in a curved position. Relax on the roll for about 15 minutes. Do this once a day; before you go to sleep is ideal—you can do it in your bed.

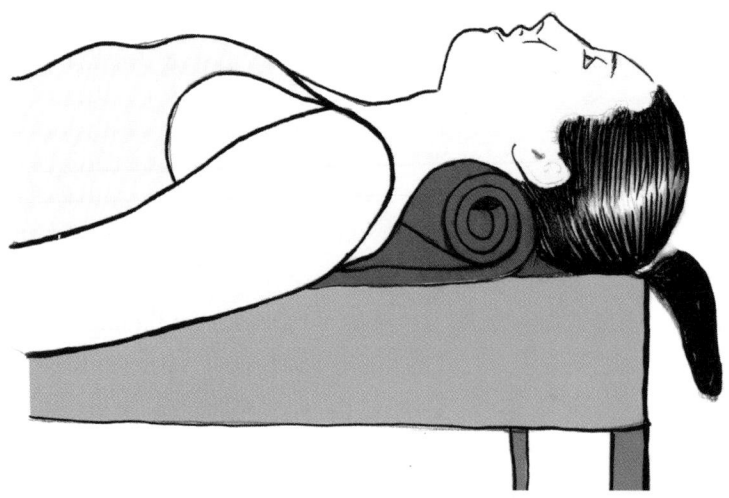

Fig.12.18. Using the Neck Roll

🍃 Using Props with the Thoracic Spine

The next area we can lengthen and open is the thoracic spine. Use a roll lengthwise on the spine, or a yoga block with the longest, thinnest edge on the spine. The placement of the block is important—it must come to the seventh cervical vertebra and slot between the shoulder blades. If it is lower than that, you may hurt your lower back. If you choose the gentler prop of the roll, it should be in the same placement, but it's less important exactly how far the bottom edge comes down on the back.

You can support your head with a pillow. I suggest lying on a secure surface so the block doesn't slip. You may also need to move your body back and forth so the block is flush to the floor. If it feels "tippy" at all, you will need to adjust yourself on the block. It usually takes a few tries to get it right.

Bring your arms back, with the elbows touching the floor if you can, to a comfortable stretch. You can also open up the knees and press the soles of the feet together for a groin stretch. Breathe in the rib cage and chest. Stay for at least 5 minutes.

🍃 Using Props with the Sacrum

You can also use a yoga block under the sacrum, the triangular bone at the base of the spine. Don't put the block any higher—you may hurt your back. Use the longest, thinnest edge widthwise across the sacrum. (You can also use a 5-inch ball.) Then straighten the legs and turn them in, internally rotating the head of the femur. Bring the legs as close together as you can.

To open up the hip joints on the inside, stretching the psoas and the groin, you could even tie your leg with a strap; you'd have to do this first before getting on the block.

🍃 Using Props with the Mid-Lower Back

For the mid-lower back, lie on your back, knees up, feet on the ground, and place a yoga block with the widest surface up under your tailbone (see fig. 12.19 on page 198). Make sure it's on the very lowest part of your spine. You can lie there relaxing your back, and the muscles will lengthen and relax after a while—maybe 20 minutes. This move can take the lower back out of spasm.

Place your yoga block on the farthest end of the spine. Hold for 20 minutes.

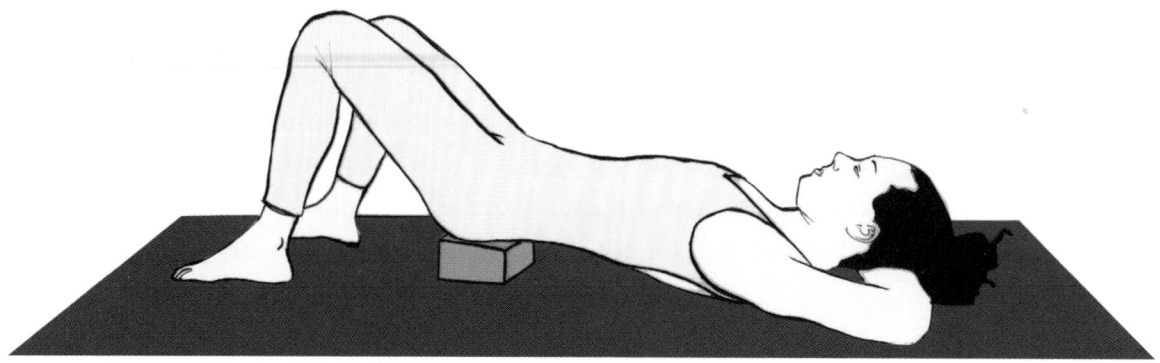

Fig.12.19. Using Props with the Mid-Lower Back

DISC HERNIATION

A herniated, bulging, or slipped disc means the jelly-like substance in between the vertebrae that provides cushioning to the spine and prevents friction has slid from its mooring, and part of it extends beyond the body of the vertebra. You probably won't know if you have a herniated disc unless it presses on a nerve. Sciatic pain may come from a disc or from a problem in the sciatic notch of the hip. So nerve pain doesn't necessarily mean that a disc is injured.

Disc herniation is incredibly common. Most people over the age of thirty with *no history of back pain* will show some disc herniations on an MRI. This odd fact does logically imply that the cause of back pain is not necessarily related to the disc. As I mentioned earlier (chapter 12), these studies have led different practitioners in various directions. On the one hand, there is John Sarno, M.D., who wrote the famous book, *Healing Back Pain: The Mind-Body Connection.* However, I have found that approaching back pain from a purely psychological perspective does not work for many people. Perhaps the location of the herniation is the crucial factor or perhaps, as one school of physical therapists believes, the strength of the spinal stabilizers, especially the deep multifidus muscle, is the most important factor in back pain. Also as mentioned earlier, Jim Johnson, P.T., wrote several excellent books with easy-to-follow exercises for back and neck pain, including *The Multifidus Back Pain Solution: Simple Exercises that Target the Muscles that Count.* He quotes studies that show that back pain is much more clearly correlated to multifidus strength than to disc herniation.

I'm more inclined to believe this; studies back Jim Johnson up, and I've never had a client who was a dropout from his program, whereas I've had a lot who failed with the Sarno program. The sad thing is that the dropouts from Sarno's program often feel like they are lamentable failures and psychologically unhealthy. It's bad enough to have that kind of pain without blaming yourself for it.

So if you have the misfortune to have herniated a disc that causes pain, here are your main options.

Option 1: Wait it out—under the care of a good health professional, of course. You probably need to rest a lot and do stabilization exercises. Swimming and biking can be fine exercise too, but probably not walking or running. Eventually—weeks to months—the bulge in the disc will break off and be reabsorbed in the body, and the nerve impingement will stop.

In the meantime, these things may help:

- Rest in a horizontal position, so the disc is not compressed
- Treatment with a good chiropractor trained in kinesiology, or an osteopath
- Stabilization exercise
- Visualization and relaxation practices
- A good nutritional program
- Fasting
- Muscle Activation Technique, a method that reestablishes proper neuro-muscular function by getting our muscles to fire properly
- Good soft tissue work (excellent acupuncture, massage, or bodywork)
- Avoidance of forward bending (which won't feel good), lifting things, carrying stuff, sitting and standing for long periods
- Be patient

Option 2: If the pain is more serious and disabling (this is mostly your call, although some nerve pressures that involve bladder or bowel control require emergency medical treatment), you can choose the more invasive approaches. Of those, traction, as in the DRX9000 treatment described below, is the least invasive. The manufacturers of this spinal compression machine describe their product like this:

> The DRX9000 is a non-surgical, non-invasive procedure that was developed for the treatment of lower back pain caused by disc herniations and degenerative

disc disease. The process is effective in relieving low back pain by enlarging intradiscal space, reducing herniation, strengthening outer ligaments to help move herniated areas back into place, and reversing high intradiscal pressures through application of negative pressure.*

Obviously, the website will tout the benefits of the DRX9000. There are drawbacks, however, especially the fact that you are moving the vertebra in one area of the spine forcibly apart without taking into account what is happening in the rest of the spine or the soft tissues. You may correct the disc situation and still be in pain, or be in pain somewhere else. I'd still try this before the third option.

Option 3: Surgery. Studies show that although surgery will relieve pain short term, the long-term prognosis is not so good. There are considerable risks, including infection, when the body is opened up. Even if you do opt for surgery, you will still need to strengthen the spinal stabilizers. The great disadvantage of any back surgery is that you will create a fusion of sorts in the spinal column that is irreparable. There will be less mobility and the spine will be permanently shorter.

You may be wondering why surgery wouldn't actually open up the spinal space instead of closing it. And sure enough, there is an experimental surgical procedure that does exactly that. It's in the beginning stages now, but I believe this does offer real hope for back pain sufferers.

If your pain is not serious enough to require constant pain medication, I would go with option 1—waiting it out—first. Whatever you decide, work with a competent health professional, and tune in to your inner wisdom—it's easy to be swayed by strong opinions when you are in a lot of pain.

*Axiom Worldwide's website: http://axiomworldwide.com/Products.aspx

13

Psoas, Hips, and Pelvis

PSOAS

The psoas (pronounced *so-as*) is the deep abdominal muscle that connects the upper and lower body, just as the scalenes connect head to torso. It is a diagonal muscle that starts at the inside of the lumbar spine and ends at the hip joint (see fig. 8.6 on page 114). The main movement the psoas facilitates is walking, but it can (and often does) substitute for the quads and the abdominals in other movements.

One sign that your psoas is doing the work of other muscles is if crunches or other abdominal exercises hurt your lower and midback. That means the psoas is contracting more than any other muscle and pulling the lumbar spine down as it shortens. That will lead to lower back problems. Usually the psoas needs to be stretched and the other deep abdominal muscles strengthened.

You need to stretch your psoas if:

1. You have a swayback (pronounced lumbar curve).
2. You wear down shoes more on the outside edge or you have turned-out feet. This distorts the hip joint, which will compromise your psoas.
3. You walk down steps with your feet turned out.
4. You have lower back pain.
5. You have weak abs.
6. You prefer to cross your legs when sitting in a chair. Especially if you favor one leg. Again, hip distortion.
7. You sometimes find it hard to breathe. Psoas is also involved with the diaphragm, and if a tight psoas pulls the lumbar spine down and in, it limits the flexibility of the diaphragm.

8. You have any knee problems or have had a knee injury. The more flexibility you have in your hips, the less stress there will be on your knee joints.

9. You sit a lot. The lumbar spine starts to compress if you spend a lot of time sitting in a chair, and the psoas will shorten.

10. You wear high heels. The forward position of the thighs will tip the weight of your torso onto the front of your psoas, near the hip joint, and create a swayback.

🍃 *Psoas Stretches*

Start by opening the groin and the quads in order to access the deeper parts of the psoas.

◈ Psoas Stretch I

1. Lie on your back, knees apart, and soles of feet together, in a diamond shape. You can vary the stretch by bringing your feet closer to your groin, or farther away. The heels should be together and in line with the perineum (fig. 13.1).

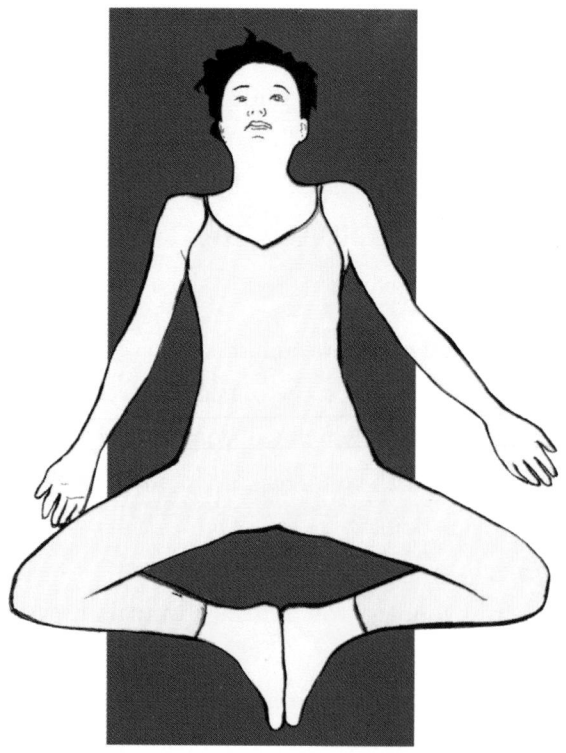

Fig. 13.1. Psoas Stretch I

Notice if one leg is closer to the ground than the other—it probably is. Then look at your feet. Join the soles of the feet together so your big toes, pads of big toes, and heels meet exactly. This will probably change your hip alignment, but it may create some muscular effort in your legs. You can tie your feet together with a yoga strap if it does.

2. If the soles of the feet are perfectly aligned, the hips should automatically become more even. If this doesn't happen and there is still a discrepancy between the two sides, place a pillow under the knee that is closer to the ground (the more open hip), until the sides are even.

3. Stay in this stretch for at least one minute, preferably longer—as long as you like—with your gaze point at the ceiling.

◈ Psoas Stretch II

1. Lie on your stomach with the soles of your feet joined together and your knees apart, in a diamond shape. Scoot your torso away from your legs by sliding it forward with your arms so the hip points (iliac crests) touch the floor, or come as close as possible (fig. 13.2).

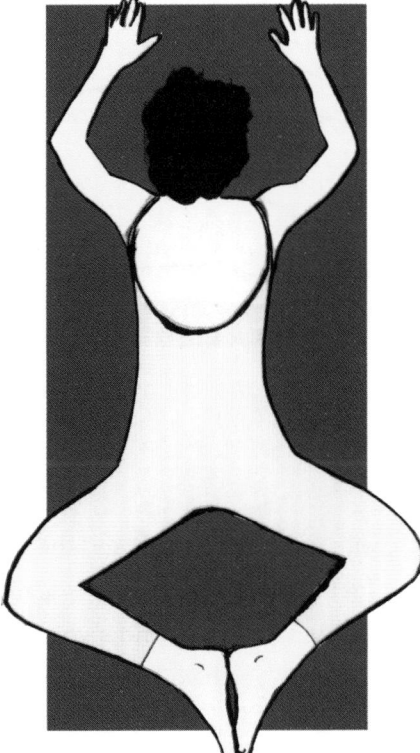

Fig. 13.2. Psoas Stretch II

2. Look down at yourself to check that the heels are in line with the groin, your torso is centered over your legs, and your knees are even. Your feet will probably be way off the ground. That's normal.

3. If you want to intensify the stretch, bring one foot on top of the other and press down. Then reverse feet. If you want still more of a stretch in the groin, bring your hands by your chest, about at the nipple line, palms down. Press your hands down into the ground and isometrically toward your feet (don't move your hands, though). You can then lift your groin off the floor, keeping the legs and feet in the same diamond shape. Your gaze point is either straight in front of you or, if you can backbend comfortably, at the ceiling. Make sure your tailbone is dropped and soft, and keep your lower back long.

4. There should be no tight or constricted feeling in the back. If there is, press more toward your feet with your hands, bringing your chest forward, and suck in your navel slightly.

5. If there is still lower-back pressure, back out of the position. Come out the way you came in: lower the groin and torso to the floor, and then move your feet and knees apart and stretch back. Then fold over your bent knees to give your back a forward or counterstretch (fig. 13.3).

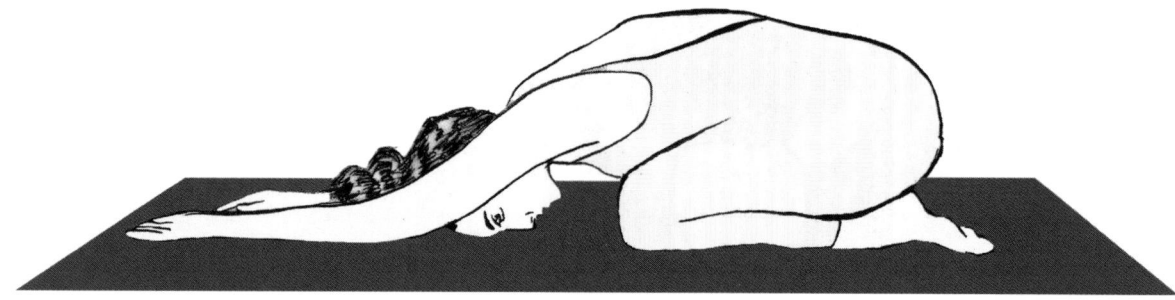

Fig. 13.3. Counter stretch

◈ Psoas Stretch III

1. Lie on your forearms and stomach, with your knees apart and the thighs at right angles to your body (fig. 13.4). Your feet should be in line with the middle part of the thigh, with the toes flexed. You may need padding under your knees. Rest on your forearms, letting the tailbone drop. Don't arch your back. Bring the tailbone back toward your feet to increase the stretch.

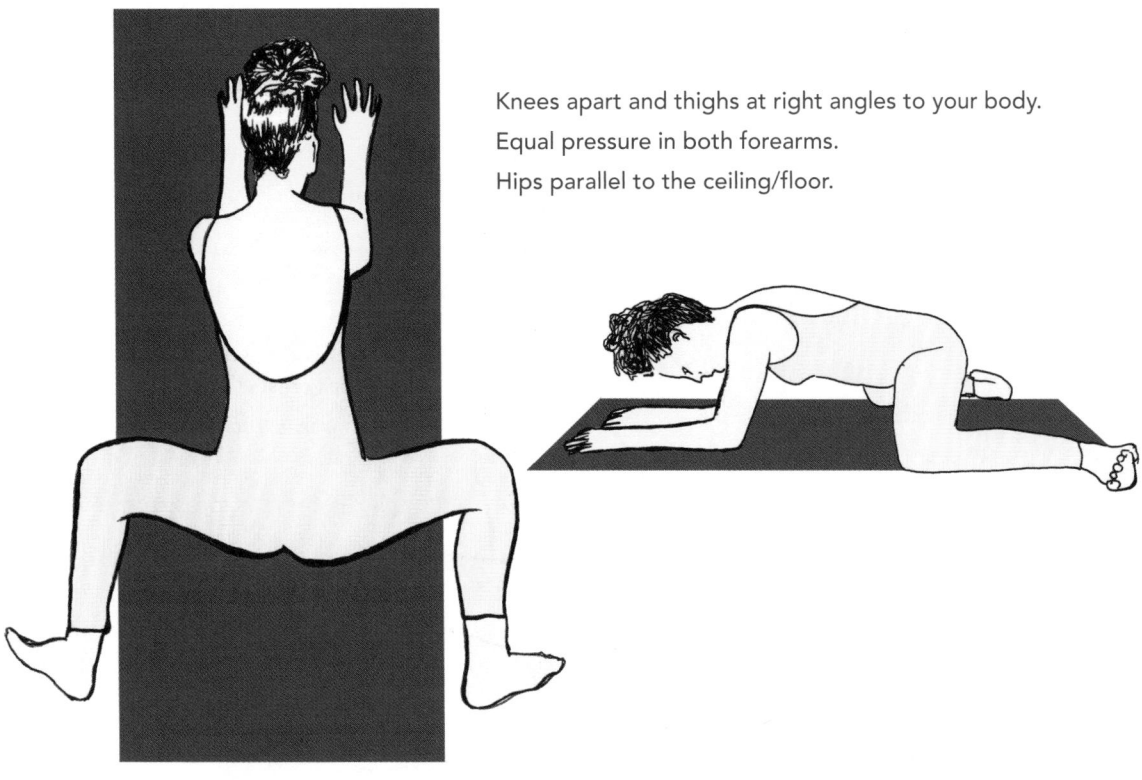

Knees apart and thighs at right angles to your body.
Equal pressure in both forearms.
Hips parallel to the ceiling/floor.

Fig. 13.4. Psoas Stretch III

2. Now look at your knees to make sure they are lined up with each other and your torso is right in the middle, not tilting over to the right or left. There should be equal pressure in both forearms. Place one hand on your sacrum to check that your hips are parallel to the ceiling. You probably will not feel an equal stretch in both groins even in a correct alignment, since it's unlikely that your hips are equally tight.

3. You can place a bolster under your groin for a supported version of this stretch. The bolster, rolled-up towel or blanket, or whatever you use should support just the groin, not the thighs, and should preferably be fairly soft, so that as you sink into it, it will open up your body.

4. If the stretch is excruciating (it can be), try it supported. Stretches that create a burning sensation in the area that is being released are stretching fascia as well as muscle—which is good, but since fascia does not stretch as readily as muscle, more support and gentleness are necessary.

❖ Psoas Stretch IV

1. To further open the psoas, start by coming into a lunge position, one leg in front of the other (fig. 13.5). Keep the knee over the ankle in front.

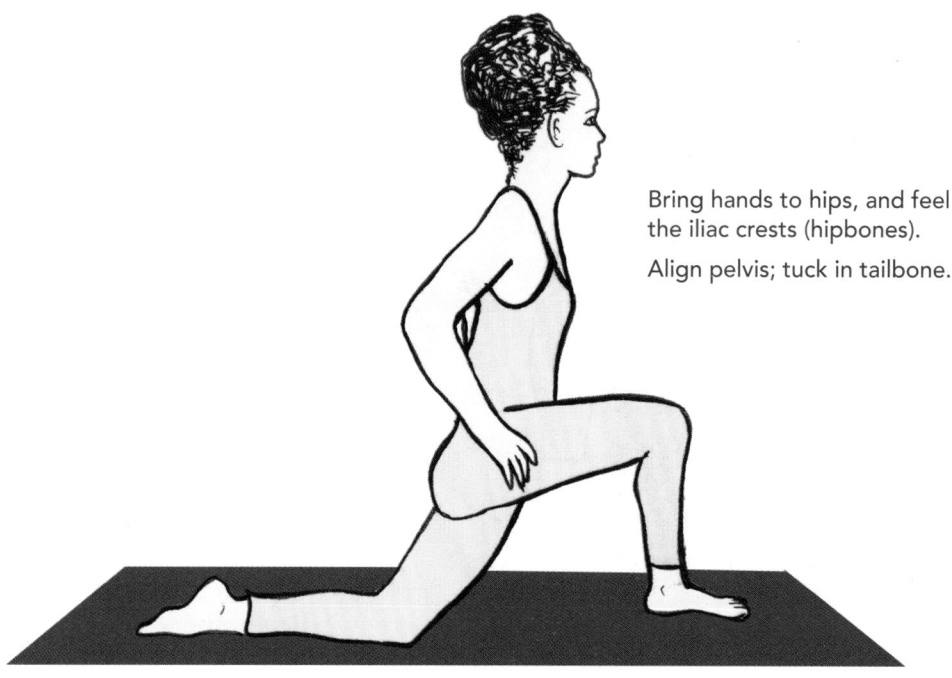

Bring hands to hips, and feel the iliac crests (hipbones).

Align pelvis; tuck in tailbone.

Fig. 13.5. Psoas Stretch IV

Bring your hands to the hips, and feel the iliac crests. You'll probably find that the hipbone on the side of the leg with the knee on the ground wants to move back away from you and may be angled down, so that the top of the crest is more forward than the bottom. This means the pelvis is tipping and rotated, preventing the psoas from opening.

2. Even up your hips, even if you can't stretch deeply any longer. Use your hands to turn the pelvis so that the right and left crests are in line, and straighten the angle of the pelvis so there is no tipping. This will mean slightly tucking in your tailbone.

3. Move into a deeper stretch slowly by dropping the hips slightly without losing alignment; you may find that, if you can keep your pelvis even, your spine now compensates, probably by arching so the front lower ribs stick out more, and the back shortens and pulls forward.

◈ Psoas Stretch V

1. Place your hand on the knee in front of you, and bring your spine into alignment by pressing back gently.
2. Pull the belly away from the thigh in front by tightening your abdominals and pulling up your pubic bone (fig. 13.6). Make sure your spine stays long, and keep your neck in line with the rest of your spine.

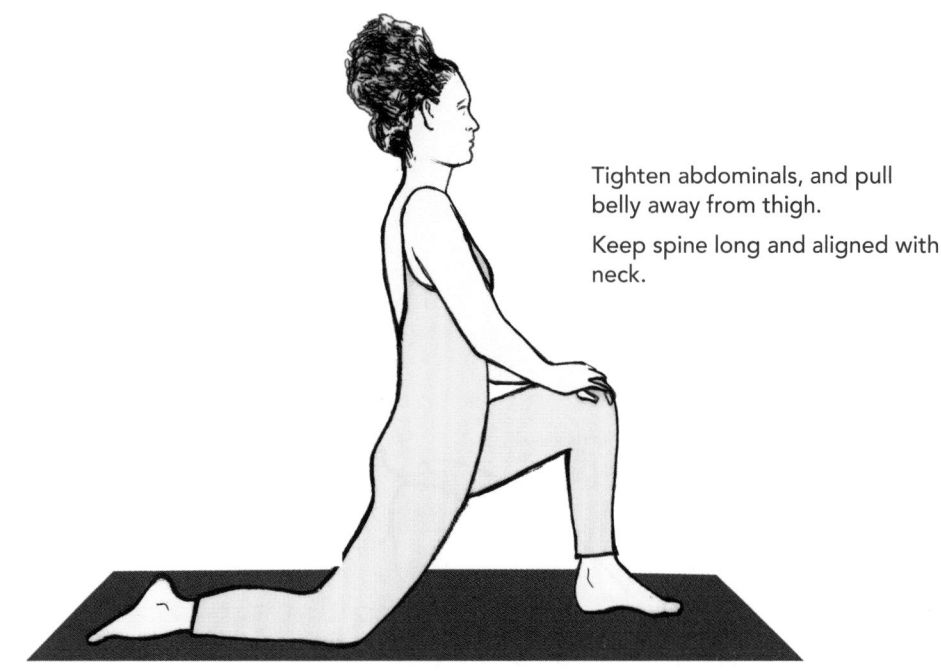

Tighten abdominals, and pull belly away from thigh.

Keep spine long and aligned with neck.

Fig. 13.6. Psoas Stretch V

🌿 Advanced Psoas Stretch

Do this one only after warming up with the previous stretches, even if you are very flexible. Make sure that you do not feel any compression, and back out of the position if you do. If the knee is uncomfortable, use lots of padding under it and stretch the quads more before you do this stretch.

1. Bring your knee back to a wall with your shin vertical and pressing against the wall. Use some padding under the knee. The knee should be pretty much flush against the wall, depending on the shape of your kneecap, but not more than 2 inches away. The shin maintains a slight pressure against the wall the whole time—this position will release your groin and protect your lower back.

2. Place the other foot in front of you on the floor, knee bent, about hip width away from the foot on the wall. Make sure the thigh is straight between hip and knee and does not angle in or out (the hip will probably want to move outward, away from your body). The ankle should be directly under the knee. Your hips and back are away from the wall, your hands on the ground (fig. 13.7).

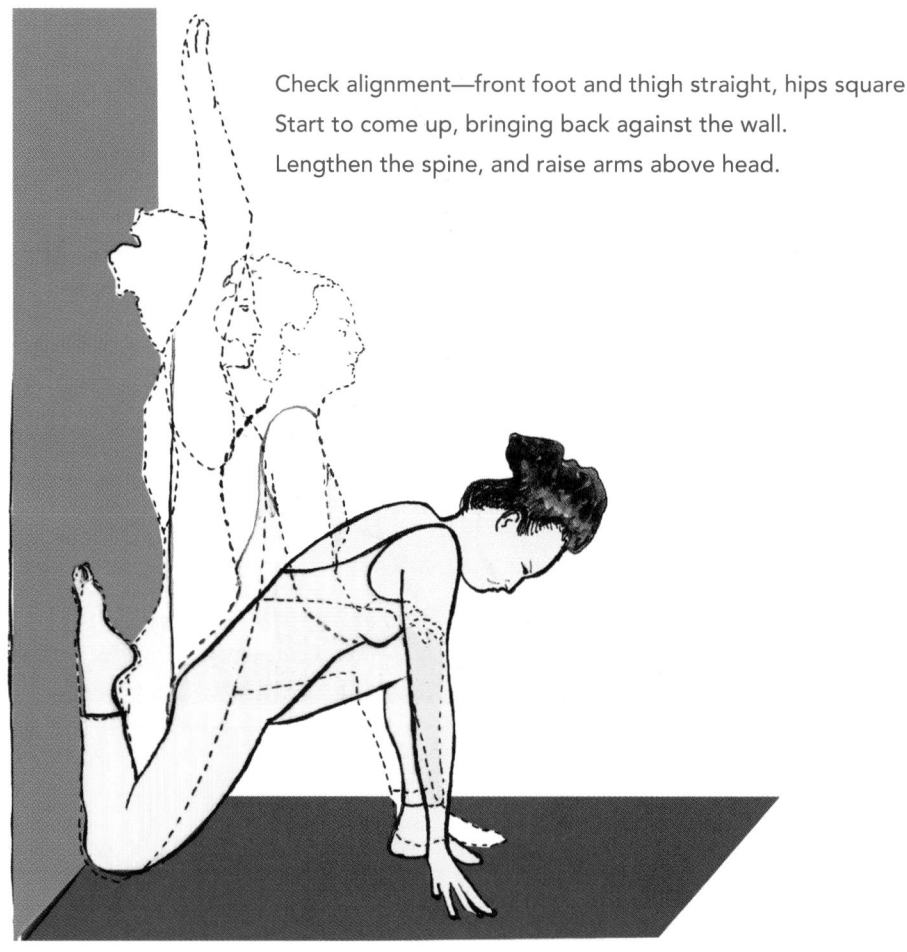

Check alignment—front foot and thigh straight, hips square.
Start to come up, bringing back against the wall.
Lengthen the spine, and raise arms above head.

Fig. 13.7. Advanced Psoas Stretch

3. Now check your alignment—front foot straight, slight pressure into the ground at the pad of the big toe, thigh straight, hips square, back shin vertical, and top of foot flat against the wall. Put padding between your foot and the wall if your foot is uncomfortable. Make sure the thighs and hips of the leg against the wall are straight.

4. Now start to come up, eventually bringing your back almost flat against the wall. First, lengthen the spine. Try to bring your hand to your front knee. If that's too difficult, you could place a chair on the inside of the knee and use that. You can also start to walk the hands back, keeping them on the ground. Make sure your torso faces front squarely. Walking the hands back can be tricky, depending on the relative length of arms and torso—you could place yoga blocks under the hands to make it easier.

5. As you move back, think of bringing the pubic bone up toward the navel, slightly tightening your lower abdominals. Keep lengthening the spine. The trick to achieving this opening successfully is in the foundation of it. Your forward foot should press into the floor, sending your pelvis back toward the wall and pressing your shin into the wall and knee and down into the floor. This will give your body the support you need to release further.

6. If this feels good to you and you can get your hips to the wall comfortably, move your front foot forward. Check your alignment, lengthen your back, thigh, and spine a lot, and move back until your back is on the wall. It should be almost flush, with a slight lumbar curve (see fig. 13.7). Lengthen your side body, and bring your arms above your head.

7. To correct an anterior tilt to the pelvis (that's when the top of the hipbones is farther forward than the bottom), tuck the tailbone under, lengthen the front of the thighs a lot, and bring the top of the sacrum to the wall. To help you, you can press the tailbone away from the wall with one hand and lift up the pubic bone with the other.

8. Now adjust your front foot forward, letting the hips dip away from the wall. You can bring your hands to the floor to do this. Push the shin of the back leg against the wall and press the front heel into the ground. Your hands can be on the floor, on blocks, or on your knee. Lengthen the spine, and move the pubic bone toward the navel to make sure your back isn't arching too much. Lengthen your side body and stretch the arms above your head, palms facing each other.

9. Square the shoulders, check alignment, and, if you want, move into a backbend with the arms by the ears. To take the backbend even farther, bring your hands to the wall behind you over your head, with fingertips pointing down, wrists on the wall, and push away from the wall with your hands. This will engage the upper back muscles, which will open up the psoas more.

10. Repeat on the other side. The gaze point is straight ahead, with shoulders squared or very slightly to the opposite side.

🍂 *Three Modified Psoas Stretches*

◈ Modified Psoas Stretch I

1. Lie on your back, and bring one knee to your chest. The other leg is straight on the floor, foot flexed and knee facing the ceiling.

2. Bring the knee on your chest to the opposite shoulder until you feel compression in the groin. Drop the hip as much as you can, letting the head of the femur stay in the socket. This doesn't feel like a stretch at all—it's more like a squeezing sensation—but it is, and it can relieve back spasms (fig. 13.8).

Bring knee on your chest to opposite shoulder until you feel compression in the groin.

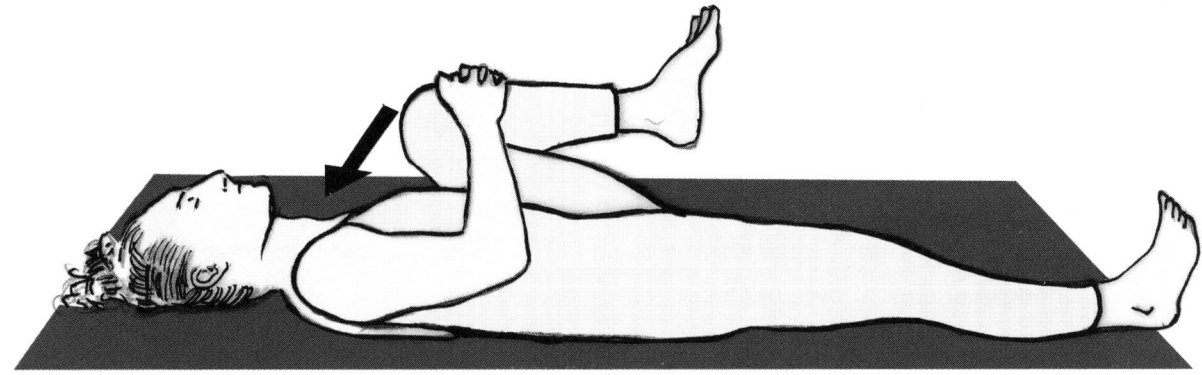

Fig. 13.8. Modified Psoas Stretch I

3. If you have any pain in the hip, place a rolled-up cloth, about 2 inches thick, in the crease of the groin. Repeat on the other side.

◈ Modified Psoas Stretch II

You can also lie on your back and bring both knees to your chest, the knees as close together as possible. You should feel some compression in the groin area. Hold your knees there, and pull your tailbone down into the floor and away from your groin, until the compressed feeling releases.

◈ Modified Psoas Stretch III

Many lower back stretches and some inner thigh stretches will lengthen parts of the psoas. The best, most complete stretch for the psoas requires a surface that you can lie on and that also has a drop of at least three feet, preferably more. A kitchen counter, a table, or even a high bed will do. Make sure it is stable before you start.

1. Lie on your back with the edge of the table at the very top of your thighs, just below the buttocks. Pull your right knee to your chest with your leg bent, and let the left leg drop (fig. 13.9). You will feel the stretch on the left side in the groin, through the abdomen, and maybe in the lower back. You can put a weight on your left leg or have someone push it down for a greater stretch.

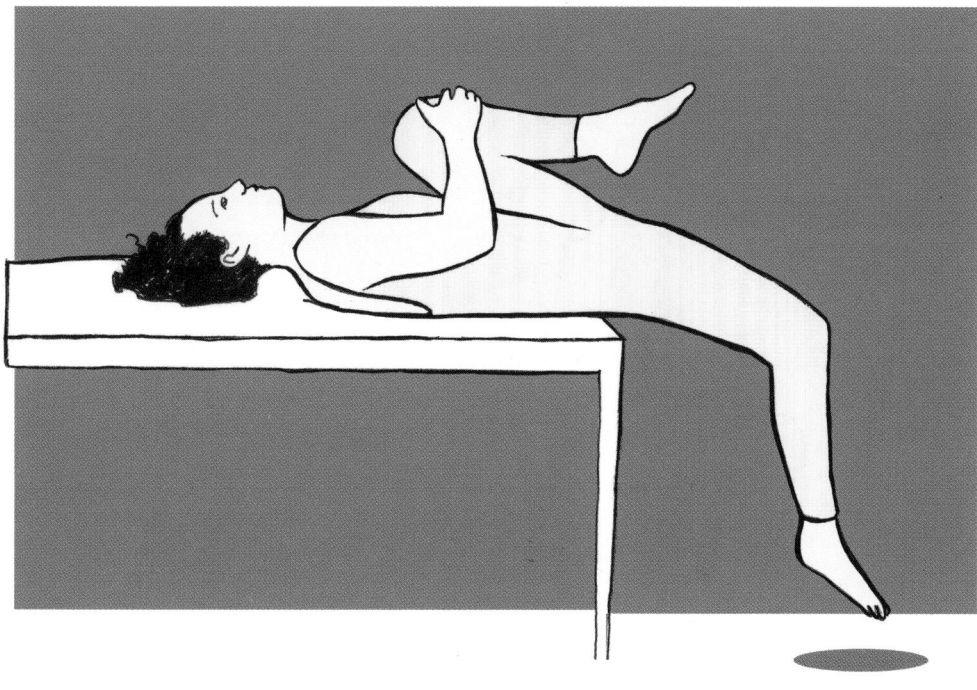

Fig.13.9. Modified Psoas Stretch III

2. Then pull the left leg to the chest, and let the right leg drop for a stretch to the right psoas.
3. Come out of the stretch by bending both knees to the chest and rolling to one side.

🍃 Psoas Strengthening Exercise

The psoas can become so tight that it actually weakens. I was always told that the psoas muscle remains strong because we use it all the time in walking. This isn't true.

The portion of the psoas that connects into the spine can become very weak if there are spinal faults that cause misalignment there. The psoas will tighten to protect the spine in that area and may become immobile and therefore weak.

1. For this exercise use a heavyish gauge of TheraBand, cut quite long. Stand with your pelvis and back against a wall, with the band looped under one foot and over the other knee (fig. 13.10).

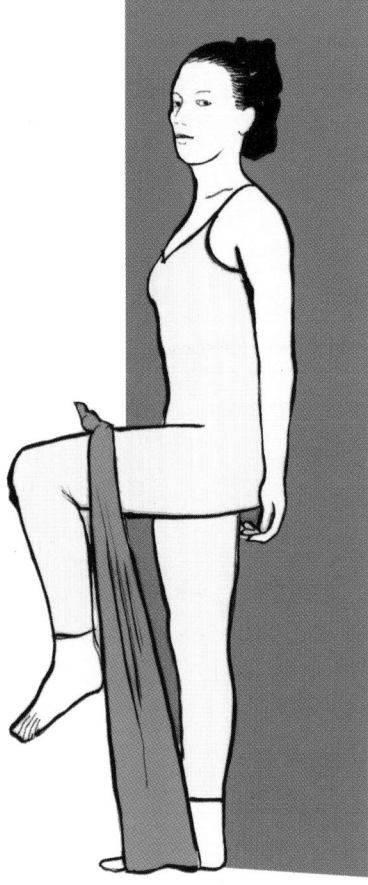

Press back against wall; lift knee as high as possible

Hold for 10 seconds; release.

Repeat until fatigued.

Switch sides.

Fig. 13.10. Psoas Strengthening Exercise

2. Press your back slightly against the wall and lift the knee up as high as you can. The knee stays bent. Do this very slowly, taking about 10 seconds, and release down. Repeat till your muscles fatigue. Then repeat on the other side.

3. Start on the weak side, shift to the strong side, and then back to the weak side again.

🍃 Psoas Exercise for Lower Back Pain

1. Sit with your legs straight out in front of you and your back against a wall. Turn the legs out (fig. 13.11). This engages the psoas. You can do this exercise with legs turned in, to engage your quads and possibly abdominals.

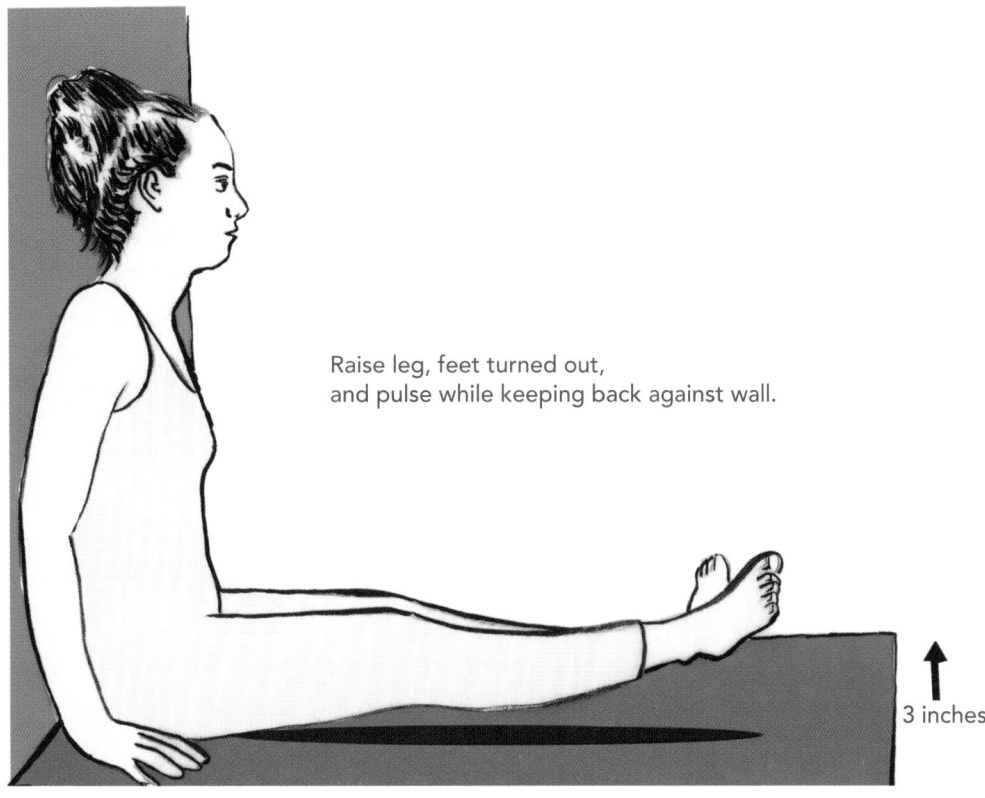

Raise leg, feet turned out, and pulse while keeping back against wall.

3 inches

Fig.13.11. Psoas Exercise for Lower Back Pain

2. Now lift and pulse one leg—making tiny movements up and down with your leg. Lift your leg only about 3 inches. Keep your back pressed against the wall.
3. If the pain is on one side, the chances are that the leg won't lift on that side. If you can't lift the leg on one or both sides, tie a strap around the leg and use the strap to pick up the leg about an inch from the floor. Now try to pulse from there.
4. Work one side until your muscles fatigue, and then work the other side. Work the weak side twice, the strong side just once. This exercise will pull up your belly and reposition your hip joints.

✿ Correcting the High Hip

This exercise will correct the problem of one side of the pelvis rotating farther forward than the other, when that distortion is caused by an imbalance in the psoas. If not corrected, this could contribute to lower back pain. You will see this imbalance show up when one leg turns out more than the other, especially when you lie on your back, and when one leg wants to step back behind the other. Usually the leg that turns out less and comes ahead of the other is the stronger one, and that is often the side we like to lean onto, the more stable side.

1. To check, lie on your back and feel your hip points. Notice if one side is closer to the ceiling than the other.

2. Now stand up, keep your feet parallel, your hips square, your toes straight, and your torso straight. Keep your hands firmly on your hip points, so you can prevent their moving, and then lift one leg with the foot flexed, not letting the leg turn out. Don't let the other hip jut out to the side or your head come forward.

3. Your head should be in line with the spine (and don't lean back or forward). Keep the hip of the raised leg dropped down and level with the other hip. In other words, the torso stays as it was when you began; the only change is in the raised leg. This alignment makes the position much harder and focuses it more in the part of the psoas closest to the spine.

4. If one leg rises up farther and you can hold the position more easily on that side, then do the exercises with the other leg. If you can barely raise either leg, do it with both legs alternately. Just raise the weak leg once with correct alignment, and hold it. You could pulse the leg slightly about an inch up and down. Try to hold 90 seconds.

5. Now stand with your back on a wall, feet hip width apart and parallel, your feet a comfortable distance away from the wall. Again, bring your hands to your hips. Hold them and your torso firmly against the wall. Now raise one leg, as before. You will notice that you want to tip to one side. Your head, shoulders, and hips will want to move. Your head may come forward, your jaw tighten.

    Your goal is to isolate the movement in the leg so that there is no shifting or tightening in your torso at all. Until you have achieved that through strengthening the deeper muscles, you can help yourself get there by pressing back against the wall, pressing the standing foot firmly into the ground, and going very slowly. Don't be surprised if it is impossible for you to raise the leg at all while you do this.

6. Alternate the freestanding leg lift with this version; you may notice the psoas on one side is stronger when you lean against the wall or the reverse. This is because you are using slightly different muscles. For the wall version, always do both sides. Pulsing is not necessary.

You may notice that the hip that was closer to the ceiling, or more raised toward your head, when you checked it lying on your back, is the weaker or stronger one. That depends on the balance of stabilizing and directly activated muscles. However, after doing this exercise, lie on your back and check your hips again, as you did before. Notice any changes. The balance of the hips should be more even now. If you get more uneven, check that: (1) your body was really still and aligned (that's the most common mistake); (2) you raised the legs equally high (if possible); (3) you are checking, or did previously check, correctly.

🍃 *Correcting Pelvic Rotation and Spinal Movement*

◈ Correcting Pelvic Rotation I

1. Stand on your heels with your arms straight out in front (fig. 13.12).

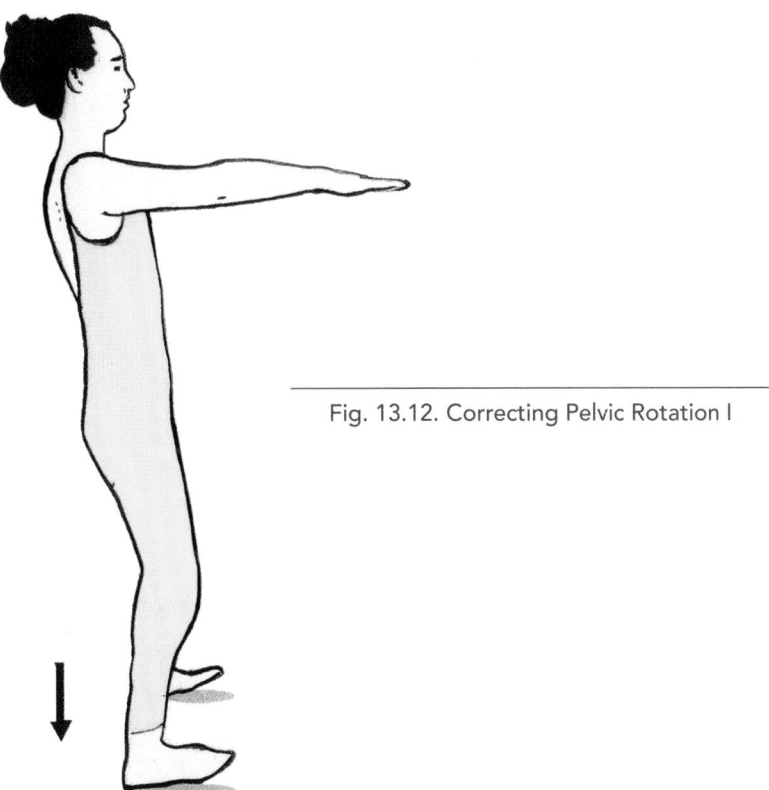

Fig. 13.12. Correcting Pelvic Rotation I

2. This is difficult for most people. If you have an anterior tilt to your pelvis (swayback), you may want to stick your behind out and lean forward to balance—which actually won't work. Instead, walk on your heels, moving as little as possible. Just focus on aiming to stop moving and simply balancing. Or you can modify by touching a wall in front of you. Do this for up to five minutes to correct the pelvic rotation.

◈ Correcting Pelvic Rotation II

1. Stand on your tiptoes with your arms at your sides (fig. 13.13).

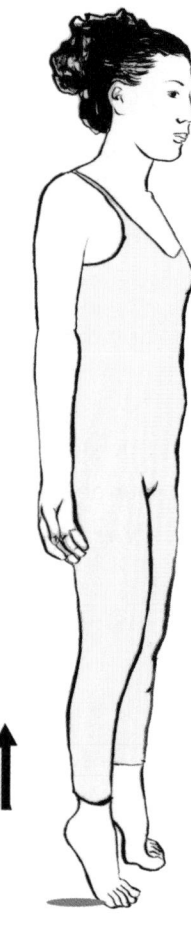

Fig. 13.13. Correcting Pelvic Rotation II

2. This is easier for most people. When it becomes more difficult (or if it is shaky right away), you will probably tend to balance by falling to the outside of your feet. Most of us rely on the outer part of the leg, which causes misalignment in the ball-and-socket joint of the thighbone. The outer portion of the pelvis

contains part of the internal rotators of the joint, so if our weight falls to the outside of the foot too much, we will tighten the hips at the inside. Press the balls of the big toes down to balance the muscles at the inside and outside of the hips.

3. The challenge here is to stay as long as you can in this position. Close your eyes for an extra challenge.

4. To balance more easily, bring your awareness to your tailbone (see fig. 2.16 on page 38). If you can keep the sacrum still—and you will only be able to do this if your torso is centered correctly over your pelvis—you will be able to stay up much more easily. To still the sacrum, imagine a quiet pond. Use your imagination, and the rest will follow.

5. Then think of lifting your rib cage, back and front, up away from your hips, lengthening the side of your body. The pelvis and hips press down slightly into the ground; the upper body rises from its stable base. The more you can achieve this, the easier it will be to move your upper body without losing balance.

LEGS, HIPS, AND PSOAS IN RELATION TO GRAVITY

Awareness and control of the psoas and the other deep pelvic muscles can help you feel how movements are supported from deep inside your body and give you a core strength that will let you consciously release tight peripheral muscles, such as your jaw, neck, shoulders, and so on.

If our lower body is not supporting us properly, we tend to pull up with our shoulders and tighten our neck muscles to keep upright, pulling away from gravity instead of releasing into it. The whole upper body should be able to relax fully and safely over the pelvis and legs, so that the upper back and shoulder muscles are free for movement. The muscles of the upper body are smaller, designed to transfer weight down the spine, not support it.

When you stand in a relaxed position, feet straight, knees soft, shoulders relaxed, you should be able to rock the pelvis back and forth slightly, using your tailbone, without engaging other muscles. You should be able to keep the knees in the same position relative to your toes (look down briefly to check), and the torso above the pelvis should be stationary. See if rocking the pelvis with the awareness of the psoas and its path through the inside of your body makes it easier to isolate.

✿ *Exploring Your Relationship with Gravity*

Try this exercise to explore the relationship of your legs, hips, and psoas with gravity.

1. Stand on one leg, and lift the other leg straight up in the air, as high as you can. Both hips must be level and even, and your torso should not change position (fig. 13.14).

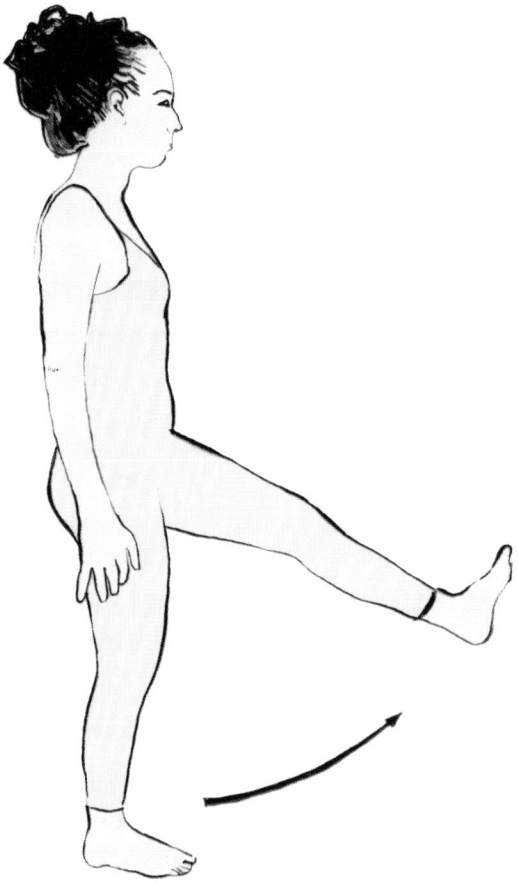

Fig. 13.14. Exploring Your Relationship with Gravity

2. The leg, for this purpose, is straight. Hold as high as you can for as long as you can. The raised leg must not rotate out or in, so keep the raised foot at a perfect right angle to the leg.
3. Repeat on the other side. Notice the differences.
4. Now stand on the original leg, and bring the leg straight out to the side, again

with the foot straight. Notice how high you can raise the leg without changing the original position of the hips.

5. Repeat on the other side, noting differences.

6. Now repeat the sequence, this time consciously using your abdominals to lift up out of the hips, while pressing your standing leg down firmly and evenly into the ground. Notice the relationship between your pelvis and the ground. Your pelvis becomes the "ground" for your torso, as the floor grounds your foot. Does this awareness change the exercise at all?

THE PELVIC FLOOR

The pelvic floor is a kyo area for the vast majority of adults. It is often not very responsive, a neurologically disconnected zone, which can lead to problems in other parts of the body, as other muscles have to take over the work of keeping us upright. You can see this if you watch people walking. Most people pull up into their pelvis, almost as though they are carrying their pelvis with their upper body. It appears stuck, not fluid and connected to their movement. It is weak, tight, disconnected, and unconscious for a number of reasons, including physical and emotional stress and trauma, shallow breathing, and the reliance we have on chairs.

There is increasing awareness of the damage that the modern sedentary, chair-oriented, lifestyle causes, and there is an attempt to address this through standing desks and various exercise systems. Chairs, particularly when sitting in them is our dominant movement pattern, become a "prosthetic pelvis" or "hip replacement." If you observe the way that many people walk as they become hunched over in old age, it looks as though they are still in the shape of the chair, as though it has become welded to the body and they are dragging it behind. This is one of the ways we lose mobility, strength, and connection to the support from our pelvis for our spine and head. Remember that the spine extends inside the skull and the skull is slotted onto the top vertebra. The weight of the head needs to be supported through the whole spine; the spine is in turn supported by the elastic, cushy muscles of the pelvic floor.

On a societal level, the pelvic floor is a deep kyo because sensation in the area, which connects to the genitals and the anus, is relegated almost exclusively to the realm of sexuality and bowel and urinary functions. These muscles are not allowed to experience much sensation in breath and movement. They are compartmentalized and often, subtly or not so subtly, regarded as shameful and tied up with any negative sexual experiences. There is a natural urge to protect the genitals; however, this does not require our becoming cut off from sensation in breath and movement or from a vital energetic and nerve center.

The deep tension around the area that I see in most people actually makes us more vulnerable, because the muscles become weak and inelastic. The pelvic floor is then unable to support the movement of the hips and smaller movements of the bones in the pelvis, which become stiff, leading to the ubiquitous lower back pain and the head moving farther and farther forward of the pelvis with age. The head coming forward draws us away from our center of gravity, and this makes us much more vulnerable to falls. Supporting the head from the pelvic floor, in addition to cultivating awareness of the tailbone as a stability point, will increase balance immensely, making both the young and elderly less vulnerable to injury.

✤ Working with Your Pelvic Floor

The first step to approaching any kyo area is to bring gentle awareness to it. Attention needs to be paid to the release and the contraction of the pelvic floor, which is a diamond-shaped area defined by four bony landmarks—the two sit bones, the pubic bone, and the coccyx (tailbone). A muscular "sling" extends across the area and divides it into two triangles.*

1. You can begin with the breath, which is in constant dialogue with the pelvic floor. As you inhale slowly and steadily, preferably through your nose, see if you can feel the muscles of the pelvic floor gently filling and descending through the bones of your pelvis.

   The downward movement (engagement) of the breathing diaphragm nudges the abdominal organs slightly downward and the pelvic floor relaxes and descends to make more space in the abdomen. Imagine the pelvic "sling" softening and gently supporting your organs. Think of the bony landmarks of the pelvis expanding away from each other as you inhale.

2. As you exhale, the breathing diaphragm relaxes upward and the pelvic floor engages very slightly to support the exhalation (the muscles are in an agonist-antagonist relationship, so conscious relaxation and engagement in the pelvic floor will help with excess tension in the diaphragm—this is crucial for singers).

---

*Bond, *The New Rules of Posture,* 58.

Try consciously engaging the pelvic floor as you exhale, this may be easier to feel if you exhale through your mouth. See if you can feel the difference between the front and the back of the pelvic floor. Release any extra tension in the back portion and feel the engagement more in the front.

I like the image that physical therapist Deborah Bowes uses in her wonderful and clear audio guide to accessing the pelvic floor.* She describes the sensation as being as if you are drawing a silk scarf up through your pelvic floor as you engage. I prefer this to the classic description of doing a "Kegel," which, however, is another way to access these muscles. I like the image of the scarf because it is gradual and more of an upward engagement; it also may be less panicky for some people. For men, it can be more helpful to imagine the perineum between the scrotum and anus drawing upward. The idea is the same; there is a relaxation as you inhale and a gradual, subtle engagement on the exhalation, especially at the end of the exhalation.

3. See if you can relax your throat and tongue, allowing your soft palate to lift slightly away from the pelvic floor as you inhale. As the pelvic floor muscles descend on the inhalation, see if you can feel how the soft palate lifts, creating more space through the breathing space and the whole body. Take 10 breaths like this, slow and steady, feeling the rhythm and relationship between the soft palate, the breathing diaphragm, and the pelvic floor.

When you are sitting, the soft palate, the muscular "roof" of your spine inside your skull, should be aligned over the pelvic floor, the muscular "floor" of your spine. Actively engage with any surface you sit on, whether it is the floor or a chair, lengthening the soft palate up from the support of the pelvic floor, pressing your sit bones slightly into your seat and lengthening through your spine. In other words, even if you are using a chair, engage your internal support, rather than allowing the chair to usurp this function. If you can sit in a full squat, this is a great stretch for the pelvic floor. If you cannot squat comfortably, you can hold onto the back of a chair and gradually ease into a modified squat.

In walking or running, imagine that the energy from the legs is being transmitted up through your pelvic floor, providing springy, resilient support for your movement. See if you can feel the ilium moving with your leg as you walk, opening up

---

*Deborah Bowes, *Pelvic Health and Awareness*.

the sacroiliac joint. This subtle movement can begin to happen as the pelvic floor muscles wake up, with profound effects through the whole body. The same rhythmic breathing pattern in step 3 of the exercise above applies in walking. See what it feels like to release into your pelvis, allowing the muscles to move, breathe, and support your whole upper body as you walk. You can incorporate pelvic floor engagement into any exercise you do; when you stretch, allow the stretch to travel up through your pelvic floor too.

Our societal kyo around the pelvic floor is being addressed by a number of people in the bodywork and movement worlds, contributing lots of valuable awareness and exercises. Please use helpful resources like Deborah Bowes's CD to guide you through awareness exercises. Working with your pelvic floor can be very emotional, so be aware of this. Any abuse or negative sexual experiences may come up. On a subtle level, there is a reconnection to your own life force that can be startling and unfamiliar. The need to control expression can result in a clamping down in this area, which may be completely unconscious. For thousands of years yogis have focused on the pelvic floor muscles as the trigger for *moola bandha*, the awakener of kundalini energy. This deep level of yoga is key to a more advanced yoga practice. As Swami Buddhananda puts it in his book, *Moola Bandha*:

> The perfection of moola bandha requires the development of an acute refinement of mental and psychic awareness that allows for the localization, isolation and contraction of mooladhara chakra. This is developed in the beginning through the physical contraction of the perineal body or the cervix as the case may be. We begin at the most accessible level, the tangible physical body. By combining physical contraction with mental awareness and visualization, we can then heighten our sensitivity on the psychic plane.*

If you already practice yoga, you can explore moola bandha and the fundamental life force of kundalini with an experienced teacher. I recommend reading *Moola Bandha* too. There is great energy locked up in the pelvis, and refined awareness and access to it can energize your creativity, spontaneity, sexuality, and your whole life.

*Swami Buddhananda, *Moola Bandha,* 65.

14

The Abdomen
and Vital Organs

MOST OF THE BOOKS I have on exercise and structural work don't mention the abdominal muscles except as a support for the back, which they are, of course, but they're a lot more. I consider the fascia and musculature in this area very important. Your vital organs (which are mostly muscle also) are housed within muscular sheaths, which hold them in the center of your body, embedded in a backing of connective tissue that is also connected to your spine.

Think about packing stuff into cardboard boxes for UPS. The molded Styrofoam backing that the objects wedge into is our connective tissue; the tape and the "peanuts" stuffing are the various muscles and fascia that keep us in our box (the skin). And just as we can receive a package from UPS that looks fine, if a bit battered from its journey, and then open it to find chaos inside, the physical journey we are on can shake up the visceral contents of our "box."

Our organs can prolapse, or move position; muscular walls can herniate; and tissues can wear away like old elastic. In evolving to the upright position, we created an uneven and rather unsound vector for gravity to work against, so in time, our organs tend to drop toward the pelvic basin. They will also drop forward as a result of our forward flexed posture (see page 32) and lack of support from the pelvic floor (see page 219).

Since blood and lymph flow, the peristaltic movement of the digestion, and the various connections between organs are all dependent on things being in the right place, the mechanical and structural aspect of organs vitally affect their function.

This is a factor that is rarely considered in our medical system, apart from the surgical repair of hernias, because we classify our bodies as containers of systems that are separate from one another, not as structures operating in the same location. We don't have this blindness in relation to any other objects in our lives—for example, you wouldn't think that part of a machine that is putting pressure on another part would have no influence on it. Classification by system is a useful way of narrowing our sights to more clearly define the function of each system as a separate unit, but it is quite unrealistic in actual practice. And we know this instinctively: "When my sinuses puff up, I can't see properly"; "When I play tennis, all that twisting bothers my stomach"; "Those Pilates mat classes have pinched in my diaphragm, I think"; and so on. I hear these kinds of complaints all the time. Now we need to take this understanding a step further and investigate how we can improve the functioning of our organs and our vital energy by working our muscles.

Other cultures understood this well. Yoga, for example, is designed to benefit the internal organs through twisting and holding positions in quite specific ways to influence glandular secretions and work peristaltic action. The Chinese located *chi*—vital energy—in the center of gravity, the *tan tien*, two inches below the belly button, and their qi gong and tai chi practices are based on the cultivation of chi by activating this and other vital centers and balancing them through muscular and breath work. In shiatsu and Japanese martial arts, the *hara* is vitally important.

You could achieve healing in the internal organs by going very deeply into these systems—and you'd achieve a great deal more in the process—but it would take years and much dedication. I've found that support of the organs to improve their function can be achieved quite easily just through some simple exercises and an understanding of how the body's core muscles work.

UNDERSTANDING THE ROLE OF CORE MUSCLES

Core muscles can be defined as any muscles that attach to the spine (there are many definitions of "core"). Since the spine is the body's main support, the muscles that control its movements directly provide most of our postural support (fig. 14.1). Take a look at the spine itself. Notice how big it is and how much space it occupies.

In the abdominal area in particular, the lumbar curve brings the front of the spine very close to the organs (see fig. 14.2 on page 226). The line that's formed by the front (anterior) of the spine, from the tailbone up to the middle of the skull, is

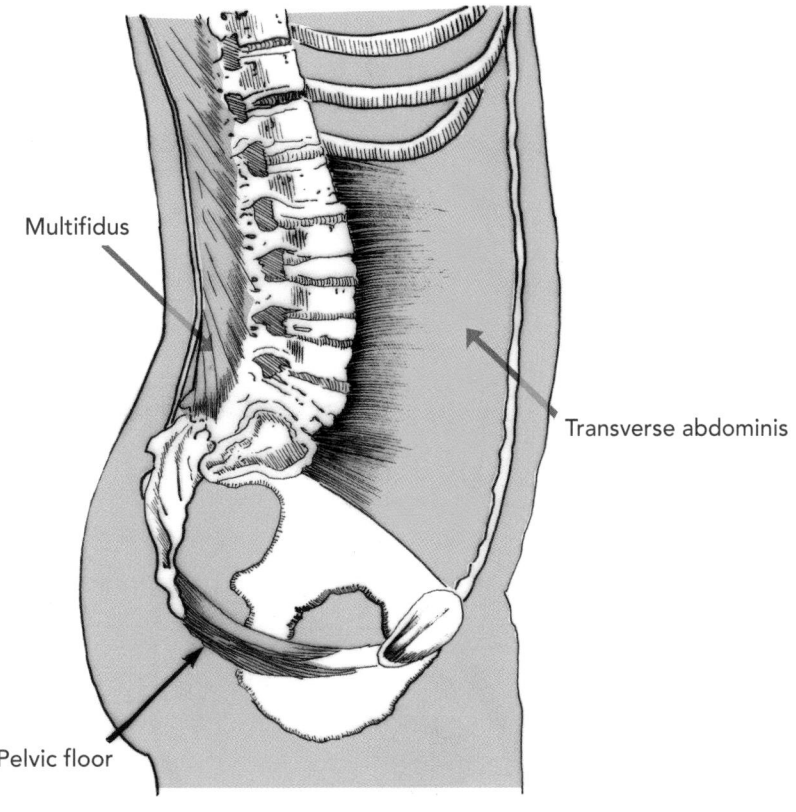

Multifidus

Transverse abdominis

Pelvic floor

Fig. 14.1. Muscles connecting to the spine

the main support of our body. Due to forward flexion (see fig. 2.11 on page 33) our organs tend to prolapse forward as we age, and the spine moves back, making our bodies thicker and creating a space between the anterior spine and the organs, where the connective and other tissues overstretch and lose tone.

People see this happening and start worrying about losing their flat stomach. They don't connect their reflux or constipation with their bulging bellies or aching backs. Instead, they'll do crunches or sit-ups or other abdominal exercises, all of which involve flexion of the abdominal muscles, rather than abdominal support. However, we seldom use abdominal flexion in real life. If you curl forward from an upright position, your abdomen is usually relaxed. So crunches and sit-ups work only a small part of the abdominal range of motion and involve primarily the most superficial muscles, rectus abdominis, and the portion of that muscle between the bottom of the ribs and the navel (see fig. 9.8 on page 138). Too much development in rectus abdominis can actually bulge out the belly, as any muscle gets bigger and thicker as

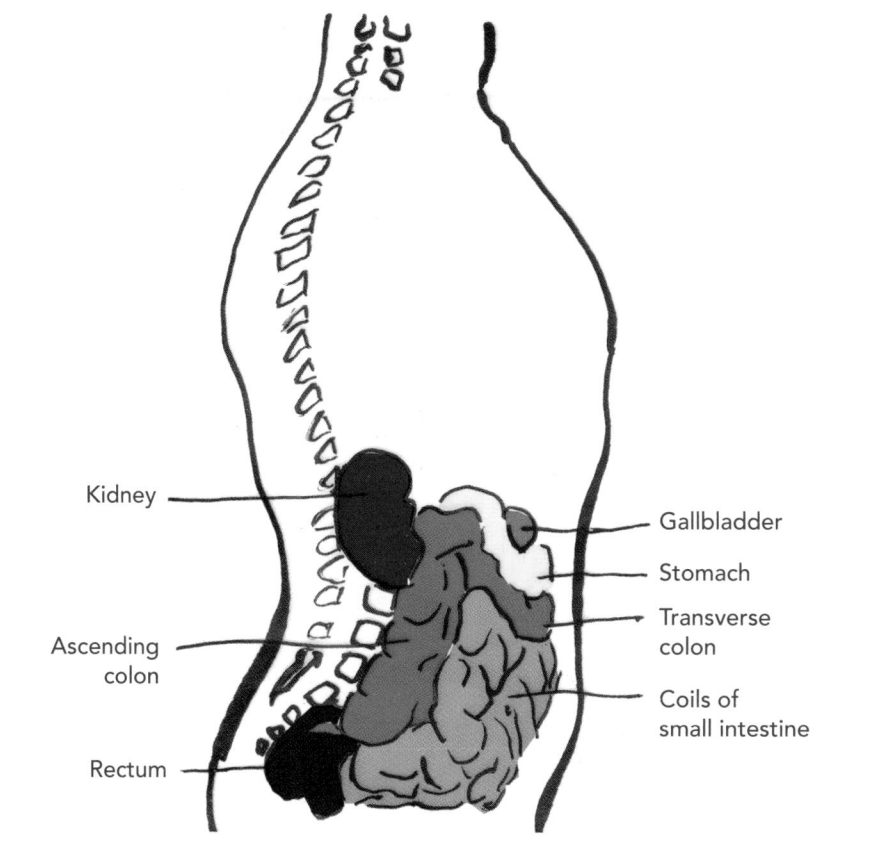

Fig. 14.2. Organs near lumbar curve of spine

it is worked. It's very difficult to stretch this area, for obvious reasons. Bodybuilding can compress the stomach and impinge on the free movement of the diaphragm on the spine, impeding breathing.

Only about 10 percent of our total abdominal strengthening work should be flexion, since that is about the amount of flexion we would normally do; 80 to 90 percent should focus on exercises that work the parts of the abdominals that pull in and support the organs and spine. This way, we'll also get a flat stomach.

EXERCISES FOR THE ABDOMINALS THAT DO NOT INVOLVE FORWARD FLEXION

While I do not include instructions for them here, two types of exercises that are very good for the abdominals are yoga and belly dancing. Yoga incorporates a lot of abdominal supportive work in all the balances and inversions. A balanced hatha yoga practice will strengthen the abdominals evenly. Belly dancing uses some unusual and really interesting abdominal moves. It was originally created to aid childbirth, so it strengthens very deep muscles. Men can do it with benefit too! The belly dancing classes I've taken all had a man or two bravely churning along.

In addition to the Plank Exercise given here, the Transverse Abdominis Exercises (pages 173-77) are also helpful.

🌿 *Plank Exercise on Toes or Tops of Feet*

Of the two options for this exercise, the familiar yoga plank posture on the toes, is the easier one, because your back muscles help out (fig. 14.3).

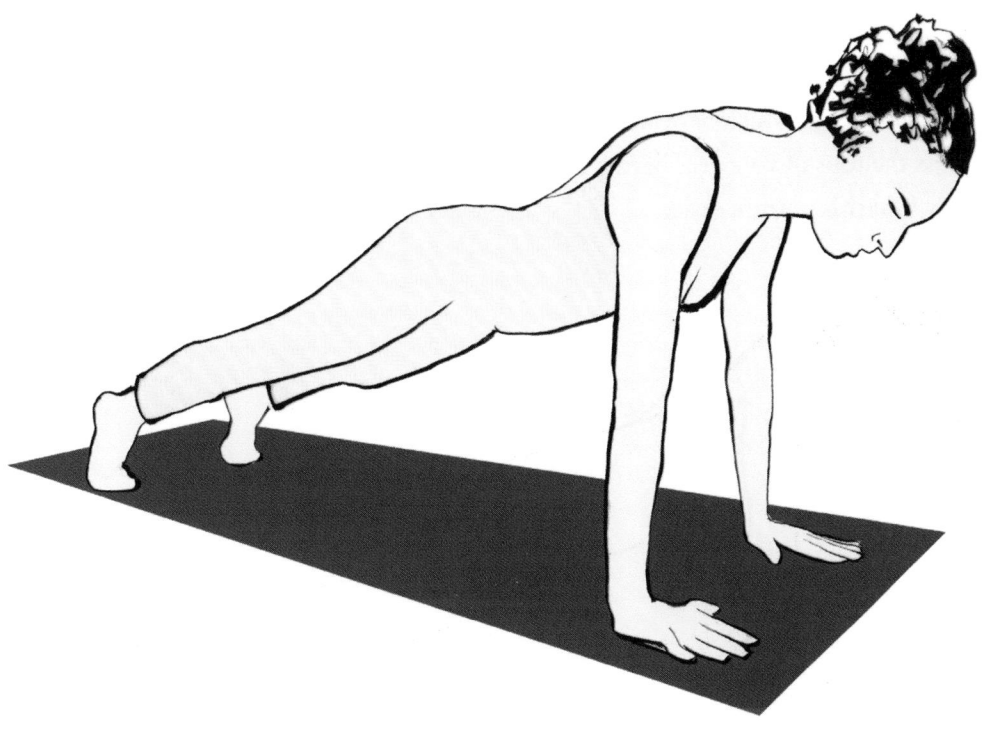

Fig.14.3. Plank on toes

1. Form a straight diagonal line with your body, with the back of the legs engaged and the heels pressing back, so the soles of the feet are perpendicular to the floor. Feet are about inner hip width apart.

2. The hard part is usually keeping the hips in a straight line with the body. They will want to drop below the level of the spine if your back muscles are weak, or stick up above if the abdominals are weaker. Think of connecting your sit bones to your heels.

3. Your shoulders must be directly over your wrists, and your upper back should drop very slightly below the level of the shoulder blades, with shoulder blades gliding down the back (almost everyone rounds the thoracic spine here).

4. Keep your head in line with your spine, soft palate in line with the pelvic floor. Your gaze point is on the floor, about 3 feet ahead of your hands. Hold for 90 seconds, or more. Focus on keeping your weight even between right and left sides, hands and feet, and on lengthening your spine.

To modify: Do the same thing exactly, but on top of your feet rather than on your toes (fig. 14.4). This will work the abdominals more (much more!). This will engage the hamstrings, which have an automatic tie-in to the lower abdominal area, so if you press the tops of your feet harder into the floor and work the hamstrings more, you may find this posture easier.

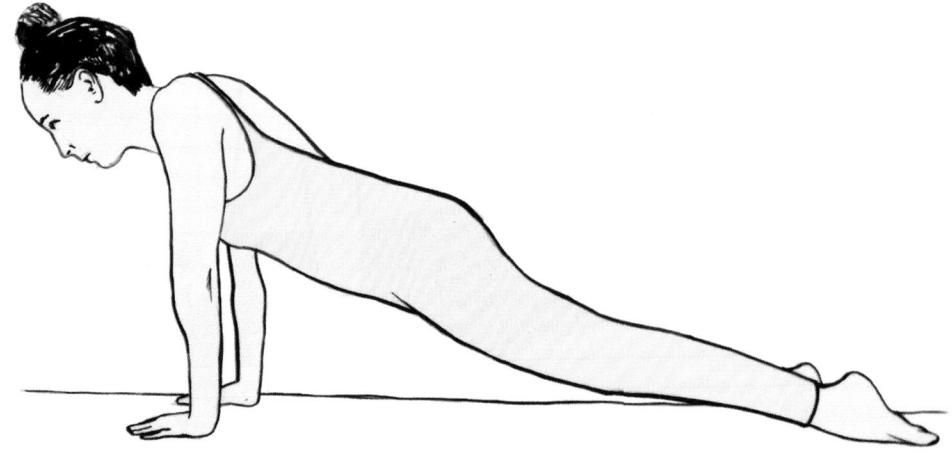

Fig. 14.4. Plank on tops of feet

RELIEVING PRESSURE ON THE AORTA

If you look at the diaphragm (see fig. 4.2 on page 53), you'll see that the various holes that run through it contain arteries and veins. So tightness in the diaphragm could put some pressures on the circulatory system, especially the aorta, the main artery of the body (fig. 14.5). When there is pressure on the aorta, the main pulse of it tends to be felt closer to the diaphragm, in the solar plexus. To feel relaxed and "normal," and for the digestion to work properly, the aortic pulse needs to be strongest about two inches below the navel, which is our center of gravity.

This important spot is the tan tien of tai chi and qi gong, the hara of the Japanese, and the kundalini center of yoga. That is where you want to feel the most heat and action in your body, rather than higher up. I can feel the position of the navel pulse quite easily when I'm touching a person who's lying on her back, but for some reason it's much harder to feel your own pulse.

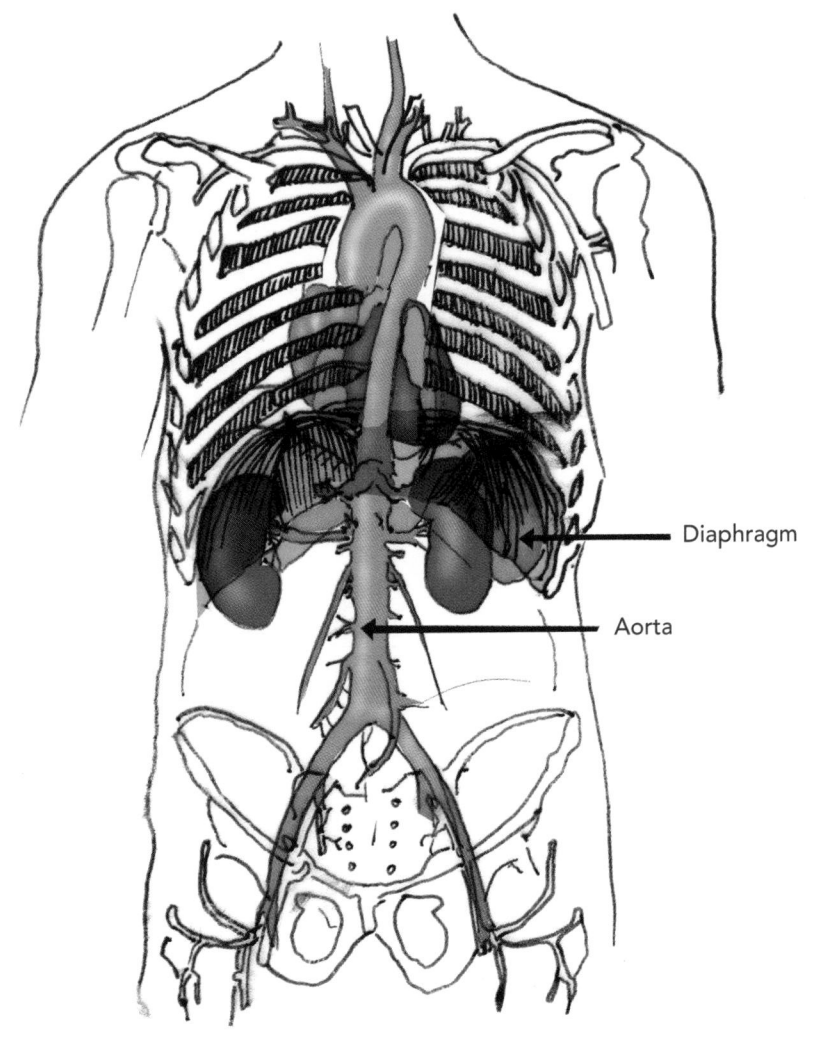

Diaphragm

Aorta

Fig. 14.5. Aorta

🍂 *Rebalance the Navel Pulse*

If you have digestive problems or feel a sensation of heat in the solar plexus (when your stomach is empty, of course), or if you just feel uncentered, your navel pulse is probably off center. To rebalance it, try this exercise, but only when your stomach is empty.

1. Sit or lie down. Lift your back ribs up—you want a slight lift in the back ribs the whole time. Imagine that a hook is attached to the back ribs, supporting and slightly lifting your rib cage away from your hips. Soften and relax the front ribs, so they drape over the abdomen.

2. Inhale, and then as you exhale, suck your navel in toward your spine. Keep this contraction, and breathe in the rib cage only. Remember, the ribs are lifted, so this should not be difficult. Keep the tight contraction throughout the exercise. If you start to lose it, pull back in. At first the contraction gets confused with your breathing, so try to separate the inhale and exhale from the sucking in of the belly.

3. With the belly held in tight, sense the inside part of your navel, where it contacts your organs. Don't touch it; just sense it. Then pull the navel down toward your pubic bone from the inside. You won't move it far—the movement might not even be visible—but you still should use as much muscular force as you can.

4. You are sitting or lying, rib cage lifted up away from your hips, abdominal area sucked in, isolating the muscles that pull down the navel. Keep going until you feel some strong sensation in the lower abdomen, maybe heat or just sore muscle. Release slowly. You should feel a pulse, or at least some heat, about 2 inches below the navel.

REFLUX

Acid reflux, heartburn, and just plain indigestion are all names for a condition that I have seen much more of in the past ten years, especially among singers. I hardly saw it at all twenty years ago. There are now quite strong and effective medications that treat this condition by shutting down the acid pump of the stomach, so less acid is produced. These medications have side effects, though, which you will understand when you learn how the stomach and diaphragm work together and what the real problems might be.

Hydrochloric acid is produced by the digestive system in the stomach to break down food and to kill bacteria and parasites. The stomach itself is well protected against acidity by its mucous lining. The problems only happen when the lining is destroyed (such as by the *H. pylori* bacteria or candida yeast) or, as reflux, when the acidity moves up from the stomach into the delicate esophageal tissue. From there it can spread through osmotic pressure, even up to the vocal folds (causing burning and injury) and the mouth (sores, infections). So with reflux, the same amount of hydrochloric acid is usually produced as in a healthy stomach—it is just in the wrong place. Some recent studies in Germany have shown that stomach secretions are even found in the fluids of the ears in some people with chronic ear infections. It's easy to see how reflux could cause the sinus and respiratory problems that singers are so prone to.

The causes of reflux are dietary, circumstance- and lifestyle-related, and structural. The first two causes are common knowledge—but the structural aspect is often not addressed and is particularly important for singers, who tend to overuse the muscles around the stomach and diaphragm.

If you look at an illustration of the relationship between the stomach and diaphragm, you'll see how vulnerable the top of the stomach is to damage (see figures 14.6 below and 4.2 on page 53 [**X-ref**]). The cardiac sphincter (a ring

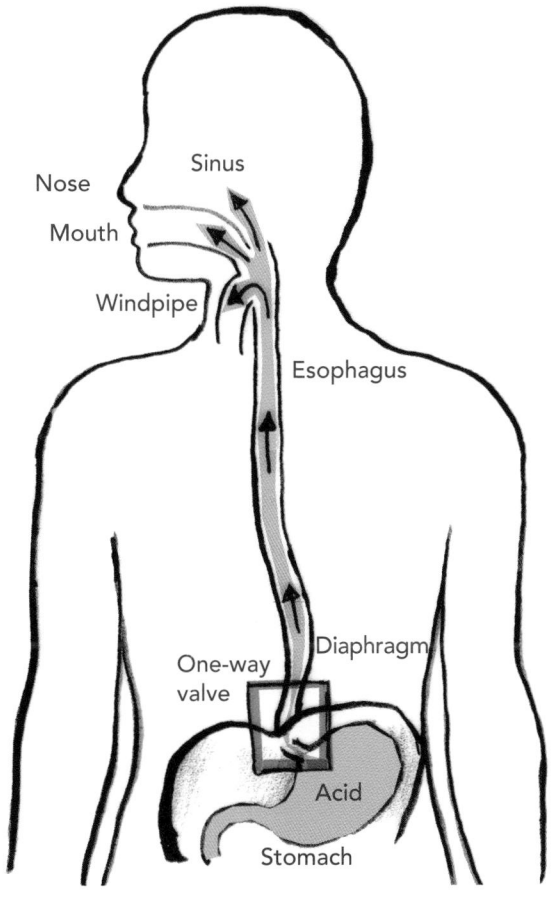

Fig. 14.6. Acid reflux and the cardiac sphincter

of muscle at the top of the stomach) needs to sit just below the level of the diaphragm—and stay there!—in order to prevent hydrochloric acid from traveling up into the esophagus. A hiatal hernia, an extreme, chronic bulge of the stomach above the diaphragm, will of course create reflux. However, if the connection is weak, the sphincter can slide up and down and cause a mild herniation, which will not be visible. The problems can be from weakness in the sphincter or from diaphragmatic tightness, or both.

Sphincter problems are caused by:

- Irritating foods, such as spices, caffeine, and alcohol
- Medications
- Too much fat in the diet, which causes food to be kept in the stomach too long
- Certain herbs, such as peppermint, which loosen the valves
- Eating too much at one time
- Eating late, so when you lie down, food is in the stomach and can push up above the sphincter
- Conditions such as candida and *H. pylori* that can weaken the valve by literally eating away at the tissue

Singers are particularly vulnerable to reflux, because moving the diaphragm energetically and contracting the upper abdominals when there is any food in the stomach can cause the sphincter to weaken through constant friction. I believe that singing is the only activity that loosens the paraesophageal ligament, which holds the stomach and esophagus in the right place. Eventually, there will be a mild hernia and the resulting reflux. You can see why the timing of performances, usually in the evening, might mean that a performer would need to stop eating at 3 or 4 p.m. This means they'll be too hungry to sleep well. Performances require lots of energy. The problems singers have are deceptive. Whereas running, gymnastics, and other activities that can weaken the sphincter are so uncomfortable if you do them on a full stomach that you stop right away, singing, since it is free of impact, doesn't feel so bad—but actually the movement of the diaphragm is much greater than in most sports.

The rate at which the stomach empties varies much more than is realized. Some people take much longer than others. Fats digest slowly; chewing food well will move it faster; and stress can cause a slowdown or a speedup of stomach mobility. Digestion might take anywhere between two and eight hours. If stomach acid is too low, digestion will be slowed.

Stomach Acidity

It's important to understand why the stomach needs to be so acidic. Then you'll have an idea why I'm so against the strong acid pump suppressors like Nexium, Prilosec, and so on. The acid medium doesn't just act locally to break down the food we eat and protect us from parasites. It also sets the relative pH of the rest of the body. The amount of acid in the stomach controls the alkalinity of the small intestine, where the food is actually assimilated. If the stomach acid is lowered, the intestine tries to balance the pH of the whole system and in the process becomes too acidic. What this means is that the food won't be absorbed properly and the larger protein particles may leak through the walls of the stomach (leaky gut syndrome), creating acidity in the tissues outside the digestive system.

So the more alkaline stomach creates more acidity in the intestine, which gives more acidity to the whole body, which upsets the natural pH balance, and can lead to inflammation in any of the systems.

The acid of the stomach also tightens the cardiac sphincter, another natural safeguard. So when you artificially lower the acid, you actually weaken the sphincter further, giving you worse reflux, since the problem is often hiatal hernia anyway. That means you can't stop taking the medication, and you can get caught up in a cycle that's hard to break. Giving the drug companies the benefit of the doubt, I don't think these medications were designed to be taken long term.

We have exactly the same neurotransmitters in the gut as we do in the brain. In fact, the gut is actually a self-contained brain, the enteric nervous system.* That's why all antidepressants affect the gut too. And that's also the reason why everything we put in our stomachs can change our neurology, moods, and thoughts. I have no evidence, but anecdotally, the medications for reflux often seem to cause depression and memory loss, or at least those problems appear to have started coincidentally with medication use.

---

*Gershon, *The Second Brain.*

TREATMENT OF ACID REFLUX
AND HIATAL HERNIA

To sum up, I believe that:

1. Most reflux is a low level, maybe undetectable, sliding hiatal hernia caused by tightness of the diaphragm or the weakness of the cardiac valve.
2. Acid medications can cause further weakness in that valve, as well as a host of undesirable side effects. A good medication will make you less reliant on it in the long term, not more dependent.

I see, so far, two useful avenues for treatment of reflux: structural and a protocol for digestion. The structural is mostly unknown, so I have come up with a few exercises, along with some dietary recommendations.

✿ Exercises to Treat Acid Reflux

◈ Strengthen the Psoas to Treat Hiatal Hernia

The diaphragm itself can't be strengthened in a way that helps hiatal hernia—at least, I haven't found it yet. This exercise will strengthen some of the fibers of the psoas that influence the diaphragm. Keeping that area strong and open is a key to overcoming hiatal hernia.

1. Lie on your back, and raise your leg about 30 degrees, keeping your other hip and leg down. Move the upper leg about 6 inches out from the centerline of the body and turn out (externally rotate) the leg—not just the foot—as much as you can (fig. 14.7). Hold for enough time to assess strength in that position.
2. Lift up to 60 degrees, and repeat the sequence, and then to almost 90 degrees, about 80 degrees. Notice when you seem the weakest on that leg, which position is the hardest to hold, and in which position you want to compensate the most by lifting the other hip, twisting, arching your back, and so on.
3. Repeat on the other side.

◈ Strengthen the Psoas with Isometrics or a Resistance Band

Now that you've found the weakest positions, strengthen them by isometric holds.

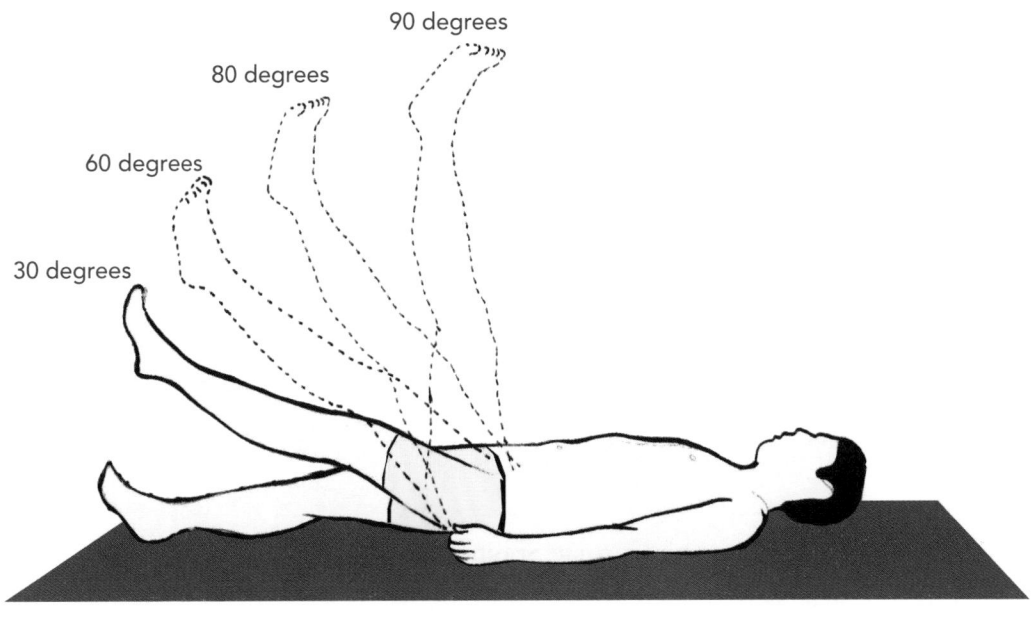

Fig. 14.7. Strengthen the Psoas to Treat Hiatal Hernia

1. If you find this enough of a strength challenge, just holding the leg in the difficult position for about 30 seconds may be enough.

2. Or you can intensify by using a stretchy TheraBand tied into a loop (fig. 14.8). You resist the band isometrically, that is, without visible movement, just pressure, for 10 seconds. Then relax completely for 5 seconds. Repeat this sequence 5 times.

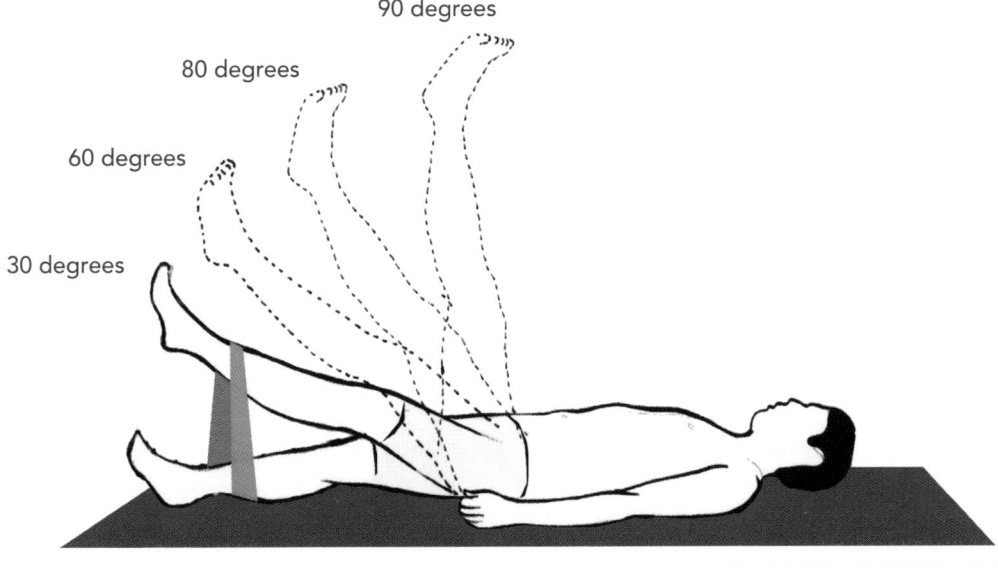

Fig. 14.8. Strengthen the Psoas with Isometrics or a Resistance Band

The other muscles that influence this area are the deeper, core abdominals, transverse abdominis, obliques, and serratus posterior, which can be strengthened with Pilates and other very consciously performed core exercises, as well as certain exercises in this book.

You also need to keep the abdomen stretched out and avoid compression in the lumbar discs. The main culprit here is sitting slumped over, especially eating slumped, so that the stomach is compressed. When you sit, keep your rib cage away (front and back) from your hips and lengthen your spine. If you are not strong enough to sit up straight without discomfort, strengthen your back and side muscles.

◈ Manually Strengthen the Cardiac Sphincter

You can also strengthen the sphincter valve, which isn't under conscious control, of course; you engage it manually. Do this on an empty stomach.

1. Stand with your back against a wall. Find the area just under your rib cage, in the front and center. Press in there—it may be a little sensitive if you have reflux. Press down toward your feet.
2. Then continue the pressure as you move down the left side of the margin of your rib cage (fig. 14.9). Repeat this move 10 to 12 times. Do this every day.

This practice will train your stomach to descend. It may even adjust the weak valve, pushing it down below the level of the diaphragm. If it does, you usually hear your stomach gurgling as the intestines reset.

Another way you can help your stomach find its right place is to drink about one and a half liters of water first thing in the morning on an empty stomach. The water should be room temperature or slightly warm. Drink it standing, and drink slowly but continuously. The weight of the water, drunk this way, and with no food in the stomach, can help the stomach descend.

◈ Acupressure to Treat Acid Reflux

There is also an acupressure point that can help reflux.

1. Find the point located on the outside of the shin, between the knee and the ankle on the stomach meridian (fig. 14.10).

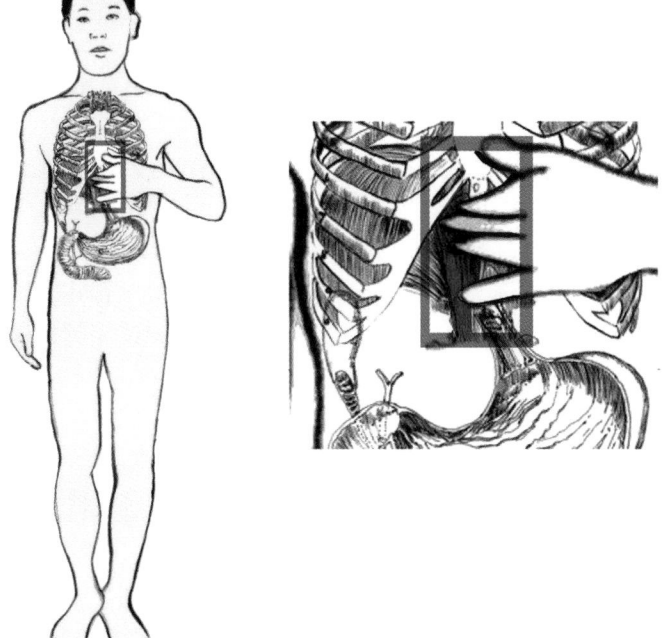

Press down
Continue pressure while sliding down

Fig. 14.9. Manually Strengthen the Cardiac Sphincter

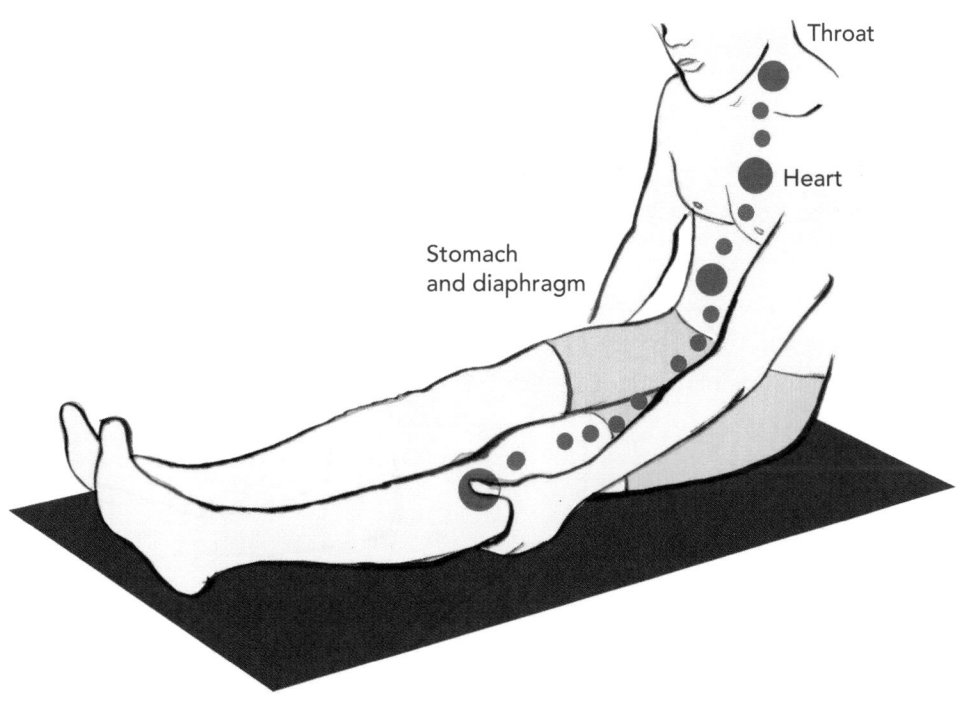

Throat

Heart

Stomach and diaphragm

Fig. 14.10. Acupressure point to treat acid reflux

2. Press it hard, or circle or rub it continuously for about a minute, once a day. If you press it for a few seconds after you eat, it may prevent reflux.

🍃 *Release the Vagus Nerve*

This exercise helps to release the tissue around the vagus nerve, the primary nerve involved in reflux and hiatal hernia. This nerve is extremely important and controls many key functions. It influences the occiput, throat, heart, stomach and diaphragm, and sacrum. It can be thrown off by problems in any of these areas, and by shock and stress. It is especially associated with trauma; it connects to the lower brain and brainstem. This exercise can help neck tension also.

1. Hold your elbows pressed firmly into your rib cage and your forearms outward, forming a right angle (fig. 14.11).
2. Bring your tongue out of your mouth and down as far as you possibly can, till the root of your tongue stretches so much it hurts a little—a good hurt. Your jaw *must* be relaxed and aligned, so think of widening the space between both TMJs. Only your tongue is working, not your jaw.

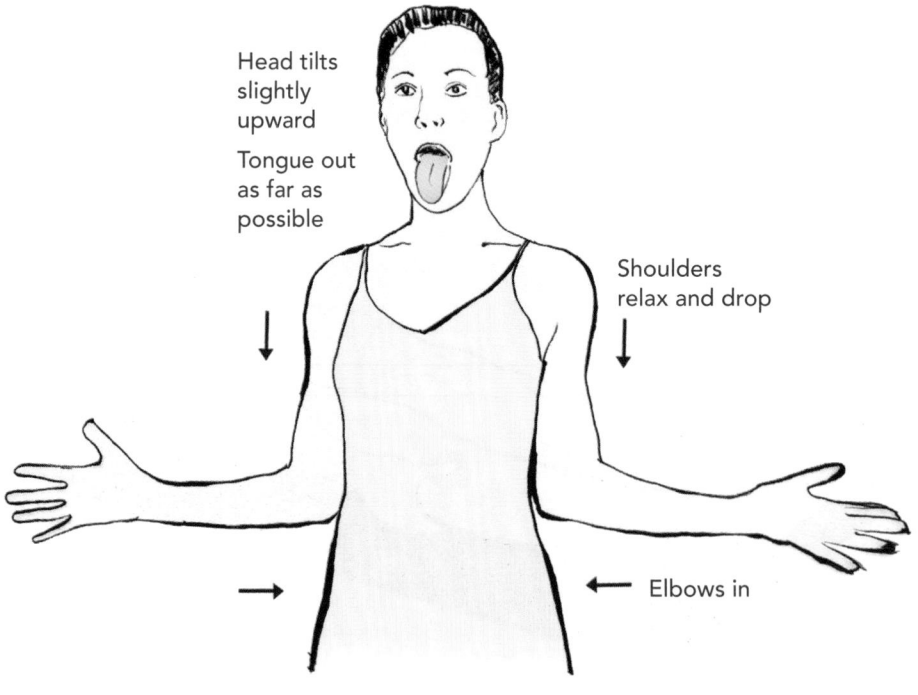

Head tilts slightly upward

Tongue out as far as possible

Shoulders relax and drop

← Elbows in

Fig. 14.11. Release the Vagus Nerve

3. Your collarbone and shoulders press down, your head tilts slightly upward. Stretch the soft palate away from the root of the tongue, increasing the stretch. Pant fast and hard through your mouth, like a dog.

4. Your tongue will want to come back in your mouth, especially if there is tension in the neck and throat. Keep stretching it out, relaxing your jaw, and panting. Do this for 5 minutes for a complete release of the vagus nerve. This is a wonderful exercise for throat tension, tight diaphragm, neck tension, and reflux.

Dietary Reflux Therapy

The other aspect of reflux therapy is digestive. That means, first of all, sticking to the reflux diet that most sufferers know: no acidic foods, dairy, wheat, sugar, coffee, spices, alcohol, chocolate, peppermint, and so on. What's less well known is that excess fats, especially cooked and hydrogenated ones, weaken the valve even more and slow the passage of food through the system. Large vitamin pills and other big tablets can cause reflux too. So can any foods you are allergic to. Get tested with kinesiology or a blood test if you don't know what they are.

Even more important than what you eat is how and when you eat. The main rule is a very simple one. Don't eat too much at once. One huge meal can slip that sphincter up, if you have a weakness there. And chronically eating too much in one sitting will create reflux too.

Chew your food well—chewing is the first stage of digestion. Most people don't chew enough, and it is a kyo that sets the stage for poor digestion. Chewing digests food with saliva so the stomach has less work to do, and it sets up a release that prepares the valves to open and close in a correct sequence, and the digestive enzymes to flow.

Digestion is strongest at noon—a time that's inconvenient for most people to eat. Dinner should be very light, and you should never eat solid food after ten p.m., no matter when you go to bed. Stomach acids are much higher between ten p.m. and two a.m., as the body is designed to clean out and eliminate during that time, when we would be asleep if we weren't surrounded by the bright lights of electrical devices. If you are too hungry to sleep, drink a smoothie or vegetable juice.

There's a protocol I've used that often helps people get off reflux medication. Go slowly, if you try this, and don't change your medication schedule without your doctor's supervision. Do this consistently for a month, and I'm sure you'll see some improvement. You can take the probiotics, enzymes, and DGL without concerns. Take as directed, since the brands are all a bit different.

- Take a good probiotic that contains a variety of organisms and includes a bifidus strain—Healthy Trinity by Natren is my favorite one.
- Take digestive enzymes as well. I like the Q-Zyme powder by Garden of Life; there are many other good ones.
- DGL—deglycerized licorice—helps heal the irritated lining. Chew these, usually two to three times a day before meals.
- Zinc and manganese can help tighten the sphincter muscles. Calcium is the most alkalizing of our minerals (remember Tums?). Magnesium eases stress. The amounts you might take of these minerals would vary—consult a health practitioner if you want to.

Bacteria and Acid Reflux

There's one other factor I think is probably an issue here—bacteria. However, it will probably take a few more years of scientific research before a bacteria is discovered that is responsible for reflux. Digestive disorders that were formerly thought to be caused by stress have been found recently to be caused by bacterial infection. Stomach ulcers are cured by antibiotics now (*H. pylori* bacteria are usually responsible), and Crohn's disease has been established to have some kind of bacterial component. Reflux may also be treated by a course of antibiotics in a few years, which doesn't mean that the structural and digestive components I've discussed aren't just as important, since the background for infection is created by the conditions in the digestive tract.

And for now, before we know exactly what kind of bacteria causes reflux, and even if it does, you need to work with it in the ways I've described if you want a more natural and safer resolution to your condition than the purple pills.

15

The Knees

THERE IS ALWAYS A TENSION when we are standing that has to do with the stress of maintaining an upright position. If that tension is in the correct muscles and does not become fixed at any point, these supporting muscles will simply be strengthened, and no chronic tension will result. However, it's not that simple. If these potentially strong, supportive muscles are weak or we are not using them properly for some reason, we will tend to lock our joints when we stand to brace against falling. The knees are the easiest joint to lock, so knee locking (hyperextension) is very common. Knee locking on one side will shift the hip on that side upward and compress the joint, so that the leg will seem shorter on that side. This pattern often begins very early in childhood, when we are learning to walk. If the early stages of development have not been completed properly, there may not be enough support in the deep pelvic muscles to balance. It's easier then to lock the knees to stand up. That may mean that those pelvic muscles never get developed properly and extra stress is put on the knee, making the joint more vulnerable to injury.

KNEE INJURY

If you have a knee injury, physical therapy will help—take advantage of it if you can. The exercises for knee rehabilitation are usually leg lifts and hamstring strengtheners. These are all fine, but since they are usually done in a lying or sitting position, there are some disadvantages.

For example, if you learn to strengthen a muscle in a sitting position, you have developed the fibers for more strength—in a sitting position. The benefits may not translate exactly to what you need the legs for, which is standing and walking.

If you exercise for general strengthening and don't have an injury, it doesn't matter that much, but if you need to relearn walking and reaccustom the knee to its usual patterns, you will also need to strengthen the muscles in the positions you will use them in.

This also simplifies the strengthening of the large muscles of the legs. You are working a number of movement pathways at the same time, using stabilizers to support yourself, as well as phasic fibers to perform the movements.

🍃 Muscle Exercises to Help the Knees

◈ Quadriceps Exercise

Take a fairly lightweight TheraBand and tie it into a loop it around a table leg or something similar, preferably in a position where you can hold the table or a wall for balance.

1. Place your right leg inside the loop at about midcalf level, facing away from the table leg. Support yourself so your weight is even, your hips are square and level, and your gaze is straight ahead.
2. Without shifting your body, lift your leg up, straight out, working the quadriceps at the front of the thigh (fig. 15.1).

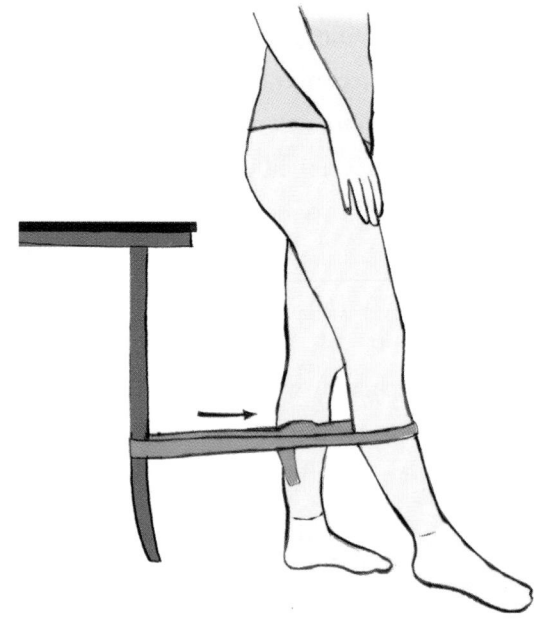

Fig. 15.1. Quadriceps Exercise

3. Keep the leg up, and pulse about an inch, moving the leg against the resistance of the band, until the muscle fatigues. Keep the leg very straight, and pull the kneecap up slightly during the exercise, if you can.

◈ Inner Thigh Exercise

1. Then turn, keeping your leg in the loop, and position yourself so your left leg moves parallel to the table leg and the inner calf of the right leg resists the TheraBand. Your left leg should be slightly behind the right. Move the right leg in toward the centerline of your body and slightly upward (fig. 15.2).

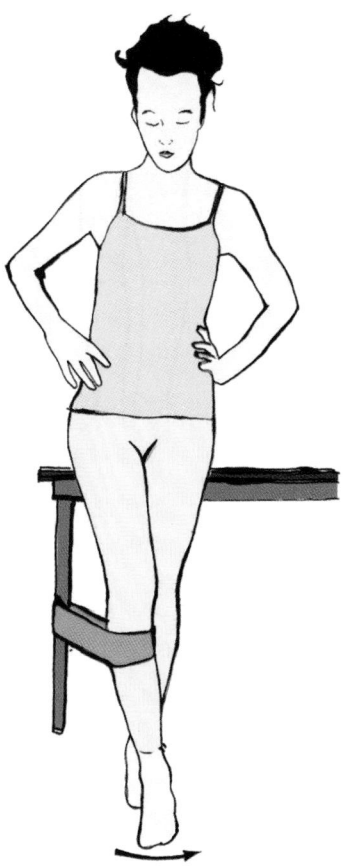

Fig. 15.2. Inner Thigh Exercise

2. You are working your inner thighs. Again, keep your body still so the stabilizing muscles get a workout too. Repeat the pulsing movements.

◆ Hamstring Exercise

1. Now turn again, leg still in the loop, so your left and right legs both face the table leg. The TheraBand will resist against the back of the right calf (fig. 15.3).

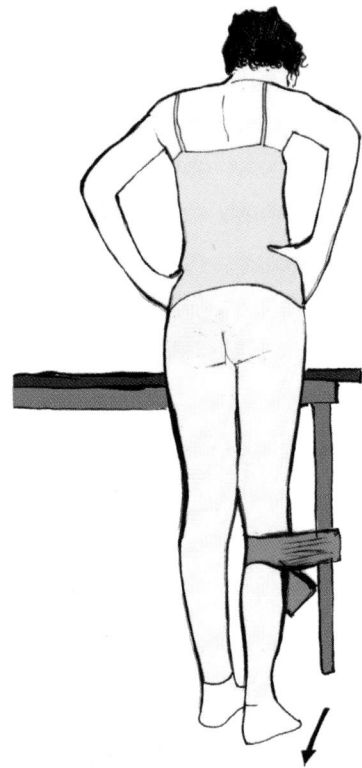

Fig. 15.3. Hamstring Exercise

2. Move the leg in the band back away from your body, working the hamstrings, repeating the small pulsing movements in the same way.

◆ Outer Thigh Exercise

1. Turn around so the TheraBand is resting on the outside of the right calf (fig. 15.4).

2. Move the right leg away from the centerline of your body to the outside, working the outer thigh the same way.

After completing all of the exercises with the right leg, put the left leg in the band and repeat the same movements. Notice which moves are difficult for you—the

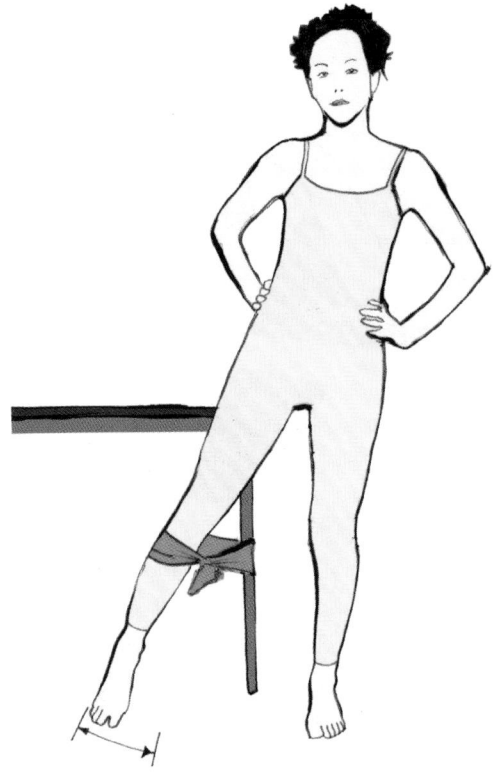

Fig. 15.4. Outer Thigh Exercise

injured side may be strong from all those physical therapy exercises, but perhaps you can't use it to stabilize when you work the uninjured leg. Repeat any of the moves that were difficult, whether from difficulty in standing in a balanced way or just weak in the consciously engaged muscles.

🍃 Meniscus Strengthener

This exercise works the muscles at the back of the knee that hold in the meniscus.

1. Lie on your back with your heels on a chair or stool (see fig. 15.5 on page 246). The height of the stool will determine the part of your hamstrings or your gluteus involved, which are worked as well as the knee, but it won't change the way you work the back of your knee much.

2. Flex your feet, press your heels down hard, and bring your hips and knees up at exactly the same time. If you do this, you'll feel the exercise behind the knees,

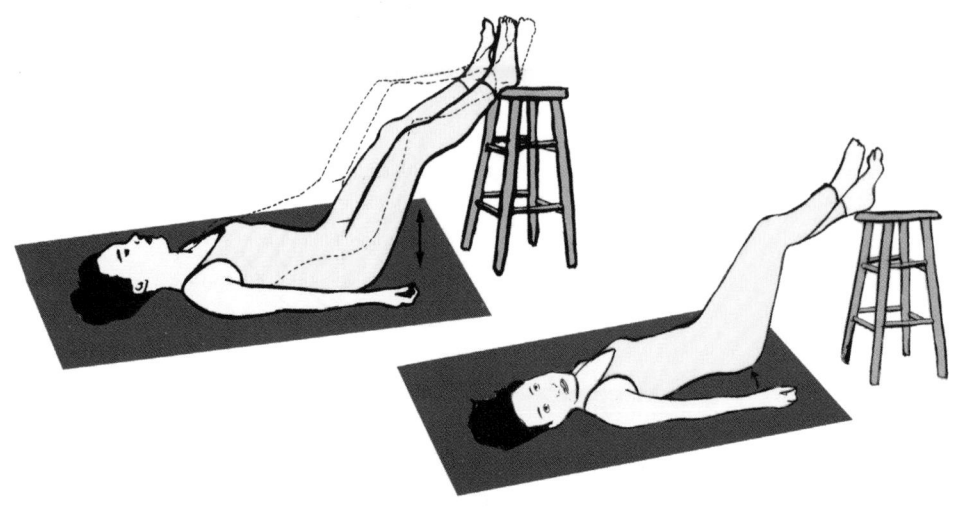

Fig. 15.5. Meniscus Strengthener

in the peroneus—stirrup muscles (see fig. 16.5 on page 256)—as well as your hamstrings and gluteus. Hold for at least 5 seconds, relax and repeat until your muscles are fatigued.

To modify: You can also work each side in the following way—and you should for a knee injury. Keep one heel down and the other leg wrapped over the working leg (as shown in fig. 15.5, right side). Start with the weak side, repeat on the stronger side, and then go back to the weak side.

✿ Calf Raise Exercise

Bring the balls of your feet to the edge of a step, somewhere you can hold on. (I use the fire exit steps in my building.)

1. Now do some regular calf raises: stand up straight with the feet parallel, hip distance apart, and the heels pressing straight down off the step. Make sure your feet are equally straight and the heel is in line with the second toe (fig. 15.6). Put equal weight on both feet as well as on the inside and outside of the feet. Stretch as deeply as you can.

2. Then slowly, to a 10-second count, raise your heels, pressing them forward. Pay attention to keeping the weight equal—you'll probably find you want to turn to

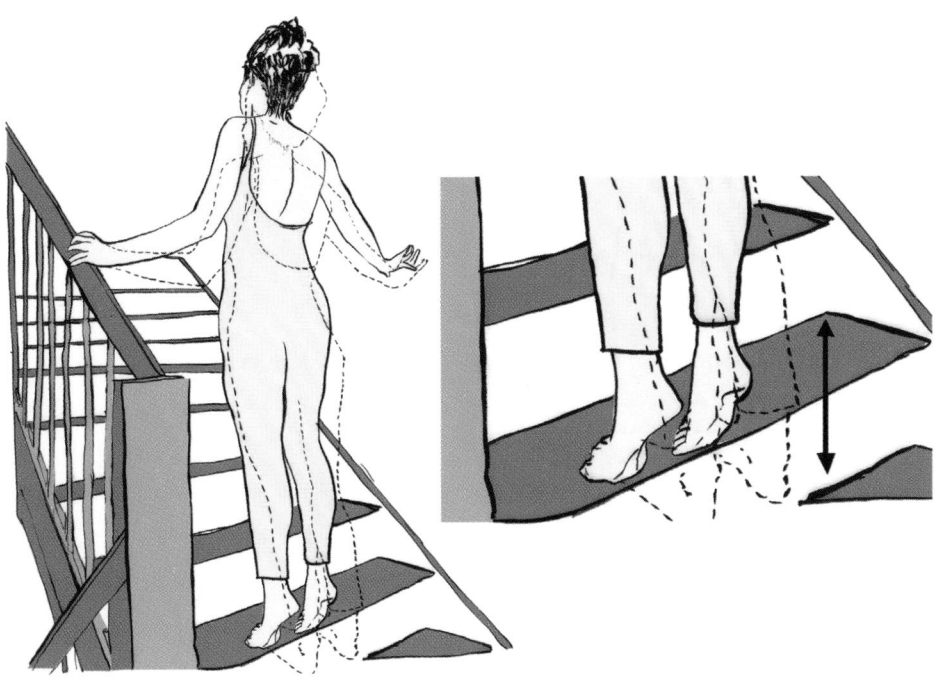

Fig. 15.6. Calf Raise Exercise

the outside of your foot. Bring your heels up as high as they will go, and keep pressing them forward. Now slowly lower. Repeat a few times, till you feel the muscles working, but not till fatigue.

3. Then turn one foot in a lot. Lift the other leg off the step, placing it on top of the working leg or just bending it. Repeat the calf raises with one turned-in leg until you fatigue. Work on keeping the leg straight and controlling the movement.

4. Do one set on the weak side, and then the strong side, and finish with the weak side.

🌿 Knee Stabilizer Exercise

This exercise strengthens the knee stabilizers in the front of the knee—vastus medialis.

1. Hold on to something in front of you. A ballet barre is ideal, but anything comfortable like a chair will do. Bend one knee up and to the side as much as you can (see fig. 15.7 on page 248).

2. Then keep the knee in the same place—don't drop it!—and straighten the leg.

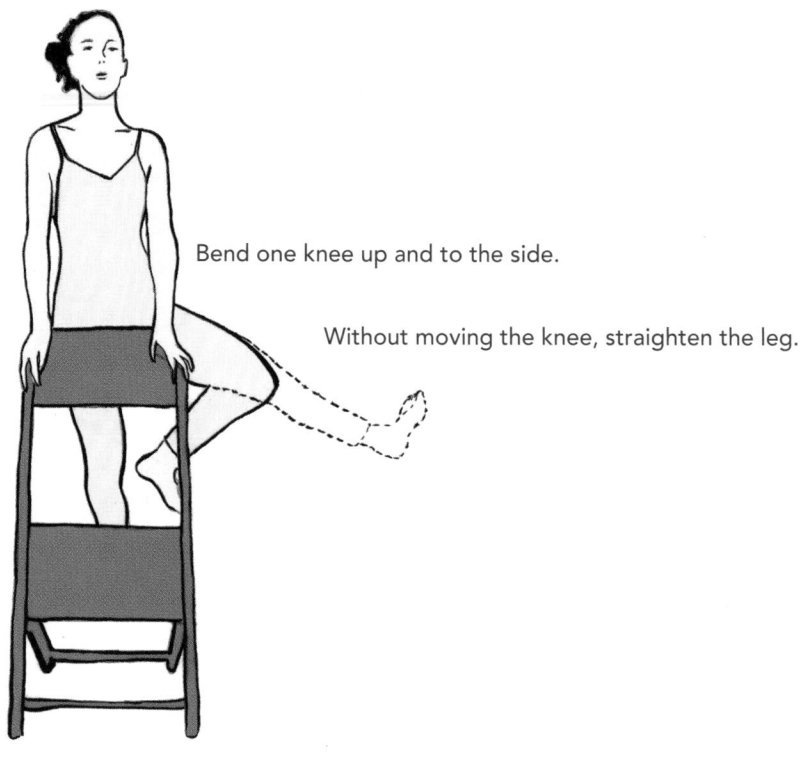

Bend one knee up and to the side.

Without moving the knee, straighten the leg.

Fig. 15.7. Knee Stabilizer Exercise

It's hard. You can bring one hand under the knee if you need to or on top of the knee so you can press up into your own hand. The knee must stay still, or you're engaging a different set of muscles. You can also drop the knee a little, but not too much. Holding it is better.

3. Bend and straighten that leg till you start to feel muscle fatigue. Really straighten it, focusing on pulling the kneecap up and in.
4. Do one set until fatigued on the weak side, and then the strong side, and then the weak side.

16

The Feet

OUR FEET ARE AN EXTRAORDINARY piece of engineering, and they are capable of a range of subtle and delicate movements, as well as supporting our weight. They tell us what kind of ground we are standing on and how secure or insecure we feel in relation to gravity. Our feet tell us about our safety, security, and the depth of contact we have with the world outside us.

Our feet can be as sensitive and capable as our hands. The electromagnetic forces of the earth, which I believe feed our nervous system's vital electrical energy, are filtered by concrete, rubber, and leather, so we feel—and we are—cut off and disconnected from life around us. Most of us respond by pulling away from the force of gravity—tightening our leg muscles and gripping with our toes, telling ourselves with these actions that we are alone and disconnected from our environment, and creating inside us a chronic, inexplicable sense of insecurity that can't be changed by psychological maneuvers.

Everyone in the industrial world has weak, underdeveloped feet, no matter how athletic he or she is. Just as our present relationship with the earth is diseased, our points of contact with the earth's surface are messed up too. Because everyone has weak feet (kyo), we don't understand how many of the structural problems and aches and pains we have are caused by this.

The two main problems our feet have—and I don't see much we can do to change this directly—are the flat hard surfaces we walk on most of the time and the shoes we wear. Some shoes are better than others, of course, but all shoes deprive our feet of mobility and sensitivity, dull them, and stiffen our joints.

THE PROBLEM WITH SHOES

One of the main problems that shoes create—all kinds of shoes, including excellent athletic shoes—is the relative atrophy of the foot muscles, compared to the legs. Actually, the best we can hope for from a good, well-fitted shoe is that it will strengthen our legs and maybe our ankles.

Start by taking a look at the shoes you wear most often. Also check shoes you give hard wear to, especially running shoes. Look at the soles, and notice how they're worn. Which shoe, right or left, is worn more? That's the side you put more weight on and lean on more. Probably the hip is higher on that side.

Then notice the front and back, inside and outside of the soles. Most people wear their shoes down more at the outside of the heel. If this is true for you, please get rid of any shoes that are worn down unevenly. If you wear your shoes down in some other way—it still may apply to you, as it applies to most people who wear shoes and walk on flat surfaces. Whenever you wear these worn-down shoes, you will distort your alignment. Inserts won't work either—just throw them away. And don't wear shoes you wore if you had an injury involving the lower body.

Running outside is a natural activity that most primitive people and animals do without thinking anything of it. So why do we need elaborate puffy sports shoes? Children run outside, and they don't hurt themselves.

Thirty years ago, before people exercised in the gym much, people my mother's age—forty-five or so—accepted the loss of abdominal tone as they got older and wore girdles. Now, fortunately, we know better and go crazy with Pilates, and so on, so we don't sag and lose muscle tone. But it never occurs to us that what we are doing with our feet is the same pattern of submission, and we are accepting unnatural and harmful restrictions on our movement. We can hide our weak, ugly feet in a way we can't conceal a sagging abdomen.

ALIGNMENT OF THE FEET

Most of us only become aware of the role of the feet when they develop serious problems—bunions, for example—and start hurting. Since we can't (presumably) go without shoes and walk on rocks continually, we need to compensate by exercising and massaging the feet. So let's look at the feet and what we can do for them.

🍃 Exercise for Aligning the Feet

In this exercise you need to have lines of some sort to provide a grid to align your feet with. A parquet floor is excellent, as are tiles or any other flooring with squares. A yoga mat with straight lines drawn in is ideal.

1. Stand with your feet inner-hip distance apart (that's the space inside of the iliac crest) and the outside of each foot completely straight. The absolutely straight line of the outer edge of the foot will probably feel pigeon-toed and maybe uncomfortable to you (fig. 16.1).

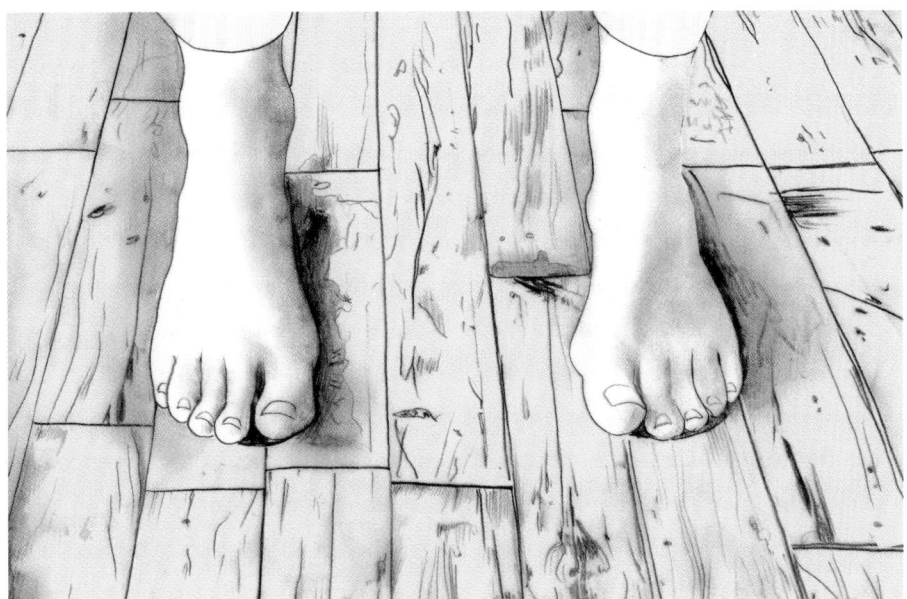

Stand with feet inner-hip distance apart; align outside of each foot with floor.

Fig. 16.1. Exercise for Aligning the Feet

2. Now press the ball of the big toe into the floor, relaxing the toes.
3. You should feel the arch of the foot "dome" up away from the floor (see fig. 16.4 on page 256). See if you can pull the heel isometrically toward the toes, working the transverse arch and the connective tissues, where injury or lack of tone can cause plantar fasciitis. Keep the toes relaxed!

4. Now keep the alignment and come up on the balls of your feet. You will probably want to roll outward on the feet—don't. See if you can balance and relax your toes in this position—if you can't balance, hold lightly on to something and try to use your foot muscles rather than your toes.

🍃 Foot Workout

You can work out the feet by isolating the movements. Think how easy it is for most of us to use our fingers individually. There are the same number of nerve endings in the toes as in the fingers. Bear this in mind as you explore the possibilities of toe movement.

1. Hold down all the toes except the one, or two, you want to explore, and wiggle them up, down, to the side, and so on, fast and slow, any way you can think of. You are simply stimulating a sleepy part of your nervous system. Work one foot well and notice if any other part of your body feels different. You can also try "fanning" all of your toes toward the pinky toe side, and then toward the big toe side. Try curling them and doing this, and then flexing them and doing this. Feet are usually a profound kyo (weakness), and bringing energy to them can take pain away from a jitsu (symptom) area—maybe your neck or back.

2. You can also massage the connective tissue that tends to build up around the ankles by stretching the front of the foot. Keeping the foot stretched out, rub the top surface of your foot and as much of your ankle as you can reach with your knuckles. Keeping this upper area of the foot loose can prevent overcompensation in the sole of the foot, which can lead to plantar fasciitis. This technique will also help if you already have plantar fasciitis. You'll find the same areas sensitive on the top of the foot as on the bottom.

The Ankle Joint

Now let's look at the part of the ankle where the shinbones, tibia and fibula, connect with the interior of the heel. This joint, because we stand on it, often gets compressed, so the bones jam in together in such a way that the full range of motion is impossible. Because you can walk without much ankle flexion, you might not notice that this has happened. Instead, compression may cause pain in the feet, legs, or hips.

The bones can also be misaligned forward, backward, or to the inside or outside—pronation and supination are familiar words to sneaker buyers and runners. Forward means that the front of the foot is higher than the back. Backward means very tight calves and Achilles tendons; chronic wearers of high heels may have this problem. Pronation means that the bony protrusion on the inside of the ankle falls inward and is not level with the rest of the inner ankle. The foot tends to roll inward; probably there will be a difference on each side. Supination means just the reverse, rolling to the outside of the foot, with the bony protuberance at the outer ankle moving beyond the outside heel. Pronation often accompanies knock-knees and tight hip flexors. Supination gives you bowed legs and tight outer thighs.

Role of the Iliotibial Band

Balance on your toes for as long as you can. Notice which part of your foot you want to roll onto when it gets harder to balance. You may wobble a bit, but most people end up balancing on the outer edges of both feet. That usually feels stronger and more supportive than the inside of the foot.

There's a good reason for this. The outside of the leg contains a long, thin strip of connective tissue, much harder and less flexible than muscle, which runs from the hip into the knee (fig. 16.2). The purpose of this strip, called the iliotibial

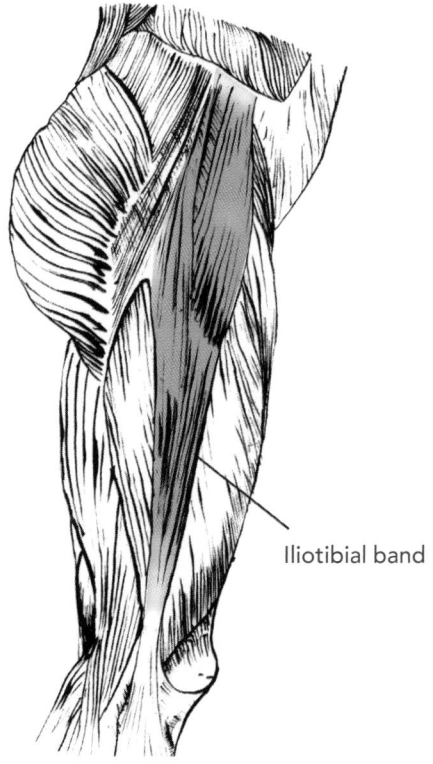

Iliotibial band

Fig. 16.2. Iliotibial band

band, is to protect the knee from rolling outward, which would injure the meniscus. So we need it, but because we don't move and stretch the outside of our legs very much, it tends to harden and get tight, pulling us away from the inner leg and the core of the body, onto the outside of the feet, the knees, and the hips. The knees can be pulled so far outward that they become vulnerable to injury. The core abdominal muscles are not used properly, and even the side of the neck can become tight. So you see that the way your feet contact the ground affects every structure in the body.

The Relationship between Feet, Knees, and Hips

Now look at the other side of the foot and notice differences. Then, with your feet parallel, observe both ankles from the front. Notice the middle front part of the ankle, where the space is between the two shinbones, relative to the knees, hips, and toes. Which toes are in a line from it, and where are they relative to one another?

Now look at your feet from the back, again with your feet parallel. You'll have to twist to see, of course, so this visual test isn't quite as accurate. You can observe the relationship of the middle of the heel to the center of the back of the knee and see whether one or both heels turn in or out.

This will show something about the relationship between your feet, your knees, and your hips—often an uneasy alliance. Ideally, these three joints work together to maintain the stability our upper bodies need for free movement. The problems many of us have when we run come from an imbalance somewhere in these areas, where the shock absorbers of feet, knees, and hips are not in line with one another. Many factors are involved here—all the material I've written on the lower body will be of some relevance.

✿ Ankle Circles

The ankle mediates between the foot, the knee, and the hip; this exercise evens out the movement of the ankles.

1. Lie on your back. Keep your kneecap pointing straight up at the ceiling and your heel as still as possible (it will move a little, but don't let it slide at all). Most important is to keep the inner malleoli (the inside of the ankle bone that protrudes slightly) aligned; do not let one rise higher than the other (fig. 16.3). Think of a connecting line drawn between them.

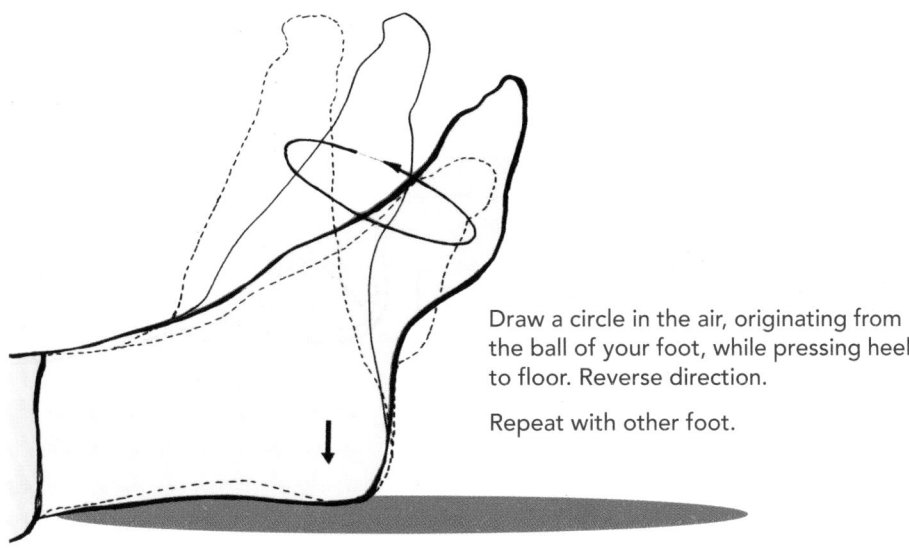

Draw a circle in the air, originating from the ball of your foot, while pressing heel to floor. Reverse direction.

Repeat with other foot.

Fig. 16.3. Ankle Circles

2. Now circle one ankle, pressing the heel into the ground. Try to use your foot to make the circle, rather than steering with your toes (they will help out, but try to minimize the movement). Think of a circle around the still line between the malleoli, originating in the ball of the foot. Make the circle as big as you can. Rotate in both directions for a minute or so.

3. Repeat on the other side. Usually, one side is stiffer or harder to coordinate. Repeat the exercise on the more difficult side. Your goal is to even them up.

We usually stand more on one foot than the other, and that ankle generally is less flexible, often dramatically so. This causes imbalance in the rest of the body. Keep your weight even on both feet, front and back, right and left. Notice the subtle shifts that can happen when you practice standing evenly on both legs.

THE ARCHES OF THE FEET

The three arches of the foot are equally important in their function, which is to support the weight of the body and act as shock absorbers (see fig. 16.4 on page 256). You'll notice that, probably due to the rolling outward that shoes encourage, many of us lose the lateral and transverse arch, only retaining the main large medial arch. Some of us lose this too.

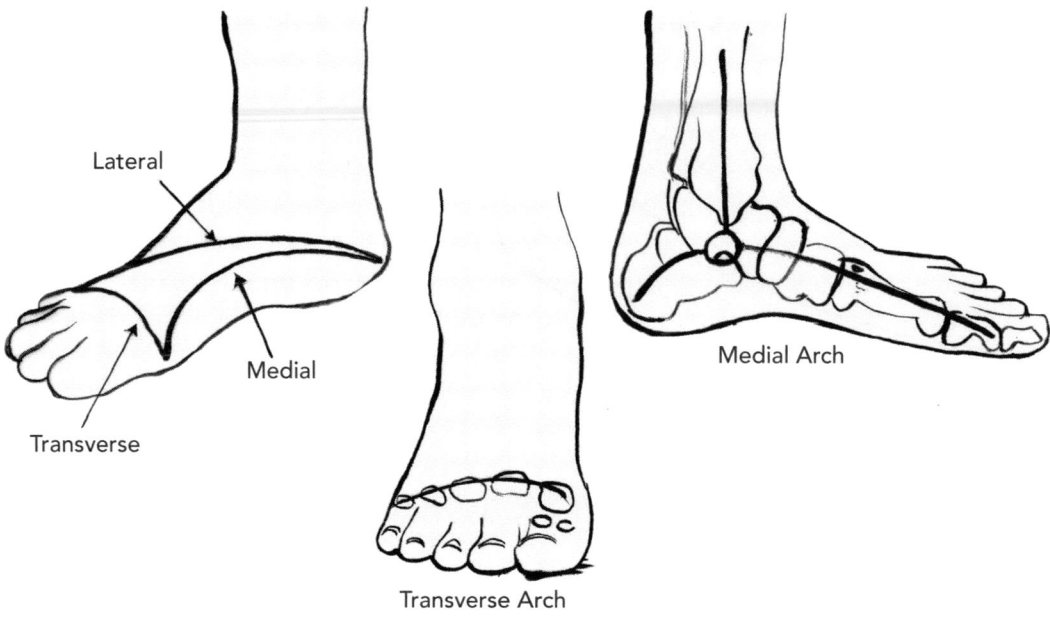

Lateral

Medial

Transverse

Medial Arch

Transverse Arch

Fig. 16.4. The three arches of the foot

🌿 Exercise for the Arches of the Feet

This exercise works the stirrup muscles that act as pulleys on the arches, toning them and lifting the small bones that compose the structure of the foot (fig. 16.5).

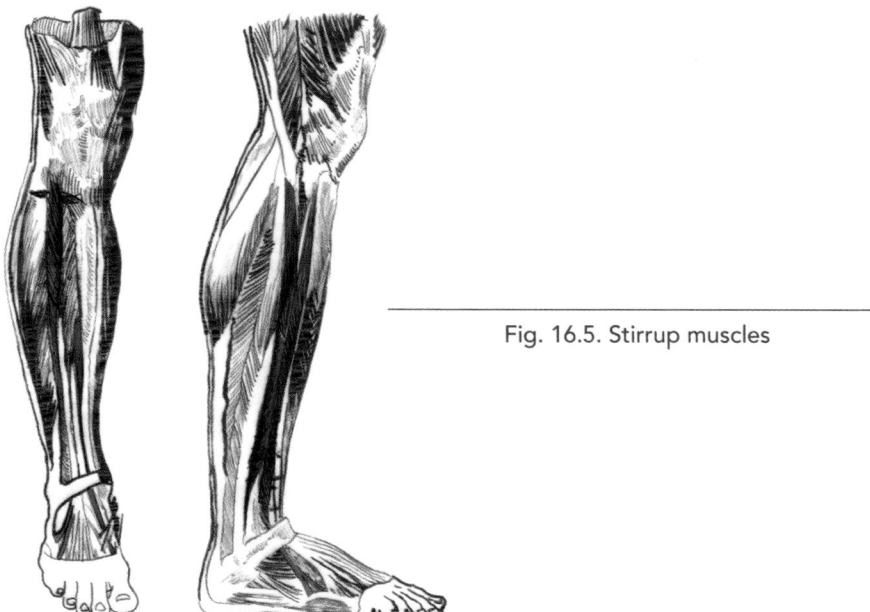

Fig. 16.5. Stirrup muscles

1. Sit in a chair with your knees and hips level, feet flat on the floor. Throughout this exercise, the inner anklebones, the knees, and (hopefully) the big toes should be together. The toes may not join if you have a bunion or hammertoes—you could place a piece of foam rubber between your toes to join them. Tie the big toes together with a rubber band. Sit up straight, keeping the big toes, inner anklebones, and knees together, and lift just the toes as high as they will go. Try to lift them together, so the outer toes come up as far as the big toe (fig. 16.6 left). Then lift up the whole foot, keeping the heels on the floor (fig. 16.6 right).

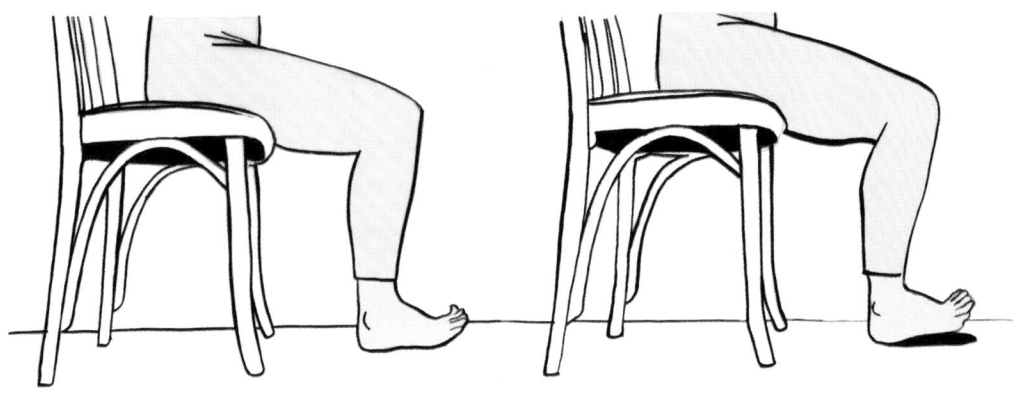

Fig. 16.6. Lift only the toes; then lift up the whole foot, heels on floor

2. Next lower just the balls of the feet, keeping the toes up.
3. Then lower the toes so your feet are back in the starting position, flat on the ground.
4. Repeat the movement—toes up, feet up, feet down, toes down. Keep each move separate and crisp, taking it for its maximum stretch. As you learn this, go slowly, concentrating on form, but aim to speed it up without losing the precision of each separate movement. Continue until your muscles are fatigued, rest 30 seconds, and repeat.

The muscles you feel working in the calves are the ones that pull up the arches of the foot. If you feel a lot of work in your groin or thighs, check that your chair is the right height—it's probably too high. This exercise tones the stirrup muscles that pull up the arch of the foot and can correct flat feet.

THE RETINACULUM

The retinaculum is a band of fascia that encircles the ankle like a collar, protecting the ankle joint from injury. Because we don't move our feet and ankles very much, due to walking on hard, flat surfaces in restrictive footwear, the retinaculum often gets very tight in one or all of its aspects.

When you stand normally, barefoot, you may feel tightness and pulling in one part of the ankle. This pulling will shift your weight over into that place, possibly creating other problems. A tight retinaculum can also pull the plantar fascia or the Achilles tendon on the other side of the foot and ankle, contributing to plantar fasciitis.

Sports tend to produce tightness in the front of the foot and shin, and weak muscles in those areas, combined with tightness, cause shin splints. If you suffer from shin splints, do the stretches below and the Achilles tendon stretch (see page 261), and then strengthen the pained shin muscles, tibialis anterior and posterior. The top of the foot gets tight mostly because we exercise wearing restrictive—supportive—footwear, which prevents full flexion of the ankle. Sedentary people who never walk usually have more flexible shins and feet—unless they drive all the time, in which case the tissue at the top of the right foot is shortened, and the ankle joint compressed on that side, from using the accelerator and brake pedals.

✍ Deep Stretches for the Top of the Foot

The sole of the foot receives attention in reflexology, and most of us have some awareness of it. Those reflex zones go all the way through the foot, from the sole to the top, so you are also working your whole body when you work the top of your foot.

1. Bring one foot up onto a table or anything that will work for you. Roughly speaking, the higher the surface, the more of a stretch you get. The raised leg must be straight to do this one properly, so if your hamstrings are too tight to straighten the leg, you'll need to modify (and work on your hamstring flexibility). The standing leg can be bent if you like.

2. Now lean forward and press your toes down, away from you, while isometrically pressing your heel down and pulling the ankle back toward you (fig. 16.7). Make sure you get both sides of the foot, and don't avoid the tight toes. You can press your feet down and to the side as well for a different stretch. To increase the stretch, you can place the heel of the foot you are stretching on a yoga block.

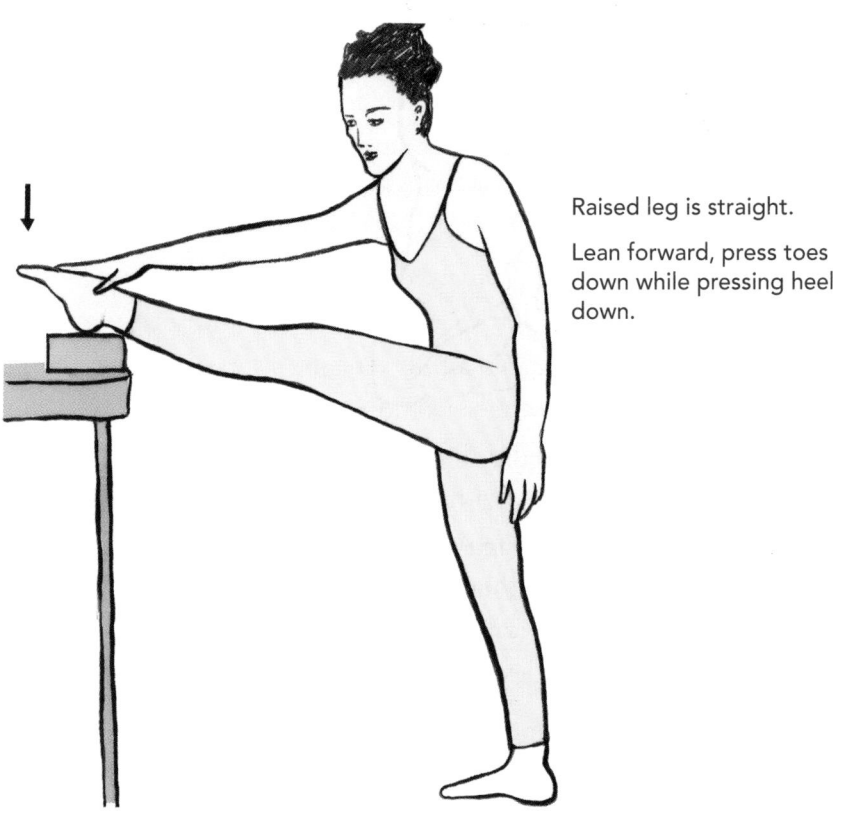

Raised leg is straight.

Lean forward, press toes down while pressing heel down.

Fig. 16.7. Deep Stretches for the Top of the Foot

3. You can also work that tight fascial collar in this position. Hold onto the foot in the stretch. Then, using the knuckles of the other hand, rub all over the top, the sides, and wherever else feels good on the foot. Then work the retinaculum around the top and sides of the ankle, all the way up to the shins.

4. When you have stretched and worked one foot thoroughly, walk around and compare the two sides of your body. Notice any differences, and then repeat on the other side.

To modify: You can just press down with your hand very lightly. Lean your body up against a wall for balance if you need to—the wall should be to your side.

If you can't straighten or raise your leg enough to open the retinaculum this way, you could sit or stand, curling the toes under, and pressing the heels forward (see fig. 16.8 on page 260). You can roll the top of the foot on the floor to stretch evenly from the outside to the inside of the foot.

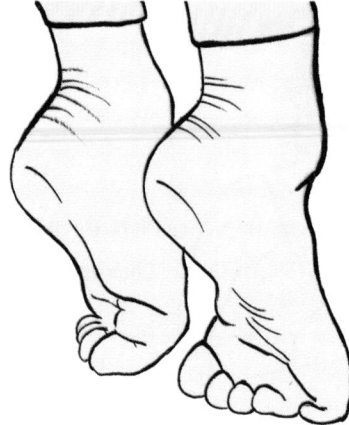

Fig. 16.8. Toes curled under

If your foot cramps, stretch the Achilles tendon and calf first. Again, walk around after you stretch your feet and notice how the rest of your body feels. You will probably have shifted your weight in some way, perhaps feeling more of the surface of your foot on the ground. You may even feel changes in your back and neck.

🍃 Runner's Stretch

If you have tight hamstrings, you can stretch the front of the foot and shin successfully in a runner's stretch.

1. With one knee bent, sit on the heel, and straighten the other leg in front of you with the foot pointed down at the floor. Bring your hand to your toes to curl them down, stretching the front of the foot (fig.16.9). You can also stretch this area

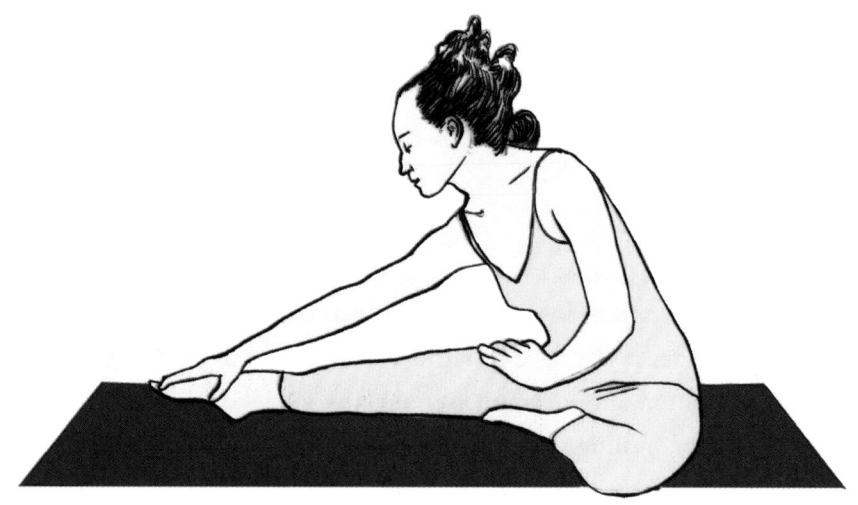

Fig. 16.9. Runner's Stretch

while standing, by rolling the top of one foot onto a soft surface and bringing the top of the ankle forward, away from the toes.

🌿 *Stretch the Achilles Tendon and the Deeper Calf Muscles*

Most of us in this nonsquatting culture have chronically shortened Achilles tendons. We do almost nothing in our everyday lives that stretches this area.

1. To determine if your Achilles tendon is shortened, see if you can squat with your hips on your heels and your feet straight out in front of you. Don't try this if it hurts your knees or hips. The feet should be placed together. If your tendon is very short you'll hardly be able to bring your hips down below knee level.

2. You may find that you have enough flexibility to come into this position, but you can't maintain your balance. Usually this is because the tendon isn't flexible enough to enable you to bring your knees forward to the place where your weight is stabilized. If so, you can hold onto something in front of you and practice gradually letting go until you can maintain your position without holding on. You need to do this barefoot.

◈ Achilles Tendon Stretch with Yoga Block

If this stretch is out of the question for you, you can bring the ball of the foot on top of a yoga block, positioning the block securely against the wall, heel on the floor with as steep an angle as is comfortable (see fig. 16.10 on page 262). You will need to be barefoot.

1. Keep the back leg straight, square the hips, and then bend the front of the knee directly forward over the ankle—no torqueing to either side. Lean forward onto the side with the bent knee to stretch. The degree of bend in the knee will determine how much you stretch your Achilles tendon and the deeper calf muscles. You will not stretch these tissues in a straight leg calf stretch.

2. You may notice that the knee tracks differently over the right and left sides, wanting to turn in or out more on one side; don't let it. The knee should track over the second toe as you look down. Alignment is important here,

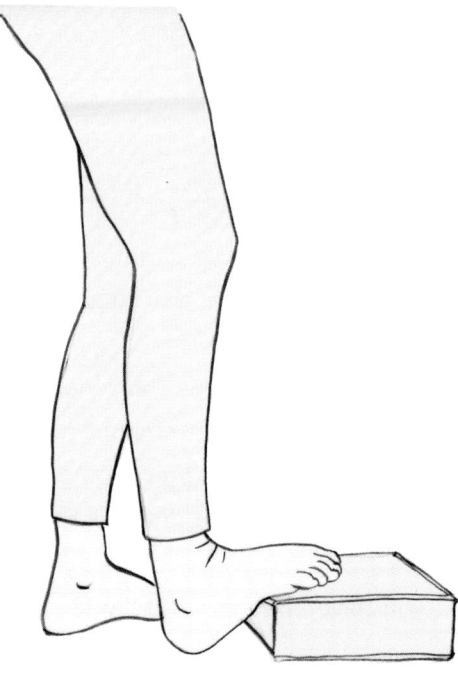

Fig. 16.10. Stretch the Achilles Tendon and the Deeper Calf Muscles

but make sure that when you correct this, your hips remain square to the front and your feet do not roll in or out. If the front of the foot prevents your knee coming forward, you need to stretch this area before you do this exercise.

◈ Massaging the Top of the Foot

While the top of your foot is stretched out in any position that works for you, you can rub that area with your knuckles. Use a small amount of cream or oil if you want. Start at the ankle, rub back and forth all around, and work the entire top of the foot. You'll probably find some real sore spots; work them until they feel released.

You are breaking down the excess granulation in the fascia around the foot and ankle, which will free up the muscles in the top and center of the foot. Since the sole of the foot gets some movement and stretch by default—through walking on it—you will balance the structure of the connective tissue this way. You can also relieve plantar fasciitis or any problem in the sole of the foot.

17

Ball Exercises

A LOT OF THE EXERCISES I do with clients are with rubber balls, the ordinary toy store kind, of different sizes and materials. The most basic exercises use the pressure of the ball and the weight of our bodies to widen muscles and release surface tension. Once the tension is released, you can start to include movements and work with combinations of pressure and movement. See my first book, *The Bodywork Manual*, for more on this. You will need two 2.5-inch balls ("Pinky" or lacrosse balls, available at sports supply stores), two 4-inch soft rubber balls (Balanced Body makes nice ones), one 5-inch hollow rubber ball, and one 7-inch hollow rubber ball (these are playground balls, available from toy stores, sports supply stores, or school suppliers).

Most of the movements in these ball exercises involve using small, interior muscles that are difficult to isolate and even to feel. These muscles tend to become progressively less available as the larger, easier-to-feel surface muscles take over their subtle functions. As the more superficial muscles become overused and tight, the movements they are involved with grow more restricted. In order to use these deep muscles consciously, we need to prevent the superficial ones from moving. Placing a ball directly on the areas we want to immobilize prevents us from using them and lets us feel when parts of the body move in precise, often unfamiliar ways.

You may find that it is difficult for you not only to feel and control deep muscles, but also to avoid using completely different parts of your body. For example, when you try to work your shoulders with small movements, you may feel the tightening in your feet or your pelvis as well. This tells you that the movements of your shoulders and your feet are somehow connected, either through fascia or in your nervous system as part of a movement pattern. You can identify these patterns as you work on the balls and learn to differentiate your movements as much as possible.

The balls also provide a kinesthetic surface for movement, amplifying the small movements, allowing you to feel more precisely what you are doing. Awareness—awareness felt and experienced in the nervous system, not just intellectual awareness—will create change without a painful effort, so even if you cannot do the exercises as well as you would like, the process itself will form new patterns that you will be able to incorporate in your everyday life.

The small, hard "Pinky" balls, or tennis balls, can be used on their own to release tension. You can work them all over the body, starting by lying on the floor and rolling them up and down alongside the spine (not directly on the spine, just next to it). You can work them into the buttocks and legs. You can sit on them; you can use them under the legs and turn onto your stomach and work them into your chest and rib cage. The head and the face also respond well to this use of the balls, you can put them inside a clean sock if you like. Put them between the hipbone and the pubic bone to release the psoas. You can raise yourself onto your hands, arching your back, and roll the balls up and down in the groin area to release those muscles more effectively. You can stand on the balls and work them into your feet. Use them any way that feels good.

It is very effective to make sounds and vocalize when you use the balls this way, in order to release completely and on a deeper level. Try to find a sound that expresses the sensation you are experiencing at that moment (this type of ball work can be quite painful) and express it as fully as possible on the exhale.

🍃 Warm-Up Exercises for the Back and Neck

You will need two 4-inch rubber balls and either a 5-inch or a 7-inch ball, whichever is more comfortable, for your neck.

These are the most basic pressure exercises for the back and neck. They are a good lead-in to just about any other sequence, and they break up some surface tension and improve flexibility in the shoulders and neck. Pain that subsides is an indication that surface tension is breaking up. If you have pain or pressure that does not go away in a short time, use softer balls; that is, older balls that have deflated a little. You can also vary the amount of pressure by changing the surface you lie on; a soft bed will provide the least resistance, a hard floor the most.

When you have finished with each exercise, roll off the balls and lie flat on your back for a minute, letting yourself become aware of any changes in your body. This practice is important with all the ball exercises, because it gives your nervous system a chance to take in the new patterns you have just given it and make them a part of your movement language.

◈ Warm-Up for the Back

Put the two 4-inch balls on either side of your spine, just touching each other. Start about waist level or a little higher, making sure your lower back is not arched off the floor, and bend your knees with your feet on the floor at a comfortable distance from your buttocks. If you find yourself tightening your back to prevent your feet from sliding down, stabilize them against a wall.

1. Make sure you are relaxed over the balls, and take a deep, comfortable breath, letting your shoulders drop back toward the ground. Then slowly move the balls up your back vertebrae by moving your feet down so your body slides over the balls. Stay longer in any place along your back that feels tight or is hard to let go of.

2. When you have slid the balls up so they are at the lowest part of your shoulder blade, which is probably lower than you think it is, start to rotate your arms as far as you comfortably can, keeping the shoulders relaxed and letting the arm rest in any position that feels tight. Let the shoulder joint fall back so that the energy of the rotation comes from the fingertips and the shoulder stays relaxed. You can rotate both clockwise and counterclockwise, once in each direction.

3. Move the balls up the spine, and rotate your arms in each position. One rotation on each side for each position of the ball is enough. When you have come up to the top of the spine and the balls cannot go any farther, raise your arms above your head so the balls slide out between your ears and your shoulders.

◈ Warm-Up for the Neck

Now take the 5- or the 7-inch ball and put it under the back of your neck. Remember how heavy your head is, about twelve pounds, and allow all of that weight to rest completely on the ball (see fig. 17.2 on page 271 for head position).

1. Make sure that all the vertebrae in your neck are touching the ball and that there is no tension in the front of your neck or your throat. Then turn your head slowly over to the right, as far as you can go without tightening the neck muscles or sliding off the ball.

2. Turn back to the center, and then repeat the same movement over to the left. If it is much harder to move toward one side than the other, repeat that movement until both sides feel the same.

You may discover, even if you are not aware of having a tight neck, that you may only be able to move an inch or so on the ball without tightening your neck. (You can touch the front of your neck if you are not sure what is happening here.) This means that you are used to supporting the weight of your head with these muscles in the front of the neck, which happens a lot if you are sitting and using your eyes a great deal, so that the head is pushed forward and is no longer supported by the entire spine, as it is designed to be. Think of rolling the back of the head on the ball to allow the neck to relax.

⚘ Basic Ball Exercises
Each of the following basic ball exercises works a specific area of the body.

◈ Basic Ball Exercise for the Legs
1. Sit with your back supported against a wall. Use the 2.5-inch solid rubber ball on the calf at the top of the Achilles tendon; this is the sensitive place at the back of the calf just below the bulge of the calf muscle. Both legs should be straight out in front of you.
2. You can use the small ball or the 4-inch ball anywhere up the back of the leg. The 4-inch should be used under the knee and at the top of the leg just under the buttock.

◈ Basic Ball Exercise for the Hips
1. Lie on your side with a ball between the hipbone and the fleshy part of the buttock; most people have a slight depression here that the ball will fit right into. The 4-inch is probably the best for this exercise, but the smallest ball will work as well and can penetrate deeper into the hip joint. Rest your weight on your elbows, with the other leg behind or in front for more intensity. Rotate your ankle from side to side, turning your foot, to work the ball deeper into the hip.
2. Lie on your stomach with the two 4-inch balls between the hipbone and the pubic bone on both sides. Rest with your toes pointed inward. Do not stay in this position longer than a few minutes, because it will put some pressure on the frontal nerves, and your legs may go to sleep.

◈ Basic Ball Exercises for the Diaphragm and Rib Cage

1. After working the pelvis, you can move the 4-inch balls straight up the abdomen until they are under the rib cage.

2. Then, when this position feels comfortable, take one of the balls out and roll the other into the middle of the abdomen right under the rib cage, on the solar plexus. If this doesn't feel like much, try the 5-inch ball. If it is too strong, raise yourself on your elbows to decrease the pressure. Expand your whole rib cage when you breathe, rather than breathing directly against the ball. You can move the ball up until it is resting against the sternum. Let your shoulders drop to the floor, palms facing upward.

3. For your rib cage, lie on your side with the 4-inch ball under your ribs. To decrease pressure, rest your weight on your elbow; to increase it, lie down so your head is resting on your arm. Start with the ball at the waist, and slowly move so it slides up toward your armpits. When we breathe, we tend not to use the ribs by the armpits much, so they can be sore. Breathe into the pressure, and work slowly.

4. When this gets easy, you can use the small ball the same way to get into the spaces between the ribs.

◈ Basic Ball Exercise for the Head

Use one or two of the 2.5-inch balls for the head. You can put the two balls in a sock and then tie the sock so the balls stay together. The sock will also prevent the balls from getting caught in your hair. For a slight elevation, use a book or a firm pillow. Place the ball or balls anywhere on your head, either lying on your side, front, or back, depending which part of the head you want to work. You can use them on your forehead and rest them on the book or pillow you are using. For the best effect try to work the edges of the cranial plates, the flat bones of the skull, with the balls.

ADVANCED BALL EXERCISES

After you get used to these basic ball exercises, and they become too easy or boring, you can start to combine small movements with the pressure of the balls, with much more dramatic results. The small, precise movements work deep muscles that are underused. The balls also allow you to feel what you are doing more clearly and will prevent you from using the surface muscles that lie directly under the ball; the ball will slide away if you do. These exercises also encourage the nervous system to learn new patterns quickly when there is input from movement and pressure simultaneously.

Learn to differentiate muscles; not engaging the wrong muscles is much more important than "doing it right." Change is created by the process of working your body in a different way, so don't worry about jerky, uncoordinated movements—that just means you are moving new muscles, and the exercise will become progressively easier as you get used to it. Making the switch from the idea that *what* you are doing is important to focusing on *how* you are doing it is probably quite different from the way you have learned any other skill, so be prepared for some resistance. Please persist—these exercises are worth it.

Advanced Ball Exercises for the Neck and Shoulders

Advanced Ball Exercise for the Neck and Shoulders I

1. Start with the 7-inch ball under the back of your neck, touching each vertebra. You should be lying on your back, with your knees bent (see fig. 17.2 on page 271 for head position). Let your neck relax so the weight of your head is completely supported by the ball.

2. Roll your head slowly from side to side, using the weight of your head to roll, not the muscles at the front of the neck or your throat. Put your hand at the place just below the throat where the collarbones meet to make sure nothing happens there. If you can move only a little before these muscles start to work, then only go that far.

3. You may find that one side moves easily, but you can barely move the other side at all. Work from the center toward the difficult side, back to the center, back again to the difficult side, until the movement is equal.

Advanced Ball Exercise for the Neck and Shoulders II

When this movement feels comfortable, turn your knees over to the right side, keeping the ball where it is. Then slide your right arm under your body and roll your head over to the right, still keeping it on the ball, so you are lying on your side with your right arm under you and the side of your neck on the ball (fig. 17.1).

1. Push the ball down to the collarbone so the whole neck is resting on it. You may feel sore, so try to relax into it for a while, and if it still feels bad, move the ball

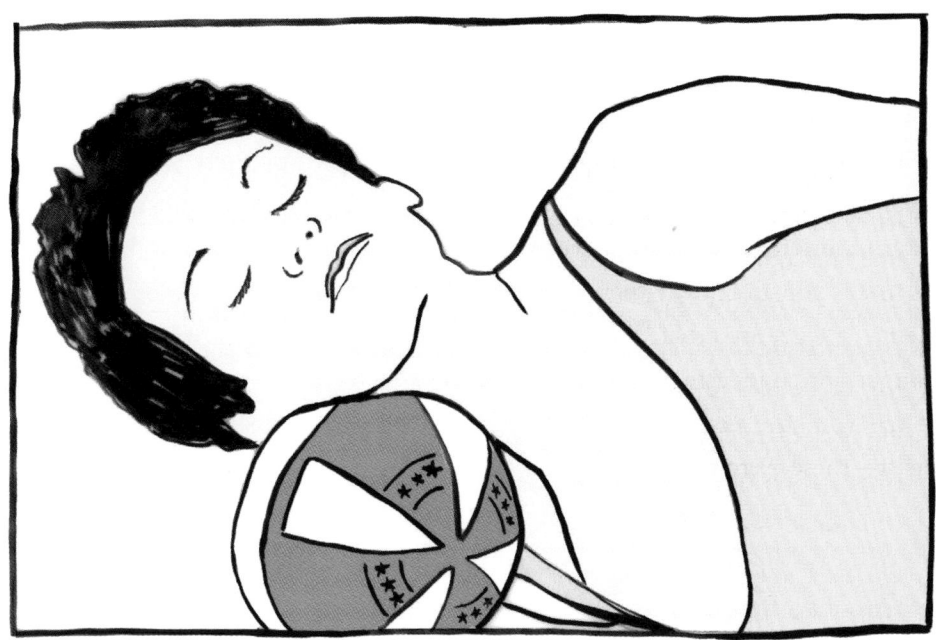

Fig. 17.1. Advanced Ball Exercise for the Neck and Shoulders II

farther toward the back of the head. The left hand can be in front with the hand resting on the floor to support you, or behind your back, whichever is more comfortable. Make sure the left side of your neck is completely relaxed as you move and that the weight of your head stays dropped into the ball.

2. Now look up as far as you can, toward the ceiling, and then move your head up in the direction you are looking, keeping your neck soft so that the movement is a rolling of the head on the ball. Then look down as far as you can toward the ball, and let the head follow. Now look down as far as you can toward your feet, still letting the head follow. Repeat this sequence a few times.

3. Then go back into the starting position and work with the first step for a while, rolling the head from side to side on the ball. You should feel a difference between the side you worked and the other one. Notice what the differences are, and then repeat the whole sequence on the other side.

4. You can intensify this exercise by reversing the eye movements so your head moves away from the direction of your eyes. In other words look toward your feet, move the head away from the feet when the stretch in the eyes becomes sore, look up, and then move the head down. Do the same for the other movement: look at the ball, head moves to ceiling; look at ceiling, head moves down.

BALL EXERCISES

269

◈ Advanced Ball Exercise for the Neck and Shoulders III
Use either the 5- or 4-inch ball for this exercise.

1. Lie on your back with the ball on the ridge at the base of the skull, just above the hairline. This hollow varies in size and shape for people, so choose the size ball that feels right for you. Relax the front of the neck and open your mouth slightly, so you do not use your chin or tighten your jaw.
2. Imagine that the circle where the ball touches your head is a clock face, 12 on top, 6 on the bottom. Keeping the circle even, push down from the spine and the back of the head very slightly, allowing the weight of the head to fall on each segment of the clock face as precisely as you can. Move clockwise and then counterclockwise. If it helps you, you can imagine a line going from the middle of the clock face to a point in the middle of the forehead between the eyes. This is the axis that your rotations should move around.

The purpose of the exercise is to allow the weight of your head to rest exactly on each number of the clock face without pushing down from the front. This is an isolation exercise, so if you find yourself using parts of your body other than the back of the neck and the base of the skull to move your head, gently stop that other part of your body and take notice of what is happening. You have identified a movement pattern in your body, a part of your body where the movement is unnecessarily hooked up with another part, and you can use that understanding to inform the way you move in your everyday life.

◈ Advanced Ball Exercise for the Neck and Shoulders IV
1. Lie on your back, knees up, feet on the floor, with the 7-inch ball under your head and the 4-inch between your left shoulder blade and your spine (fig. 17.2).
2. Your arms rest at your sides with your palms down. Imagine a magnet at your fingertips and another magnet at the wall by your feet. The magnet at the wall is pulling your arm and shoulder down toward the wall, the movement spreading all the way to the middle of the collarbone. Keep your shoulder back as you move your fingertips down, even if it means pushing down into the ball. Move your shoulder up and down in this way, your farthest-up place being where the shoulder lies when the collarbone is straight.
3. Then include a head movement, so that when the shoulder moves down, you

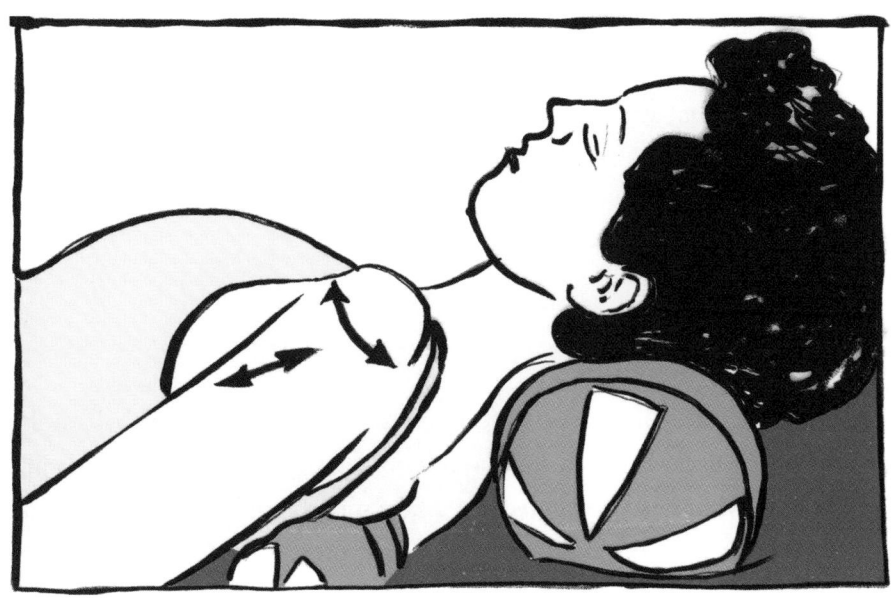

Fig. 17.2. Advanced Ball Exercise for the Neck and Shoulders IV

turn your head toward it, and when the shoulder moves up, you turn your head back to the center position. Remember to keep the front of the neck soft and do not let either movement become larger than the other. Repeat this movement for about a minute.

4. Then reverse the movement, so that when the shoulder moves down, the head turns away from it, and when the shoulder moves up, the head turns toward it. Repeat for about a minute.

5. Then go back to the shoulder movements on their own without moving the head. Notice any changes from the beginning.

6. Then repeat the whole sequence on the other side.

◈ Advanced Ball Exercise for the Neck and Shoulders V

This is the same exercise, but with a change in the shoulder movement. The 7-inch ball goes under the neck, and the 4-inch is between the shoulder blade and the spine.

1. Press the shoulder into the floor, so that you try to touch the floor with the tip of the shoulder. Release and relax the shoulder, and then repeat a few times.

2. Now bring in the head movement, so that when you press the shoulder down,

you turn your head toward it, and when the shoulder moves up, you turn your head back to the center position. Repeat this movement a few times, and then reverse it, so that when the shoulder is pushed down, the head turns away from it, and when the shoulder releases, the head turns toward it. End with the shoulder presses on their own.

3. Then repeat everything on the other side.

◈ Advanced Ball Exercise for the Neck and Shoulders VI

Lie on your back with your knees up, feet on the floor. Put the 4-inch ball on the left side of the upper back, between the shoulder blade and the spine (fig. 17.3 upper). Use a pillow for your head if you need to. Make sure the right shoulder is resting on the floor, and if it will not go down, rest a pillow on it to remind you not to move it. You are going to work your rotator cuff muscles, the four tiny muscles that are involved in the rotation of the arm, and you must carefully avoid using the trapezius, the deltoids, and the chest and back muscles, all of which are usually involved in shoulder and arm rotations (fig. 17.3 lower).

1. Isolate the front shoulder joint, which is at the very tip of the shoulder, and start to make very tiny rotations, no bigger than a dime, starting at the top, toward your head, then moving toward the floor, then your feet, then up toward the ceiling, and then back to your head again. The mistake most people make with this exercise is to make the rotations too big. They should be *tiny*. The unevenness and jerkiness will smooth out as long as you stay with the shoulder joint movements and do not allow the larger muscles to take over. Reverse the direction of the circles after a few minutes.

2. Then bend your arm at the elbow and, keeping the shoulder relaxed, make wide circles with the elbow. When these circles are completely comfortable, hold your arm at a right angle to your body and make circles about the size of a silver dollar, in both directions. After about two minutes, stretch out your arm completely and make wide rotations.

3. You can intensify the stretch by holding your arm out in the position where you feel the most stretch and rotating your wrist in both directions. Don't do this unless you have flexible shoulders.

4. Now repeat everything on the opposite side.

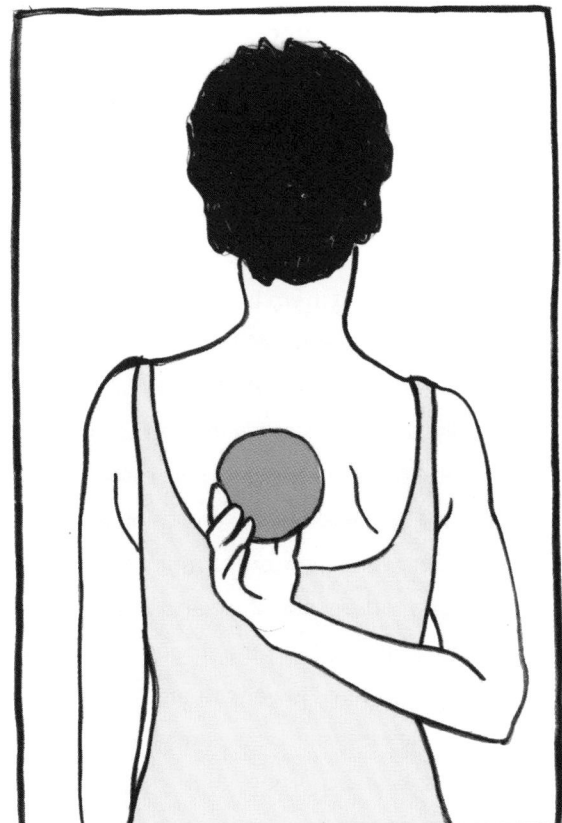

Correct position
of the ball

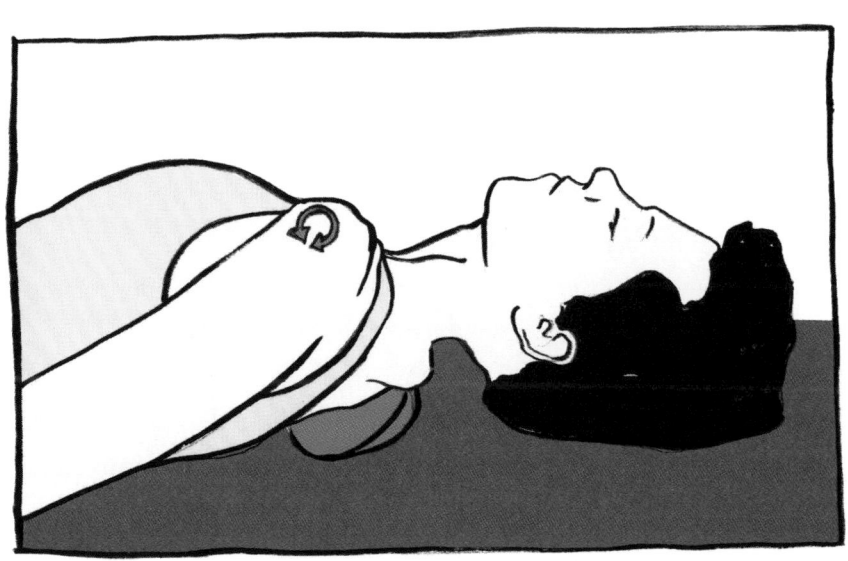

Fig. 17.3. Advanced Ball Exercise for the Neck and Shoulders VI

◈ Advanced Ball Exercise for the Neck and Shoulders VII

Put two 4-inch balls between the shoulder blades and the spine, so the balls touch. Lie on your back with your knees bent, feet on the floor. Place your arms beside you, palms down.

1. Slowly move both arms along the floor until they are at right angles to your body, palms still down. Then raise them both up so the hands are directly above your shoulder, with both palms facing outward and fingertips reaching toward the ceiling. Make sure your wrists and arms are in a line with each other. Right-handed people will tend to pull the right arm in too far over the chest because the right shoulder will want to rotate forward. You may notice that your shoulders and arms are not straight at all, even when you think they are.

2. Now raise up your shoulders so the fingertips reach to the ceiling, the movement coming from the shoulders rather than the hands, and then drop and relax the shoulders down onto the balls, keeping the fingertips up toward the ceiling.

3. Keeping the palms facing outward, lower the arms until they are about an inch from the floor at right angles to your body, and then turn your wrists a quarter circle so that the thumbs face up. Then, with the thumbs facing each other, raise both arms up and repeat the previous sequence, raising and dropping the shoulders.

4. Lower the arms, thumbs still facing up, until they are an inch or so away from the floor, and then turn the wrists another quarter circle in the same direction, so that the palms are facing up, and repeat the sequence with the palms in that position.

5. Again, when the arms are an inch from the floor, turn the wrists a quarter circle so the edge of the hand is facing up and repeat the sequence.

6. Of course, you cannot turn the wrists any farther in that direction, so repeat the sequence in the reverse direction, to complete the exercise.

Even though the movements are somewhat complicated, they are easy to do, so when you can do the exercise easily, concentrate on keeping the arms straight and even, and try to move both arms equally.

◈ Advanced Ball Exercise for the Neck and Shoulders VIII

This exercise will either work miracles for you or have no effect at all, depending on whether or not you need it. You will not feel the release right away, as you do in most of the other ball exercises, so give it a few weeks of regular practice before you decide whether to keep using it. Take a 4-inch ball, preferably slightly used and softer for better traction, and place it under the spine of your neck, touching the base of the skull at the top and the seventh cervical vertebra (the large protuberant bone at the bottom of the neck) at the bottom. Relax the neck and head over the ball, letting your head touch the floor if it goes that far. You may find it more comfortable to bring your knees to your chest to stabilize your pelvis. Having your knees bent and your feet on the floor is also fine. Try to sense each vertebra and its position as it touches the ball.

1. Press the very top vertebra that you can feel in the back, just under the skull, into the ball without using the muscles at the front and sides of the neck. You should use the muscles at the back, along the spine. Think of working the spine itself to help you isolate these muscles. You can allow your whole spine to move. This is an almost impossible isolation to achieve with mental effort alone, so you will probably find that you need to hold the muscles in the front to prevent them from working. Start at the top of the throat, under the earlobe, and press diagonally down toward the juncture on the collarbones. You may find it more effective to hold the muscle in the middle or where you feel it protrude on top of the collarbone. Work both sides at the same time as you press the top vertebra down. If you find your jaw tightening, open your mouth. If your tongue feels tight, stick it out so it cannot help you with the movement. Your head will lift slightly as you press down.

2. Now try to isolate the second vertebra, again paying attention to relaxing the front and sides of the neck. Think of lengthening the neck, imagining that a line moves from the bottom of the cervical spine through the middle of the neck and up to the base of the skull. Slowly work down, vertebra by vertebra, until you come to the lowest vertebra that you can work with (there are six in the neck you can work this way). With each one, carefully lower your neck onto the ball, keeping the contact with the spine, and try to feel each vertebra as you go down.

3. Relax for a minute in this position, and then repeat the sequence.

🍂 Advanced Ball Exercise for the Jaw

Use the small solid pink ball for this exercise. You can put it on a hard pillow, the edge of a thick hardcover book, or a rubber "donut." If you have fine hair, you may need to put the ball inside a sock so it doesn't slip. The other side of the ball should be on the ridge at the base of the skull above the hairline, where there is a hollow that the ball should fit right into (fig. 17.4).

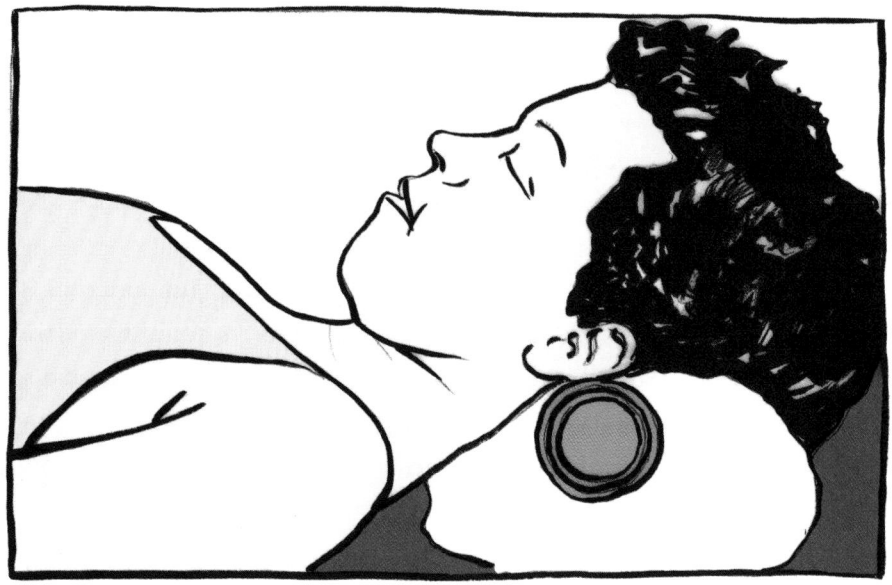

Fig. 17.4. Advanced Ball Exercise for the Jaw

1. Lie on your back, knees bent, feet on the floor. When the ball is comfortable, start nodding your head up and down, with your jaw loose and your throat relaxed, moving from your forehead. You can hold the ball in place if this makes it easier.

2. After about a minute, rest your head in the position where the chin is closest to the throat, and immobilize your lower jaw completely by holding onto your chin. The teeth will be touching in this position. Then open your mouth by opening only the upper jaw, not letting the lower jaw move at all. If this seems easy, you are probably not doing it right. Slow down—the movement is very slow—and closely observe what you are doing.

3. Sometimes it is easier to immobilize the lower jaw if you hold the top of the lower teeth, even though this means you cannot start from a closed mouth position. Think of opening and closing the mouth by leading from the nose, or visualize a band running around the head from the middle of the ball around the cheeks and under the nose. Now open and close the mouth with the strength of this band.

4. There is no need to repeat this exercise many times if you are doing it correctly.

If it is too difficult, work with a smaller range of movement, gradually increasing it as the exercise gets easier. When the whole exercise becomes easy, soften and protrude your tongue slightly, keeping it in the same place throughout the exercise.

🍃 Advanced Ball Exercise for the Diaphragm

Lie on your back with your knees bent, feet on the ground. Put two 4-inch balls on your back, directly opposite your solar plexus (fig. 17.5). The balls should be on the rib cage, not the lower back. If you feel any strain in your lower back, put a pillow under your pelvis, so there is no arch in the back. The balls should be almost touching, with the spine in the middle.

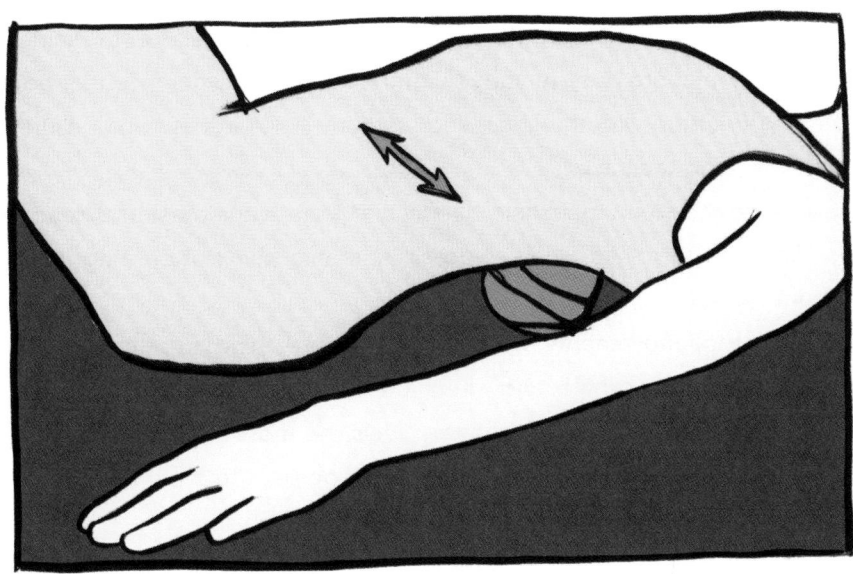

Fig. 17.5. Advanced Ball Exercise for the Diaphragm

1. Imagine that you have a belt on, and the balls are the clasp at the back of the belt. Try to move just the segment of your body that is under the belt toward the right, then back to the center, then over to the left, and back to the center again. If you are doing this correctly, you will not be able to move more than half an inch or so. Think about using the muscles at the side of the body, between the ribs. If it helps, you can imagine that a magnet on the wall is pulling your side ribs over toward it.

2. You will probably find that one side is harder to move than the other. You should work the more difficult side until both sides feel equal.

3. Remove the balls by rolling them away with your hands, keeping your back relaxed, and finish by hugging your knees to your chest to release any tension in the lower back.

❧ *Advanced Ball Exercises for the Sternum*

◈ Advanced Ball Exercise for the Sternum I

Lie on your stomach with the ball on your sternum, wherever it naturally rests (fig. 17.6).

1. Bring your hands to your shoulders, palms on the floor. Lift your chest and head up by pushing your sternum against the ball, and inhale deeply at the same time. This is like the cobra pose in yoga, with the important difference that now you are trying to lift up with the chest and sternum, while in the yoga position you are mainly using the back.

2. Still working the sternum, exhale deeply and lower your chest and head to the floor. Let the ball roll as much as possible; in fact, think of pushing it with the sternum.

3. Now repeat the movements with the opposite breathing; in other words, when you lift the sternum, exhale, and when you lower your chest, inhale.

4. Work with whichever breathing pattern feels the most strange or unfamiliar to you until you feel some ease with it, and then go back to the more comfortable pattern and notice any changes you may feel.

◈ Advanced Ball Exercise for the Sternum II

This sternum exercise is a little more subtle and harder to feel than the first one.

1. Start in the same position, with the ball under the sternum (fig. 17.6), and gently bring your arms up to your head, keeping your palms on the floor. This is easy but becomes much harder if you try to isolate your sternum without using your shoulders in the movement. You should think of the shoulders dropping and relaxing as the arms lift up, which will automatically force you to engage the sternum.

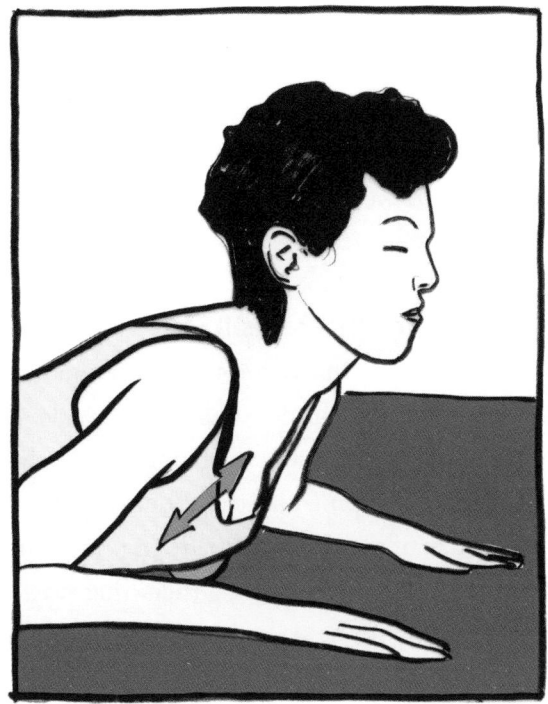

Fig. 17.6. Placement of ball under the sternum

2. When you are comfortable with this idea, you can experiment with different arm movements that work the sternum and allow the shoulders to relax.

✿ Advanced Ball Exercises for the Pelvis

◈ Advanced Ball Exercise for the Pelvis I

Lie on your stomach with one 4-inch ball in the groin area, between your pubic bone and your hipbone. If you are uncomfortable in this position, move the ball farther toward your abdomen. Then bend your knee, keeping the thigh on the floor, so that the heel faces the ceiling, perpendicular to your knee.

1. Make circles with your heel, with the foot slightly flexed, trying to smooth the circles so they feel even. The circles should be about the size of the knee. This movement originates in the hip joint and works the rotator muscles of the hips. Some people can feel this exercise in the hip joint right away; others find it harder to feel. If you have any trouble with this, touch your hip joint (in the

middle of the buttock) with your fingers to locate the movement and try to feel it from the inside.

2. To work different parts of the joint, move the knee up, farther away from the other leg, as far as you can go without changing the relationship of the knee and the heel (the heel should always be directly over the knee). Work until the movement is as smooth as you can get it, and then change sides.

◈ Advanced Ball Exercise for the Pelvis II

This exercise follows the previous one, but you can do it on its own as well. Lying on your back, place one 4-inch ball under your pelvic girdle, on the bone, a few inches to the left of the sacrum. Make sure the ball is not on the lower back. Place another 4-inch ball between the spine and the shoulder blade on the left side, in the middle of the inside edge of the shoulder blade (fig. 17.7). Your hips should be level; if you feel any effort or strain in keeping them that way, use a pillow under the right hip. Your back should not be arched at all, but should curve slightly like a hammock between the two balls.

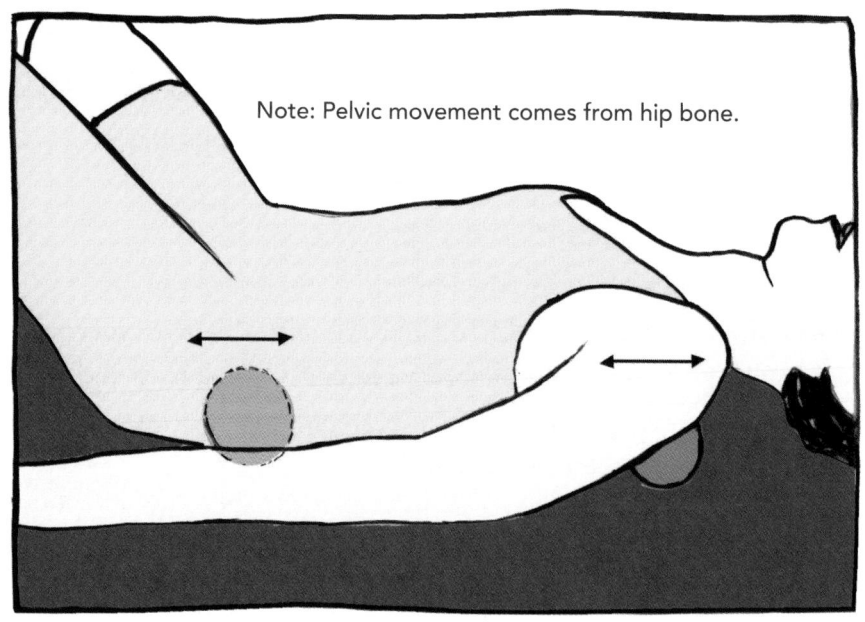

Note: Pelvic movement comes from hip bone.

Fig. 17.7. Advanced Ball Exercise for the Pelvis II

1. Now start by just moving your shoulders, as in Advanced Ball Exercise for the Neck and Shoulders IV (page 270), so your shoulders stay dropped toward the floor and your fingers move down toward your feet.

2. Then relax your shoulders and move the hipbone up and down, keeping it absolutely level so it does not rock or tilt up or down at all. Focus on isolating this movement so the only movement you feel is deep inside the pelvis. Imagine a line running from the inside of the hipbone in the middle, through the depth of the pelvis, connecting the hipbone to the inside of the sacrum. The part of the line attached to the sacrum stays still, while the part attached to the hipbone moves toward the feet and then up toward the head in a fan-like movement. The whole movement cannot be more than ½ inch. This is a very hard movement to isolate, so work with it for a while before you introduce the shoulder movements.

3. There are two ways you can combine the pelvic and the shoulder movements: opposition, where you bring the hipbone down and release the shoulder up to a position level with the collarbone, and then bring the hipbone up and move the shoulder down; and parallel, where the hipbone and shoulder move down together, and the shoulder releases up as the hipbone moves up. Make sure the movements stay the same size, as there will probably be a tendency for the shoulder to overwhelm the hip movement. And remember that you are actually isolating both the shoulder movement and the hip movement, not crunching them together from the middle of the body. Repeat on the right side.

◈ Advanced Ball Exercise for the Pelvis III

You need a chair for this one, and your knees and hips need to be level when you sit on it. Sit on the two 4-inch balls, one placed on each sit bone (see fig. 17.8 on page 282).

1. Now try to rock the sit bones on the balls without rocking the whole pelvis, while relaxing the groin and the abdominal muscles.

2. If the two sit bones feel uneven or different from each other, try to rock in such a way that the pressure of the ball can even them out. Again, this is a very small movement, not more than ½ inch.

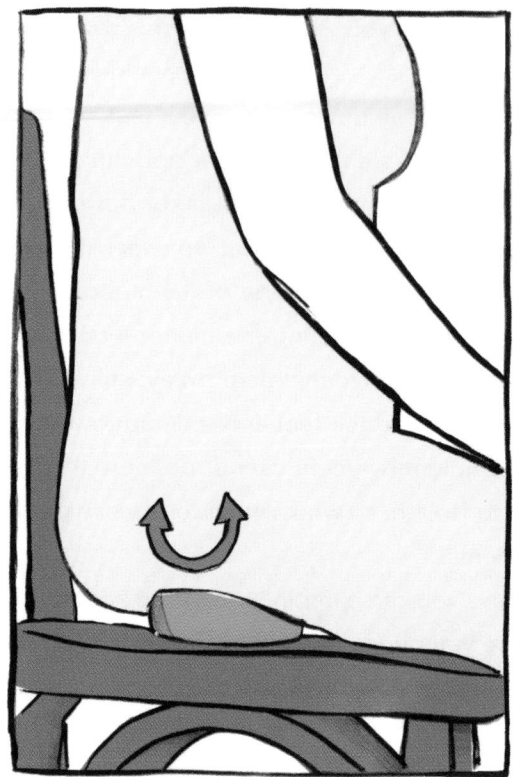

Fig. 17.8. Advanced Ball Exercise for the Pelvis III

◈ Advanced Ball Exercise for the Pelvis IV

This exercise adjusts your hips in a vertical direction; that is, you can use it if one hip is higher than the other. Don't use it unless you do feel uneven. You will need a door that has a rug on one side and two firm 4-inch balls. Be careful with this one—it's easy to fall off the balls.

1. Face the door as it is open. Place the balls a few inches from the door, and step onto them, holding the top of the door for support, or just the top and side. Put something behind the door to stabilize it if you want to. Your whole body should face the door, with no twisting, and both feet should be completely off the ground and firmly planted in the center of the balls.

2. Now press the foot on the side of the higher hip down hard into the ball until the foot is below the level of the other foot, so that the lower hip has to come up higher.

3. Release, and notice how the hips feel in relation to each other. If they still feel uneven, repeat the exercise. Be careful when you get off the balls!

◈ Advanced Ball Exercise for the Pelvis V

This exercise goes with the Advanced Ball Exercise for the Neck and Shoulders III on page 270; in fact it is the same exercise, but instead of putting the ball under the head, you put it under the tailbone (fig. 17.9).

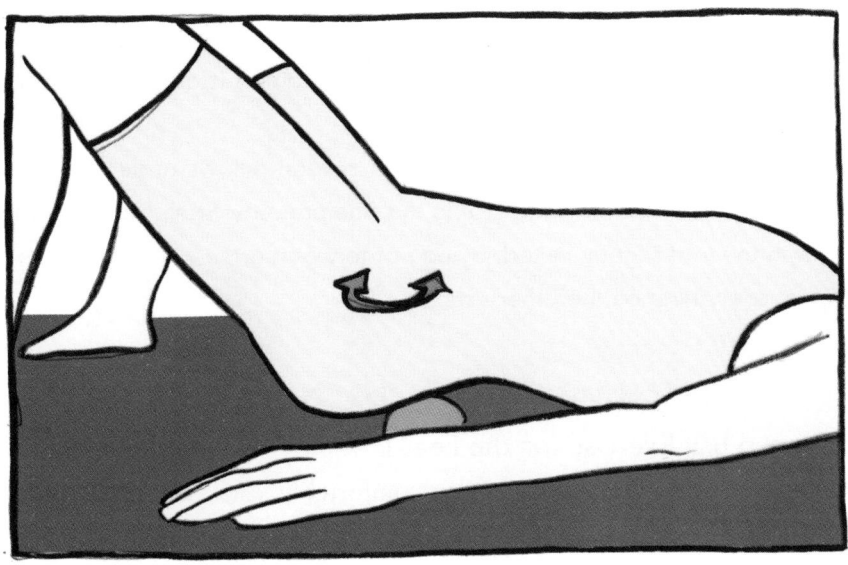

Fig. 17.9. Advanced Ball Exercise for the Pelvis V

1. Lie on your back with your knees bent, feet on the ground.
2. Imagine that there is a clock face on the sacrum, with the 12 toward your head and the 6 toward your feet. Thinking of moving only the sacrum, let the weight of the pelvis shift onto the imaginary clock face. Make sure the groin is relaxed and you are not rocking or swinging your hips.

🍂 *Advanced Ball Exercise for the Knees*

The knees, because they are hinge joints and do not have any rotation in their range of movement, are not ideal for ball work (neither are the elbows). Here is the only one I have found that is useful at all. This exercise can be used for injuries to the patella tendon if it is not painful to do.

1. Lie on your side with the top leg in front of the bottom leg, so the knee of the top leg is on the ground in front of you. Then place a 4-inch ball on the inside of that knee, raising the leg slightly by putting a pillow under the ball if you want to.

2. Start with the leg bent, and then slowly and gently straighten the leg, keeping it as straight and even as you can. The leg will probably wobble at first.

3. Then put the foot of the top leg on the floor, knee bent, and place the ball on the outside of the knee of the bottom leg (the position of the top leg is not important as long as it is not in the way).

4. Start with the bottom leg bent and gently straighten it out, just as you did in step 2.

5. Then place the ball under one knee with several pillows under the ball—you need at least a foot of elevation to do this one properly. Straighten and bend the leg with the foot slightly flexed, trying not to wobble.

6. Repeat everything on the other side.

🍃 *Advanced Ball Exercises for the Feet*

◈ Advanced Ball Exercise for the Feet I

You will need a chair that you can sit on comfortably, with your knees and hips at the same level. First, move your knees together and apart while you are sitting on the edge of the chair. Feel the place in the movement where both inner and outer thigh muscles are completely relaxed and your legs don't have to work at all. Then put two 4-inch balls under the middle of each foot (fig. 17.10).

1. Try to remember the feeling of the relaxed inner and outer thighs, so you can re-create that sensation with the balls under your feet. You can also use a mirror to make sure your feet are straight and both knees are directly above your ankles. Now, keeping your alignment, roll the ball from the second toe to the heel, first one foot, and then the other, and then both together. Don't let the movement get so big that you use your thigh muscles. You want to concentrate on using just the feet and all the muscles inside them.

2. Then rotate the ball under your foot, clockwise, counterclockwise, each foot separately, and then both together.

3. Now check your alignment with the balls under the feet, and press down gently with only your foot and calf muscles, as though you were trying to push the balls

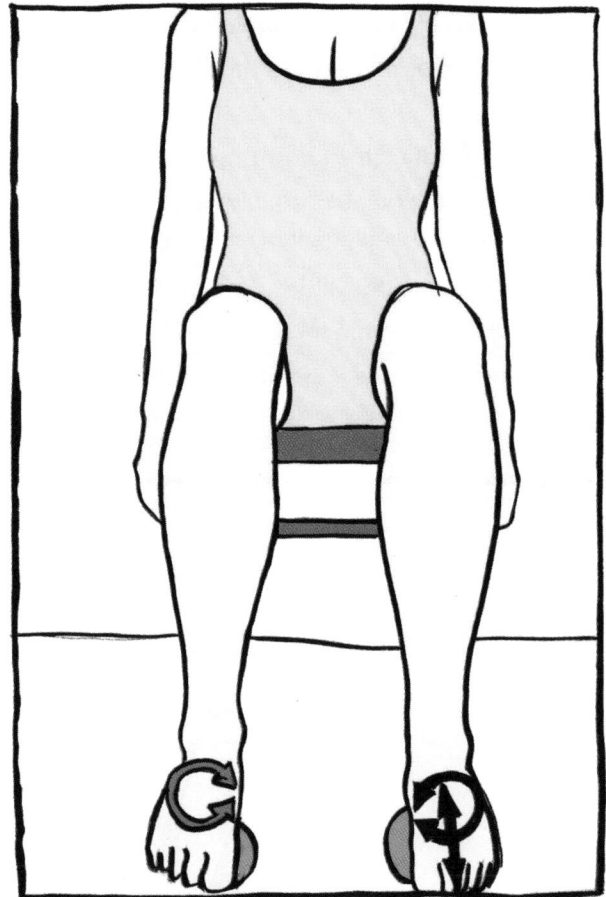

Note differences in the two sides of the body, including the feet.

Fig. 17.10. Advanced Ball Exercise for the Feet I

into the ground. Resist the temptation to use your thighs and hips. It will be a tiny movement, more of a feeling than a distinct movement.

4. Then repeat the whole sequence. You will probably feel a difference in the last pressing movement after repeating the sequence. Get up slowly!

◈ Advanced Ball Exercise for the Feet II

You will need a small futon, a mattress, or a pillow 6 to 9 inches high. It should be a fairly soft material. Place two 4-inch balls about hip width apart next to the futon or pillow. Stand with the balls of your feet on the edge of the futon or pillow and your heels on the 4-inch balls.

In this position, the balls of your feet should be about an inch higher than your heels. If not, change the futon or pillow until they are (fig. 17.11).

1. Relax, with your hands touching the futon or pillow in front of your toes (fig. 17.11). You can bend your knees if you need to, although this exercise is most effective if your legs are as straight as possible. Now visualize a line going from the crease of the buttock to the heels on both sides. Think of that line lengthening, pressing the ball into the ground. Make sure there is no movement in the front of the foot, the front of the ankle, or the toes. Let your body stay still so you are not rocking back onto the ball.

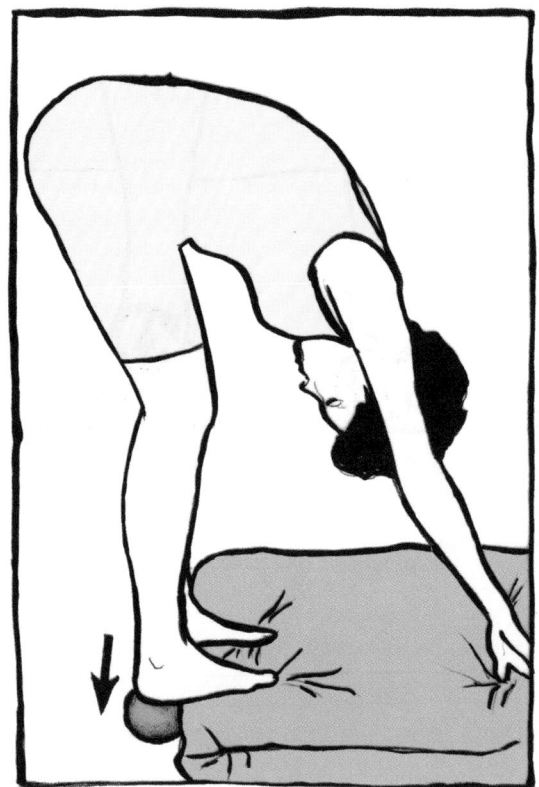

Fig. 17.11. Advanced Ball Exercise for the Feet II

2. Press gently, and then release, 10 times.
3. Now come off the balls carefully—the safest way is to come forward onto your hands first. Walk around the room, and notice any differences you feel.

18

Ergonomics

LIFTING AND CARRYING THINGS

Only two areas of the body are really designed for carrying heavy weight: your back, especially close to the spine, and the top of your head. If you can carry weight from those places, you are safer. The farther away a weight is from your spine when you lift it, the more vulnerable you are. Lots of people injure their backs lifting things incorrectly. There are two main reasons, one well known, the other not.

1. When you lift something, you should bend your knees and ankles so you are using your gluteus muscles, not your lower back. Stretching into a forward bend with straight legs and lifting weight with the back can throw the lower back muscles into spasm.
2. Don't lift with your arm bones out of their sockets. See the Shoulder section (page 155) for details of this. Keep the arms firmly in the joint, so you work the muscles of the upper back. When the shoulders are overstretched, you may not only damage your shoulders and neck but can also overstretch your lower back muscles, sending them into spasm.

When you use one arm to lift something in front of your body, pull the bottom tip of that shoulder blade down your back and drop the shoulder as you lift your arm. That way, you will use the muscles in the upper back that are designed for the job. Your arm will move as a lever against the dropped, pressed-down-and back scapula. This will create space in the shoulder joint for the head of the humerus to rotate freely (see fig. 11.1 on page 156).

The more common way is to lift the upper trapezius and raise the entire shoulder up. This is an appropriate way to lift heavy objects. However, you can see how this way of lifting allows less space for the head of the humerus to rotate and sends the shoulders up to the ears, creating tension. Only lift this way if you must lift a weight that's really too heavy for you, and keep that weight as close to the body as possible. For example, if you're in a store and you realize you have bought some things that are actually too heavy to carry, but you're stuck with them (we've all done that), raise the shoulder of the carrying arm as I describe here, and you'll protect your back and neck. Then alternate sides. If you let the heavy package stretch your shoulder down, you can cause a compensatory spasm.

When you lift things with your shoulders, expand your chest. If the chest collapses, you may injure your neck.

Carrying bags can cause many problems. Carrying any weight on one side of the body, especially if you have scoliosis, creates a distortion in the movement of the vertebra as you walk. The thoracic vertebra will not rotate properly on the side you carry your bag on. The shoulder on that side will tend to rise up and move forward to hold the bag. Usually, people carry their shoulder bags on one side only because on the other side, where the shoulder is lower, the bag slides off! If you have to use a shoulder bag, switch sides frequently.

Avoid shoulder bags completely if you have scoliosis or any right/left distortions in your spine. If you carry weight in your hand, use your biceps to slightly curl in the arm. Again, use alternate sides. A backpack is okay too, although it also prevents free rotation in the spine on both sides by pressing into the back. Make sure the straps are even and carry the backpack a little higher on your back than you would probably do automatically, so the upper back supports more of the weight.

SITTING CORRECTLY

Sitting in chairs is just about the worst habit you can get into. However, since most people spend a lot of time sitting in a chair, here's how to do so with the least damage.

Sit with your weight mostly on the front inside part of your sit bones (the bottom of your pelvic bones). Don't cross your legs. The pressure on the two bones should be equal; if it is not, shift your weight around until it feels more even. Press the sit bones slightly into the chair, lengthen your spine in one straight line and hinge forward only from the sit bones when you need to lean forward. All of your movements should be initiated from these bones. Don't fold or hinge from your waist or your C7. Keep the front and back of your body equally long.

When you need to look down and forward, you must move forward on the sit bones, maintaining the lumbar curve. Move your eyes, not your head. You can look down without compromising your neck.

Sitting tends to use the body in fragmented, tension-producing ways because the immobilized lower back and pelvis let you use the neck and arms without properly involving the back and pelvic muscles. Try to involve the whole body in what you are doing as much as you can to counteract this tendency.

Some chairs are better than others, of course. The Balans chair (fig. 18.1, top right and bottom) helps keep alignment—you can't sag or fold forward in this position— but I don't like the way your knees can't move. My own favorite is the physio ball chair (fig. 18.1, top left), which is just a big physio ball with a chair built onto it—do not use the backrest, though. Your pelvis is on the bouncy, curved surface of the ball,

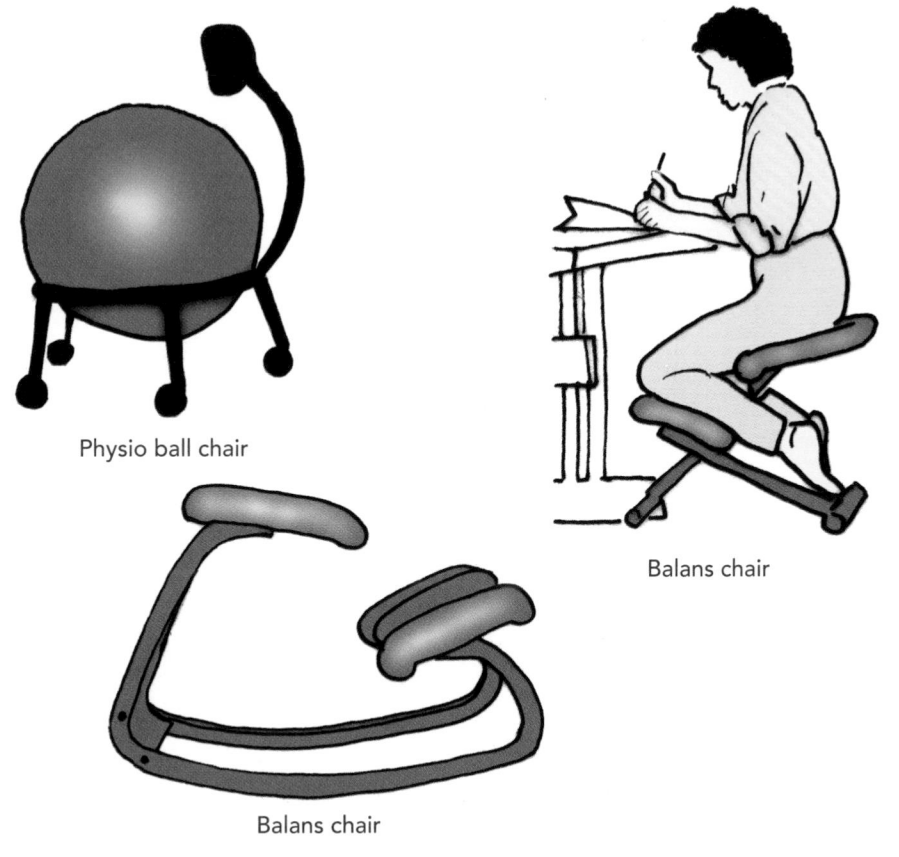

Physio ball chair

Balans chair

Balans chair

Fig. 18.1. Supportive chairs

which would engage some pelvic muscles and could actually strengthen the core. It's irresistible not to bounce up and down on the ball, which is a good break from sitting anyway and helps realign the spine as well.

If you can't change your chair, you can use a back support. I suggest the kind that you place under your pelvis, rather than the ones you lean back into, so your back stays engaged. If you have any serious back problems or a very weak back, use the supports that go in the back of the chair, such as the back support made by Therapeutica.

Sitting cross-legged on the floor (alternate the crossing of your legs, of course), follows the same general principles. Sit with the weight on the front of the sit bones, keeping the lumbar curve. Feel the diagonal line between the front of your sit bones and the bottom of your rib cage (fig. 18.2).

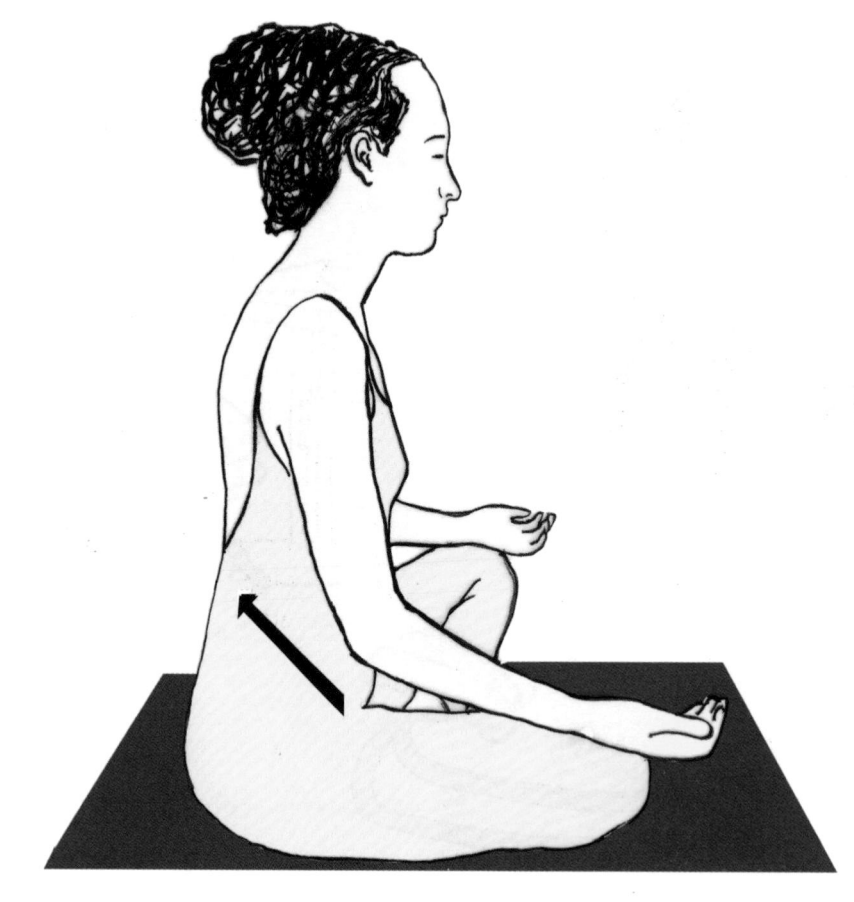

Fig. 18.2. Sitting correctly on the floor

Lengthen that line, lifting the back ribs away from the front of the pelvis. Keep that openness in the back and lift the chest, widening the collarbones. Align the soft palate with the middle of the pelvic floor. If you tip your body forward too much, your psoas is probably tight. Sitting correctly will help to stretch your groin and psoas (page 201). If your back is weak, you may want to fold forward at the waist. If your back is tight, you may want to tip back in this position. Try the Wall Hang Stretch (page 190).

BEDS AND PILLOWS

Strange things happen to the sleeping body, as you've probably noticed. Most people wake up tighter and stiffer than when they went to bed, even if they are feeling rested.

The weight of the head is as much a factor when you're lying down as when you're standing. The head will tend to tip forward if you sleep on your side or backward if you sleep on your back and will distort the neck and upper back if you are a stomach sleeper. Most people need a pillow to support the head, and possibly one of those ergonomic double-roll pillows that support the neck as well. If you sleep on your side, the most common position, make sure your pillow is hard enough and high enough to keep your head in line with your spine and prevent it from tipping forward (fig. 18.3). Soft fluffy pillows are a disaster for the neck, because the weight of the head will compress them and you will end up with a misaligned head and neck. This

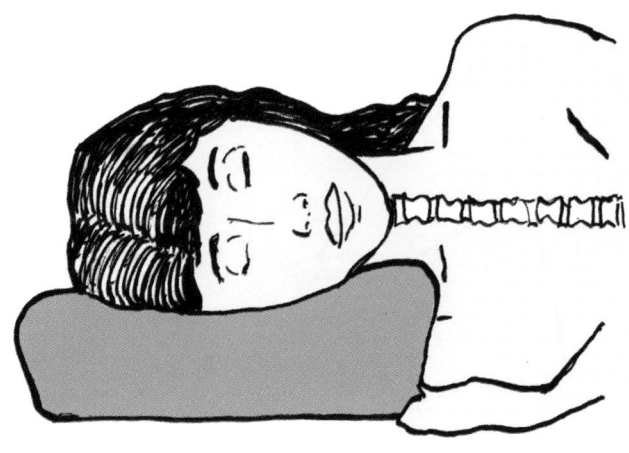

Fig. 18.3. Sleeping on your side: correct head support

configuration is the cause of most stiff necks and upper back spasms in the morning.

If you sleep on your back, you will probably want a very small, flat pillow, just so the head doesn't pull back. Stomach sleepers can use those big, fluffy pillows under their stomachs and chests, so their necks don't get twisted during the night (fig. 18.4). If you go to a hotel, throw the fluffy pillows off the bed and roll up some towels to suit your pillow needs. Rolled-up towels make excellent pillows, and they are much cheaper than the ergonomic kind.

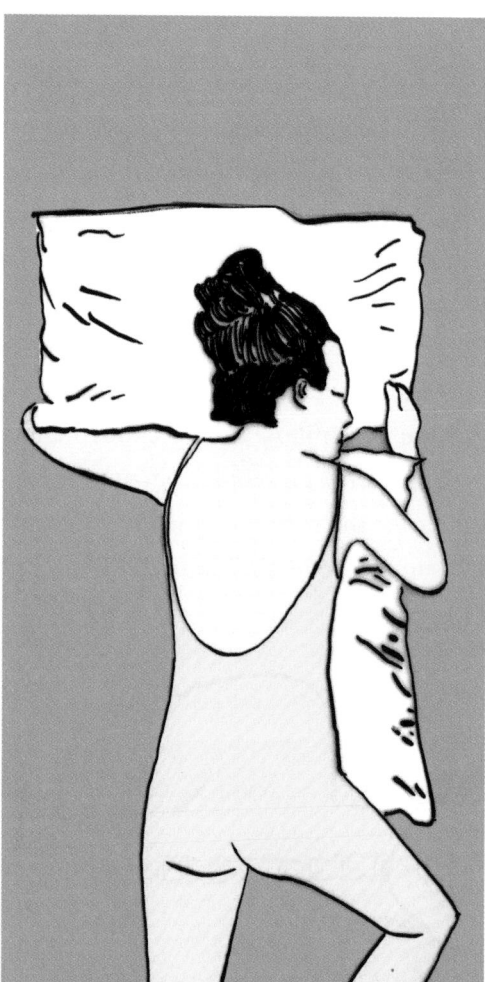

Fig. 18.4. Sleeping on your stomach

Many of my clients have bought ergonomic pillows and found that what their friends find useful doesn't work for them, so I can't suggest a universal "good" pillow. What I do recommend is testing out what kind of configuration works for you with rolled-up towels, and then, if you want, buy a similar pillow. Or just save money and stick with the towels.

If you sleep on your side, your toes curl under during the night, as the spinal muscles and hamstrings tighten to accommodate the weight of the head. This can lead to an aggravation of plantar fasciitis, which is always worse after sleep. If you have severe plantar fasciitis, you can try strapping the foot into a boot that forces it into flexion. If you don't want to resort to this solution or if the problem is not that bad, stretching the hamstrings, back, and Achilles tendons (pages 190–94 and 261 may be sufficient to alleviate the curling of the toes. Experiment to see the difference in the stretch of these muscle groups in the evening and then again right after you wake up. The upright position tends to tighten the front of the body; sleeping tightens the back.

The hands may also curl under, in the same fashion. However, the cause of this is usually pressure on the shoulder from an incorrect pillow (usually not high or firm enough). If you are a side sleeper with broad shoulders, you'll need a higher pillow.

Numbness and tingling in the arms in the morning can also come from pressure on the shoulder. Compression in the cervical spine and the upper back can cause nerve pains in the hands.

If you have knee or lower back problems, sleep on your side with a pillow between your legs, so that your knees and hips are on the same level. Or if you sleep on your back, put a large pillow or bolster under your knees, so that they are higher than your hips. Stomach sleepers can put a small pillow under their shins.

Sleep on whatever kind of bed you find comfortable. I find the idea of sleeping on metal springs disturbing and prefer futons; some people find futons extremely uncomfortable and need the support of a mattress. There are all kinds of fancy orthopedic mattresses on the market that have their adherents. This is fine, but just be aware that even expensive mattresses will need to be changed regularly. Ordinary mattresses should be thrown out after five years. They will get saggy in the middle and show wear patterns. The same goes for futons.

SHOES

All shoes are bad for the feet to some degree. I understand that you have to wear them some of the time. I also discuss (page 258) how the hard, flat surfaces we walk on deform our natural foot development. That said, here are some suggestions.

The best shoes I've found are the MBTs (Masai Barefoot Technology), developed by a Swiss engineer to imitate walking on rolling terrain as the Masai tribal people do. They have been touted as calorie burners, cellulite reducers, and so on, because they do use more muscle than regular shoes. I don't know how well they tone your legs, but they feel wonderful, and over time, they will improve your feet and balance your body in other ways too. The downside is that other shoes feel awful after you get used to the MBTs.

If you prefer a very minimal support shoe, I recommend Softstar shoes, which are designed with a very thin flexible structure and allow your feet and ankles to work. They are similar to the Five Finger shoes, which separate your toes, but I find that the toes being rigidly separated can actually give them less mobility. The toes can move freely in the Softstar barefoot shoes.

If you have to wear high heels, you will need to stretch your Achilles tendon, your hamstrings, and your psoas much more assiduously than someone who does not wear them. Wearing high heels occasionally probably won't do much damage. Wearing them habitually may distort the shape of the spine, cause organ prolapse as the viscera are pushed forward by the angle of the spine, and give you bunions. A Mexican doctor I worked with told me he attributed the high rate of reproductive organ problems in the Hispanic population he worked with to the habitual use of very high heels from adolescence onward.

People always ask me about the advisability of orthotics in their shoes. Orthotics will compensate for weakness in the foot and can help back problems caused by that weakness. In that way, they can be a real help. However, they are a crutch. The real issue is still usually the weakness in the foot, so while enjoying the relief the orthotics give you, try if possible to correct the fundamental problem with exercise and bodywork. If the orthotics don't help, *don't use them*. Supports that don't help you are not neutral in their effect on you; they are actually harmful. They can negate the natural body intelligence that will attempt to balance you and cause even more problems. This is actually a general principle of alignment—don't fix what isn't broken. Adding an unnecessary prop or support in an exercise can actually send a muscle into spasm.

So if your orthotics don't work well for you, ask your health practitioner to redesign them, and don't use them unless they make you feel better. That way, you can work on strengthening the appropriate foot muscles while your body learns from the orthotics to maintain a better alignment.

Please also see Mary Bond's wonderful book, *The New Rules of Posture* (listed in the bibliography), for more ergonomic and alignment ideas.

19

For Bodyworkers:
How to Do This Work

THE TECHNIQUES outlined in this chapter are very advanced techniques; they are based on the assumption that you already have studied massage, shiatsu, Structural Integration, or physical therapy extensively. These particular techniques are for professionals, and I would recommend studying them with a bodywork practitioner who knows them before practicing. Then you can use these descriptions as a reminder.

Bodywork can be invasive and deep. As you work, the client must be very comfortable or she won't relax fully. Sometimes people aren't aware, or are too polite to tell you, that they are not quite happy in the position they are in. Ask them. Do whatever you need to do in terms of massage/bodywork to make the body relaxed and open.

Move very slowly. Wait for the shifts in the deep body tissues as a cat waits at a mousehole.

Don't slide on the skin or hair. Aim for the center of the body. Don't overwork. Stop and change course at a 70 or 80 percent shift. Let the body complete the work.

THE CRANIUM

The skull is not just a hard, immobile, protective casing for the brain. It's a springlike system of interlocking joints—sixty-seven in total. The skull functions as:

- A part of the pump for cerebrospinal fluid, the other main section being the tailbone.

295

- The regulator of spinal stability: the sphenoid bone (see fig. 10.2 on page 151)—a horizontal diaphragm that functions as the central bone in the head—controls the position of the skull over the spine; therefore the entire body is affected by its position.
- The main system of sinus drainage. The inner cranial joints, specifically the sphenobasilar joint, function as the drainage system for the nose and ears, so cranial alignment plays a role in sinus and ear infections.
- A system of various reflex points to organs, meridians, and other structures.
- A container of fluids and electrical charges that can build up in areas of restriction and cause headaches and emotional problems. (This is my idea—no scientific proofs yet.)

When we work the cranium, we are influencing all these aspects of function and structure.

Craniosacral Work

All cranial work I use originates from cranial osteopathy, a school of cranial work that was developed mostly in Europe at the beginning of the nineteenth century by Dr. William Sutherland. Craniosacral therapy focuses on restoring the natural rhythm of cerebrospinal fluid, which moves through the membranes of the spine, the brain, and other parts of the nervous system, especially the sacrum. The sacrum is as important as the cranial structure in this work, hence the name. Under the aegis of osteopathy, two main schools developed, both of which are still evolving today, and each of which takes the theories of Dr. Sutherland in an opposite direction.

One you are perhaps familiar with already is the CranioSacral Therapy of John Upledger, M.D. This technique uses cranial releases that are extremely gentle and subtle; about five grams of pressure, the weight of a nickel, is recommended. My experience of CranioSacral Therapy is that it is very effective for babies and young children, before the cranial bones have fused. After that, there is less effect, especially if the bony structure is extremely locked up. The cerebrospinal rhythm seems to be hard to change in any lasting way if the cranial joints themselves are restricted.

In this case, the second school of craniosacral work, NeuroCranial Restructuring (NCR), a dramatic opposite to this gentle work, may be of use. NCR adjusts the sphenoid bone by insufflating a secured finger cot up the nose. Since the sphenoid is so internal, there is no practical way of influencing its movement manually, at least not directly. The technique was originally called Bilateral Nasal Specific Technique, which dates back to the 1920s or so. Dean Howell, N.D., refined the process to its present day form in the late 1980s.

This is a much more controversial treatment and, in my opinion, much more effective in correcting structural problems. It obviously could be dangerous if used incorrectly. In this book, we are mainly interested in it because NCR recognizes the primary importance of the sphenoid bone.

How to Do Cranial Fascia Work

Cranial fascia work, which is what we are going to study, is closer to NeuroCranial Restructuring, at least in intention, than to CranioSacral Therapy. We are aiming for structural shifts in cranial mobility, especially in the deeper cranial bones. You can use cranial fascia work to correct any condition where you find some locking of the cranial bones. It would be contraindicated with recent fractures of the skull, including brain surgery (wait six months before treating the cranium). You can use very gentle cranial fascia work on babies whose skulls are still open.

Our focus will be on mobilizing the sphenoid, the sphenobasilar joint, and the occiput through the cranial soft tissue structures. The distortions of the spiral rotational movements of the spine, and the balance between the pelvic bones, may be corrected in this way. At least they will be greatly helped.

🍃 Work the Outer Cranial Bones (Skull)

1. Work the entire surface of the head as one unit, paying special attention to any changes of angle in the skull, which indicate sutures in the bone. Observe areas of locking in the sutures. You can use either elbows or knuckles to "roll" over the head. Make sure you don't slide—you'll pull the client's hair, entirely the wrong kind of pain! The technique is to fix the knuckles or elbow on the surface of the scalp and then move the skin of the scalp over the deeper tissue structures. There will probably be a crunchy, grinding type of noise that the client will hear, and you may too. This crunching noise seems to indicate the presence of some toxins (lactic acid? calcium ions?) in the fascia itself, since it is more pronounced in the restricted areas of the cranium.

2. After working the whole head, making whatever observations you can about the reflex points, the jaw structure, and the spine, return to the individual blocked sutures and work them separately.

❧ *Work the Inner Cranial Structures*

The closest we can get to the deep cranial bones that govern the movements of the outer bones (primarily the sphenoid) just by using our hands is by access through the nose and mouth.

◈ Work Inner Cranial Structures via the Mouth

We can create a surprisingly large movement in the sphenoid if we approach it correctly. Once the outer cranium is loosened, get your gloves on, and go to the mouth. The movements you use are scooping and widening, as you move the flesh away from the center of the head.

1. First, go back as far as you can between the back teeth and the inner cheek. You will feel a ridge—part of the inner structure of the mandible. You want to start inside the ridge, moving up toward the top of the head first, and then scooping down. There may be no space to go that far back. Do not force. Work the rest of the mouth first, and come back.

2. Next go to the upper part of the jaw where it abuts the inner cheek. Scoop out the flesh gently, avoiding pulling at the lip. You can support the head with your other hand. Repeat on the lower jaw and inner cheek surface of that side. Pay attention to the chin area, where occipital tensions are reflected. Repeat on the other side.

3. Now go to the pterygoid muscle and the hard and soft palate, where you can influence the sphenoid (see figs. 10.1 and 10.2 on page 151). Start at the hard palate in the centerline with both index fingers and move them to the outer edge to widen. Go back into the soft palate if you can. You may feel the atlas behind the palate if the gag reflex is quiet. But don't force!

4. Now, one side at a time, go to the upper part of the pterygoid and the soft palate (the anterior of the muscle). Scoop and lengthen down. Repeat on the other side.

5. Now come back to the first position, way back inside the temporomandibular joint (TMJ), the outside of the teeth. Use both fingers, one on either side, if there is enough space. If not, don't force. Instead, noticing the rotational distortion of the mandible, bring your index finger inside the tighter joint, and very *gently* move the mandible from the lower portion to create a more ideal space. If there

is no movement, do not do this adjustment. Focus instead on the soft tissue restrictions.

This work inside the mouth is most helpful for visible structural distortions of the TMJ.

◈ Work Inner Cranial Structures via the Ears

Distortions of movement, when the jaw zigzags from side to side as the mouth opens and closes, are helped more by working the TMJ from the earholes.

1. Using both index fingers, go into the earholes about ¼ to ½ inch. Have the client open the mouth slowly, a 10-second count—just to a comfortable point—and close much more slowly, a 20-second count. Ask him to imagine little magnets attached to the teeth and visualize evenness of the bite without trying too hard to create it.
2. You, the practitioner, assist the bite correction by exerting very gentle pressure on the side that moves outward. This may change during the process of mouth closure.

This will correct the bite if the problem is restricted to the soft tissues and bones of the jaw. If there is no change, there may be an issue with the TMJ meniscus, which is not within our field—time for the dentist or oral surgeon.

◈ Work Inner Cranial Structures via the Nose

We can also approach the sphenoid through the nasal cavities.

1. With a gloved index finger, go in to the level of the first bony ring—no farther. Work one side at a time, widening the bone slightly. Support the nose if necessary. You will find most restrictions on the outer lower corner of the bony ring. Press firmly here—this is a part of the large intestine meridian, which influences sinus function.
2. You will probably discover that one nostril is much tighter than the other. See if you can equalize the relative size and strength of the nostrils. If you can, you create a significant shift in the parasympathetic/sympathetic dominance of the nervous system. Breathing though the left nostril affects the right side of the

brain and the parasympathetic nervous system; the right side affects the left brain and increases the dominance of the sympathetic nervous system (see chapter 9, Breathing).

THE ANTERIOR SPINE AND ITS ATTACHMENTS

Very little of the spine can be accessed from the back. Most of the spinal process and the muscular attachments are accessible only through the front of the body, so this is the best way to access and work with back problems, especially if there is pain or inflammation in that area. Of course, the one part of the anterior spine that can't be accessed this way is the thoracic area. Too bad—it's one of my fantasies to be able to get in there. However, you can still influence the spine by working the appropriate ribs.

🌿 *Work the Anterior Spine*

The client can be lying on his back with knees up or, especially if there is gas or other stuff in the intestines, lying on his side. The lumbar spine is extremely large and easy to find relative to the abdomen.

1. Starting at the bottom of the spine, penetrate through the layers of tissue very slowly until you feel a bony knob. When you have a bony knob (spinal process), gently scoop the muscle attachments of the psoas away from the central spine, as though cleaning it.
2. Work both sides of the abdomen, from pubic bone to diaphragm, in this way. Notice the rotational torsions of the spine. See if loosening the muscle attachments to the anterior spine changes any of the rotational torsions.

◈ Work the Rib Cage

1. When you reach the diaphragmatic tendons (crura) that attach to the spine (see fig. 4.2 on page 53), have the client breathe into the rib cage, not the belly. Ask him to focus on widening the lower ribs on the inhalation and keeping the ribs lifted away from the hips on the exhalation, so the exhalation will come from the lower abdomen (transverse abdominis).

CATHY THOMPSON'S EXERCISES

300

2. Some people have a lot of trouble doing this and will not be able to widen the ribs at all. To help them, and to work the thorax area in general, release the adhesions in the intercostal muscles (see fig. 9.3 on page 125). Press into the space between each rib as they inhale (more or less—it's useful if they can widen the ribs, but you can press anyway to stimulate the breath), and open up the rib spaces.

3. Work any conjunct or even overlapping ribs this way to release the area of the spine adjacent to them. The very sidemost portion of the rib cage will influence the back the most. Work the entire rib cage, not neglecting the armpits and including, as much as you can, the underlying breast area, avoiding any overly sensitive breast tissue. Remember the top rib, and release the upper ribs from the collarbone.

◈ Work the Cervical Vertebra

As you work the anterior spine of the cervical vertebra, pay special attention to C6 and C7 and the occipital area. Side position will get you in the farthest—and with the client's chin pressed up you can approach the top vertebra. Prone position with the head hanging down and supported (chest raised from table) will be relatively painless. Work the edges of the hyoid cartilage very gently to free the larynx.

THE ORGANS

Organs are as much a part of structure as muscles, bone, and other tissues. Back pain and other structural problems can be caused by disease—but it can easily be just a misplaced or malfunctioning organ. It's important that you, as a practitioner, have some awareness of this so you can recommend a medical checkup if you sense a possible problem. Meanwhile, you can correct many of these problems.

The most common system to cause structural trouble is the digestive. This makes sense when you think of it as essentially a long, somewhat bunched-up tube of muscle loosely attached to the connective tissue around the spine. I find more individual variation in the intestines and stomach in terms of shape and length than other organs.

The stomach and the transverse colon are the usual culprits (see fig. 19.1 on page 302).

The most common organ correction you will need to do is to pull down the

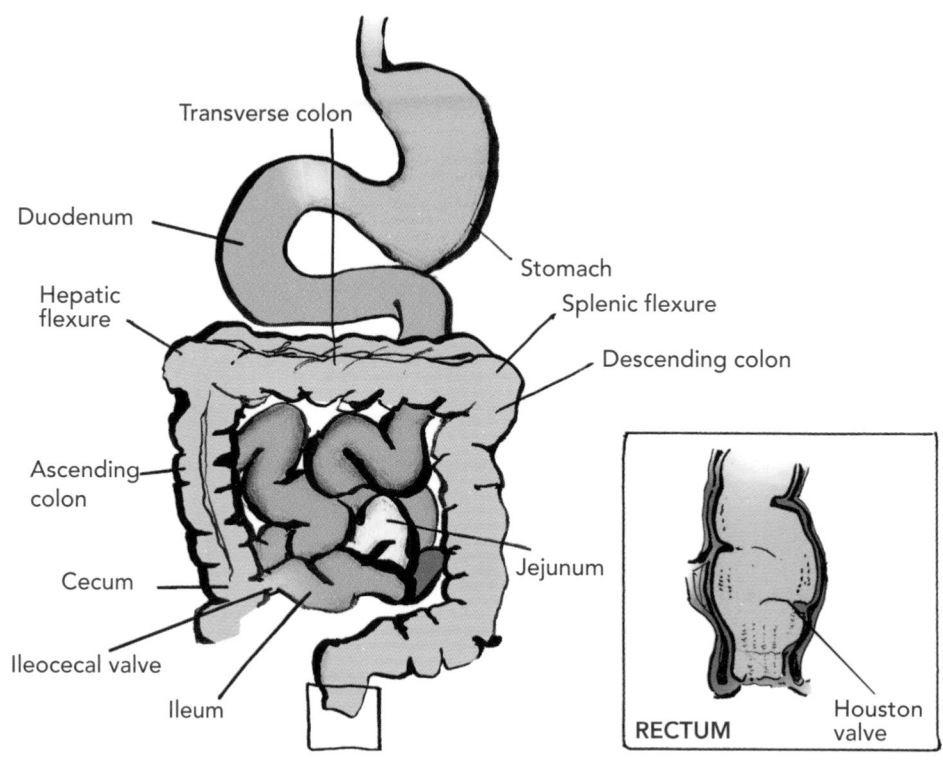

Fig. 19.1. Stomach, intestines, rectum

stomach to correct a sliding hiatal hernia. The hole the esophagus goes through in the diaphragm can easily weaken with repeated insults in the form of large, indigestible meals, lying down right after eating, or even athletic activities. Part of the stomach then can push above the level of the diaphragm, causing reflux, as the stomach acids are forced through pressure into the esophagus. One reason antacids are so bad is that the problem is almost always a sliding hiatal hernia, not high stomach acid (see Reflux section in chapter 14, page 230, for more in-depth discussion).

🌿 Pulling Down the Stomach

To correct the stomach, have the client lie on her back and breathe into the rib cage, while she visualizes the sides of the ribs widening. This will open the diaphragm and make your job much easier. You then pull the stomach down with your fingertips, either from below the xiphoid process or to the left and under the rib cage.

1. Scoop first, then pull. Start off lightly and increase the pressure until you hear a gurgling sound or feel the stomach drop. Indications that the stomach is correctly placed are rumbling, gurgling sounds; release of pressure in the solar plexus; and the client taking a deep breath.

2. If you are not successful, try releasing the rib joints around the sternum or working in the psoas.

3. Or you can have the client stand with her back against the wall and try working the area that way. This position will drop the transverse colon out of the way, making the stomach correction a little easier (but less comfortable for the client).

🍃 *Pulling Down the Transverse Colon*

The transverse colon varies in length a lot. Sometimes it gets "bunched up," and pockets of gas get stuck there.

1. Palpate the colon clockwise, from the ileocecal valve to the rectum, pulling down the transverse colon as you go.

2. Then come back to the ileocecal valve, which is usually halfway between the navel and the edge of the pubic bone (see fig. 19.1). Push your fingertips down into the valve, which may be jammed shut or too open. Either way, find the opening of the valve and continue pressing it; eventually you will feel a sensation around your fingers as though a small mouth is opening and closing around them. If that happens, the flexibility of the valve is restored.

3. Then go to the hepatic flexure (see fig. 19.1), simply massaging that area with variable pressure. This can correlate with back problems on the right side and is prone to congestion and toxicity.

4. Then check the transverse colon again, and go back down to the descending colon. The Houston valve (see fig. 19.1) gets stuck as often as the ileocecal and can be treated the same way.

Almost all abdominal pain is gas, fortunately. Hard pockets of gas can put pressure on the internal organs and even the psoas, causing much pain. Pockets can be broken up by light tapping (strumming) on the abdomen.

Umbilical hernias can't be corrected through bodywork, but I have helped mild inguinal hernia by working the associated muscles around the inguinal ligaments.

PLACEMENT OF THE NAVEL

According to Chinese medicine, the navel should be evenly placed, central and perfectly round. You can check yourself for this while standing; you can check a client when she is either lying down or standing. Some people have injuries on one side of their body only. Notice if the navel is displaced to that side or the other. The muscles involved in pulling the navel off center are all the spinal muscles, particularly the psoas. However, I've found that working very gently (at first) around, but never in, the navel in a clockwise circle about six inches in diameter can help place and center the navel more correctly.

THE PELVIC FLOOR

The "floor" of the upper cranium perfectly echoes the pelvic floor—the sphenoid, sphenobasilar, and occiput repeat the formation of the pubic bone, pubococcygeus, and sacrum. You could think of the spine as an intermediary between these two balance points.

🍃 Pelvic Floor Work

The key to successful pelvic floor work is to go very slowly and work a long time in each place. Prepare the client well before entering the anus for pelvic floor work. Describe what you're going to do and what kind of sensations the client might feel. It is definitely an end-of-session maneuver.

1. First, have the client lie on his or her back, with legs up, feet on a table. Work under the pubic bone gently, especially paying attention to the attachments of transverse abdominis on the sides of the bone. When the pubic bone moves well, have the client lie, unclothed, prone, with one knee up toward the hip (fig. 19.2).

2. Standing diagonally across from the raised leg, insert a gloved, lubricated thumb in the anus. Do not insert farther than the first sphincter, about 1 inch on most people. Bring the thumb down and outward into the pelvic structure, working the internal rotators of the femur and anus levator. You will feel the bottom of the pelvis. Notice the distance from the centerline of the pelvic floor.

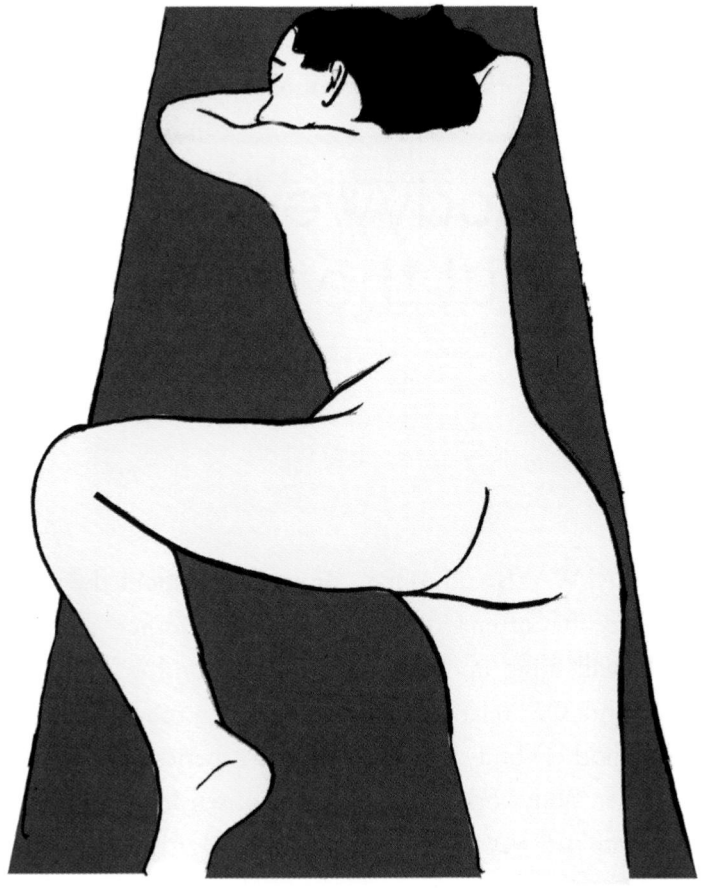

Fig. 19.2. Pelvic Floor Work

3. Then have the person straighten both legs, and move to the inner edges of the sacrum, supporting the exterior of the sacrum with the other hand. Free up the line of the sacrum carefully.

4. Then have the client raise the other leg, and work the pelvis as you did on the other side.

Much energy can be freed up by pelvic floor work. You are, after all, touching the seat of kundalini and stimulating that upward movement of energy. Structurally, your aim is to free up any restrictions in deep pelvic movement and equalize the space between the right and left segments of the pelvic floor.

Bodywork Is
about the Mother

MY MOTHER ALWAYS said to me, "Bodywork is about the mother." When I repeat this to clients, they often look at me in dismay. "Mother" is obviously a loaded topic. Bodywork will bring up whatever one's relationship to intimacy involves, which can be painful. Our relationship to intimacy, to touch, begins in the womb. The inside of our mother's body is our first sensory experience of our own bodies and the body of another. Bodywork is an awakening of sensing one's own body in new ways and opening up pathways that have been unfelt.

However damaged or healthy we may feel the mother relationship is, there is always opportunity for healing, as we are in a constant state of destruction and renewal. Whether we are conscious of it or not, we are engaged in a process of birthing ourselves, of regenerating our cells. In this way, we are our own mother. Bodywork gives us tools to do this consciously; otherwise we would continue to repeat old patterns and habits.

I had the good fortune of learning the practice of bodywork directly from my mother, in the ancient apprentice tradition. The process of writing this book was a part of that learning. My mother left it with me, for me to continue the work she had begun. There were many days that it felt like a burden. However, on reflection, it is the greatest gift she gave me. She left me with a method to take care of myself, to heal my own grief, and share the process with my clients. She left me with a mothering tool kit.

The Thompson Method of Bodywork is also "mother" in the sense that it is a source. A springboard to help propel you forward and learn more about yourself and to apply the ideas you have read to other modalities of healing and expression. I hope you enjoy incorporating Cathy Thompson's philosophy into your life and work and perhaps even create more material from hers, developing and regenerating. And the cycle of birth continues.

TARA THOMPSON LEWIS

Bibliography

Bond, Mary. *The New Rules of Posture*. Rochester, Vt.: Healing Arts Press, 2007.

Bowes, Deborah. *Pelvic Health and Awareness*. Learning For Health CD; http://www.learningforhealth.com/pelvichealthcds.cfm.

Buddhananda, Swami. *Moola Bandha*. Munger, Bihar: Yoga Publications Trust, 2000.

Franklin, Eric. *Pelvic Power*. Hightstown, N.J.: Elysian Editions, 2003.

Gershon, Michael D. *The Second Brain*. New York: HarperCollins, 1998.

Johnson, Jim. *The Multifidus Back Pain Solution*. Oakland, Calif.: New Harbinger Publications, 2002.

Masunaga, Shizuto, and Wataru Ohashi. *Zen Shiatsu*. New York: Japan Publications, 1977.

McCoy, Scott. *Your Voice: An Inside View*. Gahanna, Ohio: Inside View Press, 2012.

Pert, Candace. *Molecules of Emotion*. New York: Simon and Schuster, 1997.

Rolf, Ida P. *Rolfing*. Rochester, Vt.: Healing Arts Press, 1989.

Sarno, John E. *Healing Back Pain*. New York: Warner Books, 1991.

Staugaard-Jones, Jo Ann. *The Vital Psoas Muscle*. Berkeley, Calif.: North Atlantic Books, 2012.

Index